Narrative Theory and Therapy in the Post-Truth Era

Recep Yılmaz
Ondokuz Mayis University, Turkey

Bozkurt Koç
Ondokuz Mayis University, Turkey

IGI Global
PUBLISHER of TIMELY KNOWLEDGE

A volume in the Advances in Linguistics and Communication Studies (ALCS) Book Series

Published in the United States of America by
IGI Global
Information Science Reference (an imprint of IGI Global)
701 E. Chocolate Avenue
Hershey PA, USA 17033
Tel: 717-533-8845
Fax: 717-533-8661
E-mail: cust@igi-global.com
Web site: http://www.igi-global.com

Library of Congress Cataloging-in-Publication Data

Names: Yılmaz, Recep, 1982- editor. | Koç, Bozkurt, 1970- editor.
Title: Narrative theory and therapy in the post-truth era / Recep Yılmaz, and Bozkurt Koç, editors.
Description: Hershey PA : Information Science Reference, [2022] | Includes bibliographical references and index. | Summary: "This book focuses on the structure of the narrative and the possibilities it offers for therapy as well as the Post-Modern sources of spiritual conflict and how to benefit from the possibilities of the narrative while healing conflict, offering research on new concepts and models to be created"-- Provided by publisher.
Identifiers: LCCN 2022007240 (print) | LCCN 2022007241 (ebook) | ISBN 9781799892519 (hardcover) | ISBN 9781668458587 (softcover) | ISBN 9781799892526 (ebook)
Subjects: LCSH: Narrative therapy. | Narration (Rhetoric)--Psychological aspects. | Truthfulness and falsehood. | LCGFT: Essays.
Classification: LCC RC489.S74 N363 2022 (print) | LCC RC489.S74 (ebook) | DDC 616.89/165--dc23/eng/20220318
LC record available at https://lccn.loc.gov/2022007240
LC ebook record available at https://lccn.loc.gov/2022007241

This book is published in the IGI Global book series Advances in Linguistics and Communication Studies (ALCS) (ISSN: 2372-109X; eISSN: 2372-1111)

British Cataloguing in Publication Data
A Cataloguing in Publication record for this book is available from the British Library.

For electronic access to this publication, please contact: eresources@igi-global.com.

Advances in Linguistics and Communication Studies (ALCS) Book Series

Abigail G. Scheg
Western Governors University, USA

ISSN:2372-109X
EISSN:2372-1111

Mission

The scope of language and communication is constantly changing as society evolves, new modes of communication are developed through technological advancement, and novel words enter our lexicon as the result of cultural change. Understanding how we communicate and use language is crucial in all industries and updated research is necessary in order to promote further knowledge in this field.

The **Advances in Linguistics and Communication Studies (ALCS)** book series presents the latest research in diverse topics relating to language and communication. Interdisciplinary in its coverage, ALCS presents comprehensive research on the use of language and communication in various industries including business, education, government, and healthcare.

Coverage

- Media and Public Communications
- Sociolinguistics
- Computational Linguistics
- Graphic Communications
- Cross-Cultural Communication
- Dialectology
- Interpersonal Communication
- Language Acquisition
- Semantics
- Youth Language

IGI Global is currently accepting manuscripts for publication within this series. To submit a proposal for a volume in this series, please contact our Acquisition Editors at Acquisitions@igi-global.com or visit: http://www.igi-global.com/publish/.

The Advances in Linguistics and Communication Studies (ALCS) Book Series (ISSN 2372-109X) is published by IGI Global, 701 E. Chocolate Avenue, Hershey, PA 17033-1240, USA, www.igi-global.com. This series is composed of titles available for purchase individually; each title is edited to be contextually exclusive from any other title within the series. For pricing and ordering information please visit http://www.igi-global.com/book-series/advances-linguistics-communication-studies/78950. Postmaster: Send all address changes to above address.

Titles in this Series

For a list of additional titles in this series, please visit: http://www.igi-global.com/book-series/advances-linguistics-communication-studies/78950

Handbook of Research on Communication Strategies for Taoo Topics
Geoffrey D. Luurs (Murray State University, USA)
Information Science Reference • © 2022 • 602pp • H/C (ISBN: 9781799891253) • US $265.00

Basic Communication and Assessment Prerequisites for the New Normal of Education
Victorița Trif (University of Bucharest, Romania)
Information Science Reference • © 2022 • 287pp • H/C (ISBN: 9781799882473) • US $195.00

Critical Perspectives on Social Justice in Speech-Language Pathology
RaMonda Horton (Midwestern University, USA)
Information Science Reference • © 2021 • 355pp • H/C (ISBN: 9781799871347) • US $195.00

Rationalist Bias in Communication Theory
Leonard Shedletsky (University of Southern Maine, USA)
Information Science Reference • © 2021 • 355pp • H/C (ISBN: 9781799874393) • US $215.00

Innovative Perspectives on Corporate Communication in the Global World
María Dolores Olvera-Lobo (University of Granada, Spain) Juncal Gutiérrez-Artacho (University of Granada, Spain) Irene Rivera-Trigueros (University of Granada, Spain) and Mar Díaz-Millón (University of Granada, Spain)
Business Science Reference • © 2021 • 319pp • H/C (ISBN: 9781799867999) • US $215.00

Rhetoric and Sociolinguistics in Times of Global Crisis
Eda Başak Hancı-Azizoglu (Mediterranean (Akdeniz) University, Turkey) and Maha Alawdat (Kaye Academic College of Education, Israel)
Information Science Reference • © 2021 • 419pp • H/C (ISBN: 9781799867326) • US $195.00

Handbook of Research on Representing Health and Medicine in Modern Media
Gülşah Sarı (Bolu Abant İzzet Baysal University, Turkey)
Information Science Reference • © 2021 • 618pp • H/C (ISBN: 9781799868255) • US $265.00

Strategies and Tactics for Multidisciplinary Writing
Kemi Elufiede (Carnegie Writers, Inc., USA) and Carissa Barker Stucky (Carnegie Writers, Inc., USA)
Information Science Reference • © 2021 • 222pp • H/C (ISBN: 9781799844778) • US $195.00

IGI Global
PUBLISHER of TIMELY KNOWLEDGE

701 East Chocolate Avenue, Hershey, PA 17033, USA
Tel: 717-533-8845 x100 • Fax: 717-533-8661
E-Mail: cust@igi-global.com • www.igi-global.com

Editorial Advisory Board

Table of Contents

Detailed Table of Contents

between the narcissistic narrative in the advertisement and the consumer affects the consumer and how this interaction will be evaluated from a psychoanalytic point of view. This chapter offers the reader an analytical discussion to open these issues.

The Bolsheviks seized power in Russia with the October Revolution of 1917 and began the process of establishing a new society. Propaganda is used to influence the public in this process, and posters were an important tool in the propaganda toolbox. The archetypes of "otherness" in Soviet propaganda posters are the subject of this research. The goal of this research is to discover how otherness archetypes are used in the narrative structure of Soviet propaganda posters. To accomplish this goal, the study will conduct a review of pertinent literature and examine the characteristics and transformation of the Soviet Union's marginalizing images on posters. Additionally, the study will identify marginalizing elements and the manner in which they are used.

Violence shown in the media, and especially in television programs, manifests itself as an alarming narrative element. Establishing a narrative through violence is an important marketing tool for the television industry with its language that appeals to the general public. In television broadcasts, and especially in television dramas, violence is treated as a profitable theme for the broadcaster. Since violent programs are a subject that attracts viewers, television organizations also increase the dose of violence in their broadcasts. Along with the increase in violence in society, the role of the media's narrative of violence in directing the audience is starting to be discussed. At this point, the presentation of violence within the framework of the post-truth approach of the violence narrative presented in television series gains importance. In this context, the chapter examines how the presentation of violence through television series is blurred and affects the public opinion by highlighting emotions and various interests within the framework of the post-truth approach.

Today's technological developments have enabled the digitalization of communication and transform it into different forms. With the said digitalization, individuals have had the opportunity to communicate very quickly, exchange information, produce content, and access information about their environment much more. Besides many opportunities brought by digital transformation are reflected to individuals, it reflected to the field of news media, which provides information flow to individuals. The reflection of digitalization in the news media emerged as a result of especially distributing and producing information very quickly and reaching large masses. The acceleration of the flow of information has made it necessary to focus on the concept of truth. So that, as a result of the intense information flow in the 2016 US

Presidential Elections and the Brexit referendum in England, the production and distribution of news in the post-truth era has become questionable. From this point of view, the truth of the information produced in the news media will be examined in this study.

There are many ethical violations in the news of violence against women, which is frequently encountered in television journalism. In these ethical violations in the news of violence against women, statements that especially women are shown as victims, marginalized, objectified, and legitimizing violence are frequently encountered. The use of violence in the news also makes the issue of the reality of the news and how the reality is reflected problematic. Reality in the news is a recreated reality. In this study, the way the media handles the news of violence against women is analyzed according to Teun Van Dijk's critical discourse analysis theory through the news of violence suffered by Emriye Metegül. The aim of the research is to examine the news of violence against women in television news through the violence suffered by Emriye Metegül, to see unethical acts through the news, to examine the news by explaining how the representation of women is presented.

Today, dozens of cameras are placed at various points on the football field, making sure that no detail is overlooked. The positions are reviewed using the video assistant system (VAR). However, despite the existence of live broadcast cameras and their technology-integrated structure, there is a position to be discussed after the match; the truth is reinterpreted. As Umberto Eco emphasizes, live-action, where television time and real-time are closest to each other, is not a mere repetition of an event, but an interpretation. In the chapter, the poetics of truth in football is discussed in the historical and technological process.

FoMO (The fear of missing out) was noticed by marketers and started to be used on consumers. FoMO is an anxiety disorder that is defined as not being aware of exciting things when not being looked at, or missing out on the experiences of others. Although the FoMO effect has a negative meaning, businesses manage to use this concern to their advantage. Limited production, shortage of products in stock, short-term discounts, showing the number of people interested in the same product, promotions offered as opportunities not to be missed are among the efforts of businesses to persuade consumers through FoMO. It is seen that the literature on FoMO in the field of marketing is limited. This study aimed to examine the relationship between FoMO and consumption and to evaluate the relevant literature. For this purpose, the findings, results, and evaluations obtained by examining the experimental and conceptual studies in the relevant literature were synthesized.

The place where most of us face the perception of reality in the pre-internet social life consists of a miraculous glowing box in the focal point of our rooms. Television is perhaps one of the most basic media tools that create our perception of reality by using the power of sound and image. The urge to believe what you see continues to make us addicted to this device. Television audience surveys in Turkey show that Turkish people watch television for an average of 4.5 hours a day. Considering that the average person works 8 hours a day and sleeps 8 hours, it is understood that people spend more than half of their free time in front of the television. With the use of the internet in all areas of social life, an average of 3 hours of leisure time consumption of people is devoted to social media. This situation reveals that television has a very serious competitor in directing our perception of reality. This study is about the construction of reality in the Survivor program, which is the most consumed competition program on Turkish television.

This study is aimed to show how the gender characteristics attributed to women reflect in the advertisement narratives and how these construct through narratives. The first part of the study is presented the concept set related to the subject. In the second part, an analysis by adhering to the conceptual framework is drawn by the literature review. In this section, television commercials, which are first in Turkey, are analyzed despite the upward trend in digital media and advertising investments. In the 2019 Crystal Apple advertising competition, 16 commercial films that received the Crystal Award in the TV and Cinema category were determined as a sample. In the study, the paradigms that form the basis of the qualitative research approach are accepted. In addition to the narrative analysis method, it also supported content analysis. The research results reveal the essential components of the advertising narrative, the roles attributed to women in television advertisements, and how they are constructed through narrative.

Today, the reaction of the masses towards the lies of the politicians brings together a new process rather than the politicians lying to the masses. In the post-trust era, the insignificance of the truth, politicians reflecting the lies as if they were the truth, and the masses believing in such reflections represent such a process. In this era, politicians render excuses to cover up the truth without having any feeling of guilt. There are spin doctors that work to enable the politicians to realize these purposes. The purpose of spin

Story theory, an intermediate-level nursing theory, was developed by nursing theorists Smith and Liehr. According to theorists, stories express who people are, where they are, and where they are going. Story theory can be used when one wants to understand what is most important to an individual with a health problem. The purpose of story theory is to reveal and evaluate the story of individuals as a basis for systematic data collection and analysis in the practice and research dimension of the nurse's health promotion process. While mostly qualitative analysis is used in the analysis of the story, quantitative analysis is also used. Liehr and Smith point out that stories should be used more in nursing in order to develop nursing knowledge.

The authors present their work with parents of addicted children, some of whom died as a result of their addiction. Stuck in pain, guilt, shame they often experience a discomforting lack of understanding from those around them. Behind their worries is often the wish that things would go well for their children. Under the pressure of cultural parenting discourses feelings of guilt became 'toxic'. Subsequently any sense of a viable future got lost. In order to restore a sense of a viable future, the authors drew on narrative ideas. They organized a three-day hike with parents. A life review interview was applied to highlight their efforts, involvements, decisions, responses, and 'unique moments'. The interviews were recorded, and as such, the process was documented. Finally, 'outsider witness practices' were installed. The conjecture that this fourfold 'stage setting' could help these parents to entertain new perspectives on the future proved to be promising.

Narrative therapy can be understood as part of a narrative continuum where generative story threads are interwoven into a mandala of transformational practices. Individual and social transformation is elicited by narrative practices that reinforce narrative coherency. Through engagement with narrative methods, phases of narrative practice and inquiry are analyzed, revealing the emergence of narrative concrescence within an integrated narrative framework. Autoethnography, narrative therapy, narrative mediation, narrative conflict resolution, and transformational learning using "transformagram portfolios" can be understood as connected storying practices contained in mediatorship. This holistic approach to narrative methods creates linkages that further the generative potential of narrative practices as illustrated in case studies. By reinforcing narrative coherency in the noosphere, "narrative truth" can be generated and used as a guiding force in a post-truth era.

Creative arts therapy, like dragon-riding, is poly-sensory and paradoxical. This variegated practice frequently falls prey to reductive research processes. Yearning for less dissonance between the what and how of research and greater congruence between the skill sets practiced in research and therapy, the author began exploring arts-based research and autoethnography. These methodologies now entangle under the investigational umbrella-term abr+a (arts-based research through autoethnography). In this chapter, the abr+a-dragon's tail is grasped for an escapade that: explores abr+a as performed by several researchers; revisits workshops facilitated at Whitecliffe (Aotearoa, 2017-2021), the BAAT/AATA Conference (London, 2019), and the ANZACATA Symposium (Brisbane, 2019); and theory-builds by tracing presence, poiesis, process, partnerships, pixellation, playfulness and psyche within abr+a. The intention is to express abr+a's emergent poietic-praxis and contribute to international intersectional conversations about creative research practices appropriate to therapy within a post-truth era.

The phenomenon of migration appears as an incontrovertible reality of social life today as it was in the past. While social, cultural, political, economic, etc. factors constitute the causes of migration, they are seen as the psycho-social dynamics most affected by migration. In this study, the narratives regarding the migration process of the Balkan immigrants living in Samsun were evaluated from a social psychological perspective in the context of the post-migration adaptation process. The narratives of the Balkan immigrants were examined in depth using thematic analysis method. As a result of the analysis, the narratives were evaluated within the framework of the themes of "basic needs," "cultural characteristics," and "acculturation." It has been determined that with the effect of features such as cultural similarities, sense of belonging, empathy, and cooperation, Balkan immigrants mostly do not experience problems in the adaptation process relatively different from other migration processes.

Foreword

René Guénon, in *The Depression of the Modern World*, says, "Instead of trying to raise himself to the level of truth, modern man wants to lower the truth to his level." Since 1927, in all the years that have passed, the philosopher's determination has come to a very different point. The era we live in is now called post-truth. Whether this naming will create a barricade in front of the erosion of humanity's value or eradicate it is not a matter we can answer yet.

The book you hold in your hands is precious because it contains a bipolar approach. On the one hand, it focuses on the conflict situation created by the post-truth and its story-based triggers. On the other hand, the possibilities offered by the narrative for therapy are tried to be made understandable. As discussed in the book, the narrative presents us with both the main instrument of many problems and the key to the solution: Triggers ranging from advertisements that increase narcissistic tendencies to the distortion of truth in the news are reflected in many areas, from the VAR system to entertainment programs. The solution, on the other hand, seems to be possible with therapy methods and the possibilities offered by the narrative to these methods. I think it is helpful to work. I congratulate the editors and contributors.

Yavuz Ünal
Ondokuz Mayıs University, Turkey

Yavuz Ünal *graduated from Ondokuz Mayıs University Faculty of Theology in 1988. After working as a teacher at the Ministry of National Education between 1988-1990, he started to work as a research assistant at the Department of Hadith at the Faculty of Theology of Ondokuz Mayıs University in 1990 and completed his master's degree in 1993 and his Ph.D. in the Institute of Social Sciences in 1997. He became Associate Professor in 2002 and Professor in 2008. He served as the Member of the Supreme Board of Religious Affairs between 2008-2015; the General Secretary of the 4th in 2009 and 5th in 2014 of the Religious Council; Dean of the Faculty of Theology at Ondokuz Mayis University between 2009-2012 and at Ordu University between 2013-2016; Vice President of Religious Affairs between 2016-2017, and the Ministry of Foreign Affairs Netherlands Religious Services Consultant between 2017-2018. He was appointed as the Rector of Ondokuz Mayıs University on 13 August 2020. Unal, the coordinator of the 'Hadith Project on Themes', which was published in 7 volumes and held with the participation of 105 scientists supported by the Directorate of Religious Affairs in 2006, is currently being carried out in 2016 by 40 academic and field expert participants and presented with the participation of President Recep Tayyip Erdoğan. Unal, who has 6 published works, has chapter authorship in various books, articles, and papers published in international and national refereed journals, articles written in various encyclopedias, especially the TDV Islamic Encyclopedia, and editors in various journals, symposiums, and workshops. He has served as Chairman of the Board of the Ordu Theology Foundation, Board Member of Samsun Branch of the Ensar Foundation, Chairman of the Board of Directors of the Netherlands Religious Foundation, Chairman of the Board of the International Muslim Communities Solidarity Foundation and is currently the Chairman of the Board of Directors of the Faculty of Theology Education and Research Association (İFEAD), of which he is the founder. He was awarded the "Service to the Islamic Culture of the Century Award" presented by President Erdoğan in 2014. He speaks English and Arabic, is married, and has four children.*

Foreword

"Truth is hard to tell because, in fact, there is only one truth, but this truth is alive; Therefore, its face changes constantly, like that of a living thing." / Franz Kafka

Post-truth is defined as the fading of the objective reality and influencing the public opinion, with the personal feelings and various interests of the masses gaining weight in the face of an objective reality. Serbian American playwright Steve Tesich, who was the first to use the concept of post-truth, states in his article that a significant part of the American people accept the political propaganda made by the Bush government as real without questioning it. Philosophically, these debates continue. However, this concept increases its visibility with the prevalence of communication technology today rather than in the past. This concept and conceptualization manifests itself with the end of modernism and the emergence of postmodernism. What we mean by the end of modernism covers the period up to the first half of the 20th century. Whether we call this period postmodernism or late modernism, the existing phenomenon is that it has reached a dizzying stage with technology.

The fact that information reaches individuals at a dizzying speed and that each person can write without any obstacles by creating a blog or a social platform can increase the complexity. Namely, if you are a researcher, a scientific article you have written will only be read in certain academic circles. If you are an amateur researcher or conspiracy theorist, you can easily deliver various nonsense produced via YouTube or any other social platform to millions of internet users. If you are an ordinary internet user, how will you learn how to do research or how to find the right information? How to reach qualified resources? How will we reach processed and controlled information by getting rid of superstitions or raw information stacks? If this phenomenon has existed since ancient times, why has this conceptualization and awareness been put forward by researchers today? We can also ask: Why did this phenomenon occur today?

Google will save the pages you have followed with its smart features and will bring you the views you have always liked. The truth is not important here, the important thing is that personal interests and benefits become important, and people respond to their wishes. According to Hannah Arendt, the phenomena we call reality are never independent of our personal characteristics and our perspective on events. The concept of post-truth is mostly used for the 21st century and represents an age in which mass media present the lie by making it hyper-reality. Post-truth is used for a period in which the lie itself is presented as if it were true, and even those who lied ignore and persistently defend these lies. With this concept, some concepts such as rationality, reasonableness, and common sense become ineffective and the senses gain weight, and even scientists cannot keep up with this. "While in the past, lying was only used to deceive the opposing party and to gain profit from it, today it can also be done in the name of deceiving all the masses.

This book emphasizes the mental destruction that today's people are exposed to due to both rapid technology and other factors and the necessity of treatment. Additionally, the work succeeds in examining and highlighting the sources and effects of psychological traumas of the masses relating to their mental conflicts from different perspectives, based on scientific approaches, adds a different dimension to the related field. The study, which includes different perspectives based on scientific approaches, adds a different dimension to the field. Communication and Psychology academicians could get the best of it as a reference book. Congratulations to the editors, and contributors for their hard work.

M. Nurdan Taşkıran
İstanbul Medipol University, Turkey

M. Nurdan Taskiran *was born in Istanbul, Turkey. She got her MA in English Literature and Language and a Ph.D. in Communication Sciences. She has worked for Marmara University for 16 years and Kocaeli University for 14 years and three years for Samsun Ondokuz Mayıs University Communication Faculty. Now, she is an emeritus professor working for Istanbul Medipol University, School of Communication since 2017. She has articles in Turkish and English on visual semiotics including films, tv serials, and advertisements. She likes reading articles on media literacy, visual rhetorics and animal communication. She is married with two children.*

Preface

Narrative theory origins go back to Plato as an approach that tries to understand the story's abstract mechanism. After separating theory, mimetic, and diegetic elements, it continued its fundamental development until Aristotle, Finnish School, Saussure, Russian Formalists, Prague School, German Scholars, Anglo-Saxon Formalism, and French Structuralism. Narratology has spread beyond the literary world, from visual narrative to artificial intelligence. -After a quarter of a century from named the field by Todorov in 1966. In this context, narrative therapy is one of many fields of narrative that emerged in the 1990s. The approach that emerged with white and Epston has turned into a rich research field that feeds many disciplines. "Narrative and Therapy in the Post-Truth Era" aims to make a solid contribution to studies examining the interaction between narrative and therapy. The book focuses on the one hand, on the structure of the narrative and the possibilities it offers for therapy; on the other hand, on the actual sources of spiritual conflict and how to benefit from the possibilities of the narrative while healing them.

In this context, *Narrative Theory and Therapy in the Post-Truth Era* is designed as three sections: "Dominant Triggers of Conflict in the Post-Truth Era," "View of the Entertainment and Marketing Worlds," and "The Possibilities of Narrative in Conflict Resolution." Now let's have an outlook over the contents of chapters in sequence.

WHAT THE POST-TRUTH ERA MEANS: A SHORT GLIMPSE

The concept of post-truth, which came to the fore with the political developments in 2016, is one of the most discussed issues today. Post-truth emerged as a concept related to politics. When used in this way, the term implies that seeking the truth is no longer considered appropriate by politicians. This concept essentially defines the political tendencies that devalue the factual. Although it emerged in politics, it began to be used in other fields. Especially with the developments such as Trump's election victory in 2016 and Britain's Brexit referendum, the use of the concept has increased. Post-truth, which expresses the fact that the concept of truth has become controversial, has been chosen as the word of the year this year. This study will define the concept of post-truth on which books, articles, and theses are written. In addition, a brief introduction will be made to the reasons why today's world is called the post-truth age.

GRANDIOSE MIRRORS OF THE SELF: THE NARCISSISTIC NARRATIVE IN ADVERTISEMENTS

Advertising narratives mostly use narcissistic discourses while appealing to the self of today's people to provide identification and transfer between the consumer and the brand. The study focuses on advertisements that promise to complete the lack of spiritual structure that the consumer's ego needs, and desires based on a narcissistic narrative. The article's main question is how the promise of completion in the advertisement is realized through the egocentric structure in the advertisement narrative and how it is included in the story. Another focal point of the work is how, and within which themes the transference between the narcissistic narrative in the advertisement and the consumer affects the consumer and how this interaction will be evaluated from a psychoanalytic point of view. This chapter offers the reader an analytical discussion to open these issues.

ARCHETYPES OF OTHERNESS: AN INVESTIGATION OF THE NARRATIVE STRUCTURES OF POSTERS IN THE CONSTRUCTION OF SOVIET IDEOLOGY

The Bolsheviks seized power in Russia with the October Revolution of 1917, and began the process of establishing a new society. Propaganda is used to influence the public in this process, and posters were an important tool in the propaganda toolbox. The archetypes of "otherness" in Soviet propaganda posters are the subject of this research. The goal of this research is to discover how otherness archetypes are used in the narrative structure of Soviet propaganda posters. To accomplish this goal, the study will conduct a review of pertinent literature and examine the characteristics and transformation of the Soviet Union's marginalizing images on posters. Additionally, the study will identify marginalizing elements and the manner in which they are used.

THE NARRATIVE OF VIOLENCE IN THE FRAMEWORK OF THE POST-TRUTH CONCEPT IN TELEVISION SERIES

Violence shown in the media, and especially in television programs, manifests itself as an alarming narrative element. Establishing a narrative through violence is an important marketing tool for the television industry with its language that appeals to the general public. In television broadcasts, and especially in television dramas, violence is treated as a profitable theme for the broadcaster. Since violent programs are a subject that attracts viewers, television organizations also increase the dose of violence in their broadcasts. Along with the increase in violence in society, the role of the media's narrative of violence in directing the audience is starting to be discussed. At this point, the presentation of violence within the framework of the post-truth approach of the violence narrative presented in television series gains importance. In this context, it will be tried to examine how the presentation of violence through television series is blurred and affects the public opinion by highlighting emotions and various interests within the framework of the post-truth approach.

INFORMATICS TRUTH: NEWS MEDIA IN THE POST-TRUTH ERA

Today's technological developments have enabled the digitalization of communication and transform it into different forms. With the said digitalization, individuals have had the opportunity to communicate very quickly, exchange information, produce content and access information about their environment much more. Besides many opportunities brought by digital transformation are reflected to individuals, it reflected to the field of news media, which provides information flow to individuals. The reflection of digitalization in the news media emerged as a result of especially distributing and producing information very quickly and reaching large masses. The acceleration of the flow of information has made it necessary to focus on the concept of truth. So that; as a result of the intense information flow in the 2016 US Presidential Elections and the Brexit referendum in England, the production and distribution of news in the post-truth era has become questionable. From this point of view, the truth of the information produced in the news media will be examined in this study.

REPRESENTATION OF VIOLENCE AGAINST WOMEN IN TELEVISION NEWS: THE CASE OF EMRIYE METEGÜL

There are many ethical violations in the news of violence against women, which is frequently encountered in television journalism. In these ethical violations in the news of violence against women, statements that especially women are shown as victims, marginalized, objectified and legitimizing violence are frequently encountered. The use of violence in the news also makes the issue of the reality of the news and how the reality is reflected problematic. Reality in the news is a recreated reality. In this study, the way the media handles the news of violence against women is analyzed according to Teun Van Dijk's Critical Discourse Analysis theory through the news of violence suffered by Emriye Metegül. The aim of the research is to examine the news of violence against women in television news through the violence suffered by Emriye Metegül, to see unethical acts through the news, to examine the news by explaining how the representation of women is presented.

TRUTH IN FOOTBALL FROM THE "HAND OF GOD" TO VAR

Today, dozens of cameras are placed at various points on the football field, making sure that no detail is overlooked. The positions are reviewed using the Video Assistant System (VAR). However, despite the existence of live broadcast cameras and their technology-integrated structure, there is a position to be discussed after the match, the truth is reinterpreted. As Umberto Eco emphasizes, live-action, where television time and real-time are closest to each other, is not a mere repetition of an event, but an interpretation. In the chapter, the poetics of truth in football is discussed in the historical and technological process.

NOT IGNORING THE FOMO (FEAR OF MISSING OUT) EFFECT: AS A NEW WAY TO PERSUADE CONSUMERS TO BUY

FoMO (The fear of missing out), It was noticed by marketers and started to be used on consumers. FoMO is an anxiety disorder that is defined as not being aware of exciting things when not being looked at, or missing out on the experiences of others. Although the FoMO effect has a negative meaning, businesses manage to use this concern to their advantage. Limited production, shortage of products in stock, short-term discounts, showing the number of people interested in the same product, promotions offered as opportunities not to be missed are among the efforts of businesses to persuade consumers through FoMO. It is seen that the literature on FoMO in the field of marketing is limited. In this study, it is aimed to examine the relationship between FoMO and consumption and to evaluate the relevant literature. For this purpose, the findings, results and evaluations obtained by examining the experimental and conceptual studies in the relevant literature were synthesized.

TRUTH TRYING TO SURVIVE: REALITY PERCEPTION IN SURVIVOR PROGRAM

The place where most of us face the perception of reality in the pre-internet social life consists of a miraculous glowing box in the focal point of our rooms. Television is perhaps one of the most basic media tools that create our perception of reality by using the power of sound and image. The urge to believe what you see continues to make us addicted to this device. Television audience surveys in Turkey show that Turkish people watch television for an average of 4.5 hours a day. Considering that the average person works 8 hours a day and sleeps 8 hours, it is understood that people spend more than half of their free time in front of the television. With the use of the internet in all areas of social life, an average of 3 hours of leisure time consumption of people is devoted to social media. This situation reveals that television has a very serious competitor in directing our perception of reality. This study is about the construction of reality in the Survivor program, which is the most consumed competition program on Turkish television.

THE CONSTRUCTION OF THE SOCIAL ROLES ATTACHED TO WOMEN IN TV COMMERCIALS THROUGH THE NARRATIVE

This study is aimed to show how the gender characteristics attributed to women reflect in the advertisement narratives and how this construct through narratives. The first part of the study is presented the concept set related to the subject. In the second part, an analysis by adhering to the conceptual framework drawn by the literature review. In this section, television commercials, which are first in Turkey, are analyzed despite the upward trend in digital media and advertising investments. In the 2019 Crystal Apple advertising competition, 16 commercial films that received the Crystal Award in the TV and Cinema category were determined as a sample. In the study, the paradigms that form the basis of the qualitative research approach are accepted. In addition to the narrative analysis method, it also supported content analysis. The research results reveal the essential components of the advertising narrative, the roles attributed to women in television advertisements, and how they are constructed through narrative.

SPIN DOCTOR IN THE POST-TRUTH ERA: *OUR BRAND IS CRISIS* MOVIE EXAMPLE

Today, the reaction of the masses towards the lies of the politicians brings together a new process rather than the politicians lying to the masses. In the post-trust era, the insignificance of the truth, politicians reflecting the lies as if they were the trust and the masses believing in such reflections represent such a process. In this era, politicians render excuses to cover up the truth without having any feeling of guilt. There are spin doctors that work to enable the politicians to realize these purposes. The purpose of spin doctors is to manipulate the media and the public opinion and to reveal the aspects of events to benefit their own political targets rather than as these events are. In this study, the "Our Brand Is Crisis" movie will be considered in the context of spin doctor tactics usage in the post-truth era. The purpose of this study is to reveal the cinema representation of the spin doctor tactics in the post-truth era and to discuss the spin doctor concept and tactics with sample scenes.

YOU'RE NOT THE PROBLEM! THERE'S ALWAYS AN EXCEPTION: COMPARISON OF NARRATIVE THERAPY AND SOLUTION-FOCUSED BRIEF THERAPY

In this study, narrative therapy, and solution-focused brief therapy, which are the postmodern psychotherapy methods, are compared in terms of similarities and differences. In the study, primarily theoretical information about narrative therapy and solution-focused short-term therapy, which differs from traditional psychotherapy methods, the techniques used and information about therapeutic application processes are given. Then, narrative therapy and solution-focused short-term therapies are compared in terms of similarities and differences. As a result, although narrative therapy, which is a postmodernist and social constructivist psychotherapy method, and solution-focused short-term therapy, which is a postmodern, inductive and constructivist psychotherapy approach, have great similarities in terms of both theoretical and therapeutic processes, they also seem to have some differences.

THERAPEUTIC STORYTELLING: HOW CAN WE USE STORIES MORE EFFECTIVELY?

Therapeutic storytelling aims to find the psychological difficulties experienced by the individual through creative narratives, uses problem-solving skills, and offers alternative ways based on narrative therapy. In therapeutic storytelling, questions about the meaning attributed to the story, the hero and metaphors that can be asked to the client, and the circular question forms of systemic interventions related to others important to the person are similar. In both forms of these interventions, subjective reality is reconstructed and so, therapeutic storytelling can be used eclectically with systemic interventions. In this chapter, a sample intervention template for systemic based therapeutic storytelling has been offered. Moreover, an exemplary hypothetical case of the systemic-based storytelling intervention pattern is presented. As a result, instead of focusing directly on the client's own life story, using storytelling intervention in a less threatening environment for the client through other stories may activate the client to gain insight and different viewpoints.

THE HEALING EFFECT OF THE STORY: GATHERING THE NARRATIVE DATA OF PATIENTS USING STORY THEORY

Story Theory, an intermediate-level nursing theory, was developed by nursing theorists Smith and Liehr. According to theorists, Stories express who people are, where they are, and where they are going. Story theory can be used when one wants to understand what is most important to an individual with a health problem. The purpose of Story Theory is to reveal and evaluate the story of individuals as a basis for systematic data collection and analysis in the practice and research dimension of the nurse's health promotion process. While mostly qualitative analysis is used in the analysis of the story, quantitative analysis is also used. Liehr and Smith point out that stories should be used more in nursing in order to develop nursing knowledge.

PARENTS IN THE GRIP OF PARENTAL GUILT: NARRATIVE PATHS TO REDISCOVER A FUTURE

The authors present their work with parents of addicted children, some of whom died as a result of their addiction. Stuck in pain, guilt, shame they often experience a discomforting lack of understanding from those around them. Behind their worries is often the wish that things would go well for their children. Under the pressure of cultural parenting discourses feelings of guilt became 'toxic'. Subsequently any sense of a viable future got lost. In order to restore a sense of a viable future the authors drew on narrative ideas. They organized a three days hike with parents. A life review interview was applied to highlight their efforts, involvements, decisions, responses and 'unique moments'. The interviews were recorded and as such the process was documented. Finally 'outsider witness practices' were installed. The conjecture that this fourfold "stage setting" could help these parents to entertain new perspectives on the future, proved to be promising.

INTERWEAVING NARRATIVE METHODS INTO A MANDALA OF TRANSFORMATIONAL PRACTICES

Narrative therapy can be understood as part of a narrative continuum where generative story threads are interwoven into a mandala of transformational practices. Individual and social transformation is elicited by narrative practices that reinforce narrative coherency. Through engagement with narrative methods phases of narrative practice and inquiry are analyzed, revealing the emergence of narrative concrescence within an integrated narrative framework. Autoethnography, narrative therapy, narrative mediation, narrative conflict resolution, and transformational learning using "Transformagram Portfolios" can be understood as connected storying practices contained in mediatorship. This holistic approach to narrative methods creates linkages that further the generative potential of narrative practices as illustrated in case studies. By reinforcing narrative coherency in the noosphere, "narrative truth" can be generated and used as a guiding force in a post-truth era.

ABR+A: THE ARTS OF MAKING SENSE – THE DISCOURSE OF DRAGONS

Creative arts therapy, like dragon-riding, is poly-sensory and paradoxical. This variegated practice frequently falls prey to reductive research processes. Yearning for less dissonance between the what and how of research and greater congruence between the skill-sets practiced in research and therapy, the author began exploring arts-based research and autoethnography. These methodologies now entangle under the investigational umbrella-term abr+a (arts-based research through autoethnography). In this chapter, the abr+a-dragon's tail is grasped for an escapade that: explores abr+a as performed by several researchers; revisits workshops facilitated at Whitecliffe (Aotearoa, 2017-2021), the BAAT/AATA Conference (London, 2019) and the ANZACATA Symposium (Brisbane, 2019); and theory-builds by tracing presence, poiesis, process, partnerships, pixellation, playfulness and psyche within abr+a. The intention is to express abr+a's emergent poietic-praxis and contribute to international intersectional conversations about creative research practices appropriate to therapy within a post-truth era.

REWRITING A LOST STORY: THE TRUTH IN THE NARRATIVES OF BALKAN IMMIGRANTS

The phenomenon of migration appears as an incontrovertible reality of social life today as it was in the past. While social, cultural, political, economic etc. factors constitute the causes of migration, on the other hand, they are seen as the psycho-social dynamics most affected by migration. In this study, the narratives regarding the migration process of the Balkan immigrants living in Samsun were evaluated from a social psychological perspective in the context of the post-migration adaptation process. The narratives of the Balkan immigrants were examined in depth using thematic analysis method. As a result of the analysis, the narratives were evaluated within the framework of the themes of "basic needs", "cultural characteristics" and "acculturation". It has been determined that with the effect of features such as cultural similarities, sense of belonging, empathy and cooperation, Balkan immigrants mostly do not experience problems in the adaptation process relatively different from other migration processes.

Recep Yılmaz
Ondokuz Mayıs University, Turkey

Bozkurt Koç
Ondokuz Mayıs University, Turkey

Acknowledgment

The completion of this editorial book could not have been possible without the participation and assistance of so many people from IGI Global. Especially, behind scene contributors, Jan Travers, and Elizabeth Barrantes deserve our sincere appreciation for their valuable and timely guidance, kindness, and tolerance.

We would also like to express our deep sense of gratitude to M. Nurdan Taşkıran, and to Yavuz Ünal who wrote wonderful foreword(s) for our book, and to Editorial Advisory Board (EAB) members; Cengiz Batuk, Ayşenur Büyükgöze-Kavas, Bahar Dervişcemaloğlu, Abdullah Nuri Dicle, Selim Eren, Ercümend Ersanlı, Hatice Kumcağız, and Niyazi Usta; their remarkable suggestions and supervising helped shape the book perfectly.

Special thanks go to individual chapter authors for their scientific contributions; Betül Başer, Luc Van den Berge, Nursel Bolat, Sereney Cantimur, Ömer Çakın, Nilay Tan Çakır, Özlem Delal, Deborah Green, Mehmet Akif Günay, Elif Şevik İnal, Ufuk İnal, Gamze Mukba, Aybike Tuba Özden, Tomas Van Reybrouck, Susan Mossman Riva, Esennur Sirer, Güven Soner, Sena Şahin, Aysu Gül Şanlı, Onur Şen, Doğan Güneş Temli, Eren Trabzon, and Sabine Vermeire.

To our parents, our children, and our wives, colleagues, and others who in one way or another shared their support either morally or physically thank you.

Recep Yılmaz
Ondokuz Mayıs University, Turkey

Bozkurt Koç
Ondokuz Mayıs University, Turkey

Section 1

Dominant Triggers of Conflict in the Post-Truth Era

Chapter 1
What the Post-Truth Era Means: A Short Glimpse

Özlem Delal
https://orcid.org/0000-0002-3653-5838
Ondokuz Mayıs University, Turkey

ABSTRACT

The concept of post-truth, which came to the fore with the political developments in 2016, is one of the most discussed issues today. Post-truth emerged as a concept related to politics. When used in this way, the term implies that seeking the truth is no longer considered appropriate by politicians. This concept essentially defines the political tendencies that devalue the factual. Although it emerged in politics, it began to be used in other fields. Especially with the developments such as Trump's election victory in 2016 and Britain's Brexit referendum, the use of the concept has increased. Post-truth, which expresses the fact that the concept of truth has become controversial, has been chosen as the word of the year this year. This study will define the concept of post-truth on which books, articles, and theses are written. In addition, a brief introduction will be made to the reasons why today's world is called the post-truth age.

INTRODUCTION

The concept of "post-truth" which came to the fore with the political developments in 2016, is one of the most discussed issues today. Although the first use of this concept, which expresses the trivialization of truth, was in the 1990s, the origins of discussions about truth go back to much earlier times. Since ancient Greece, thinkers and philosophers have thought about the issue of truth and researched what the truth is and how to reach the truth. There have always been thoughts, explanations, and discussions about truth and truth.

However, in 2016, Oxford Dictionaries chose "post-truth" as the word of the year. Oxford Dictionaries, which chooses the word of the year according to the most used word every year, announced that the use of the concept of post-truth increased by 2000% in 2016.

So why did truth debates flare up so much in 2016? The answer to this is explained through 2 events this year. The first of these is the election victory of Trump in the USA. Trump has lied countless times

DOI: 10.4018/978-1-7998-9251-9.ch001

during the election process and has built his election campaign on lies. The exciting thing is that these lies worked; Trump left the election with a victory. In the same year, many lies were told during the referendum (Brexit) to learn the public's preference for leaving the European Union. Millions of people believed these lies (Belge, 2018). As these developments show, the concept of post-truth was first used in political discussions. However, over time, the truth debates were reflected in different fields, and a new era entered the field of truth.

In this study, which is a short introduction to what this period called "post-truth" is, the concept of post-truth on which books, articles, and theses have been written will be defined. In addition, a brief introduction will be made to the reasons why today's world is called the post-truth age.

TRUTH AND BEYOND

The word parrhesia first appears in Greek literature in Euripides and has been used continuously in Ancient Greek literature since the end of the 5th century BC. The word is also found in texts written at the end of the 4th and 5th centuries AD. The word has three forms: noun form parrhesia; the verb form is parrhesiazomai (or, to put it better, parrhesiazesthaf); and the word parrhesiastes, which is not used very often and does not appear in classical texts. It is possible to find this last form of the word only in the Greco-Roman period. Parrhesia is often translated into English as "free speech". Parrhesiazomai or parrhesiazesthai means to use parrhesia. Panhesiastes, on the other hand, describes the person who uses parrhesia, that is, who speaks the truth (Foucault, 2001, pp. 9–10). Parrhesiastes says what is true; because he knows that thing is true, and knowing that thing is true is because that thing is true. The Parrhesiastes not only is honest and says what he thinks; at the same time, his thought is truth (Foucault, 2001, p. 12).

What is the truth that Foucault defines as telling the truth? There are many definitions of the concept of truth that have been considered since the birth of humanity. Frolov defined truth as reflecting truth and reality in thought (Frolov, 1991, p. 199). Real refers to situations or events that "exist not imaginary but actually, not mental but physical" (Chandler & Munday, 2018, p. 152). Thoughts about this reality constitute the truth.

Reality refers to things outside of human existence and is not dependent on human existence.

Like nature, earth, universe, and planets. On the other hand, truth is closely related to human existence and thought. Truth is the knowledge attained through human existence and consciousness (Zabcı, 2021, p. 15).

The prefix "Post" indicates after a particular event or situation (Alpay, 2017, p. 25). However, the prefix post, which assumes a different role than this general usage in the concept of post-truth, refers to a stage where the word it comes before becomes unimportant and irrelevant (Oxford Advanced Learner's Dictionary, 2016).

Although the concept of "post-truth" was first used by Steve Tesich in an article in Nation in 1992, it came to the fore in 2004 with the book "Post-Truth Age" written by Ralph Keyes. While the original word "post-truth" was translated into Turkish, definitions such as "beyond truth", "post-truth", "post-truth", "over-truth", "beyond reality" were emphasized (Alpay, 2017, p. 25). The agreed-upon concept has often been "post-truth".

Oxford Dictionaries have defined post-truth as "a situation in which objective truths are less influential than emotions and personal convictions in determining public opinion on a particular issue". Post-truth is most clearly associated with the emphasis on lying, with persistent accusations of lying and disclosure of the lie. Although it is nearly impossible to prove that there are more lies or liars today than in the past, there is an observable discourse claiming that there is more about lying because lies exist (Harsin, 2018, p. 11).

Keyes (Keyes, 2017, p. 266) also explained the concept of post-truth through the concepts of lie and deception. According to him, deception has become commonplace in all levels of contemporary life. People have spoken words that are not true since they had the words to speak. Lies have been told for a long time. However, before, lies were told with anxiety and embarrassment. Now people can lie without feeling guilty. Lies are often told that we do not even realize how much we lie. This issue has come to the fore today because lying has become a norm rather than an exception.

FOUNDATIONS OF THE POST-TRUTH ERA

At the beginning of the 2000s, technological developments began to take place more in life, and the reflections of these developments against the truth began to emerge over time (Özçelik, 2021a). These reflections, which contribute to the trivialization of truth, were classified by Alpay (2017) under the headings of postmodernism, new media order, decreased trust in democracy, and populism.

Postmodernism

Postmodernism, one of the essential foundations of the post-truth era, has many different types and definitions. However, when evaluated in general terms, postmodernism advocates a view that rejects the objective reality independent of human perception. He claims that knowledge is formed by filtering class, race, and gender variables. It is also possible to say that postmodernism, which replaces the truth with the concept of "perspective" (Kakutani, 2018, p. 40), is roughly an opposition to modernism or a reaction to modernism (Bulut, 2021, p. 112).

In order to understand what modernism is, it is necessary to look at the concept of the traditional period first. The traditional period refers to when a divine power seeks the source of knowledge. The church usually controls the production and distribution of knowledge during this period. In this period, not the opinions of people but the orders of God are essential. However, this situation has changed with the transition to the modern period. The human mind has become the source of knowledge. However, essential projects of the modern era such as development, progress, democracy, and human rights could not be implemented. Postmodernism has emerged as an opposition to these ideal and definitive judgments of modernism (Demir, 2018, pp. 166–180).

While modernism glorifies science, postmodernism carries science into an ideological environment and places it in the same status as ideological discourses (Bolat, 2019, p. 42). According to postmodern thought, there is no such thing as truth. All truth claims are the political ideology of the person who made them. All claims to information are statements of authority. Since there is no such thing as truth, the person who claims to know something is trying to put the other person under pressure (McIntyre, 2019, p. 119). In postmodern thought, truths are mentioned, not truth. Postmodernity, which approaches all concepts such as absoluteness, objectivity, and universality attributed to the truth with skepticism, has become one of the most important actors of the post-truth period (Bulut, 2021, p. 113).

Contributing to the trivialization of truth, this actor points to an uncertain period. Postmodernism, which does not have a clear definition of its own, is a system dominated by uncertainty and disorder. The existence of truth in this system was also questioned, and the belief that truth could be reached through reason was shaken. In such a period when everything, including knowledge, has become relative, it is no longer possible to talk about a single truth. Everything changes according to the subject's point of view. The truth is now lost, and the important thing is not to reach the truth but to reach the more aesthetic one (Alpay, 2017, pp. 36–38).

New Media Order

One of the deepest roots of the post-truth era is the cognitive biases we encounter at every stage of human evolution. Psychologists have been experimenting that we are not as rational as we think for many years. One of the main characteristics of human psychology is that it tends to avoid mental unrest. It is not pleasant to think something negative about oneself. The fact that something we believe is not true also creates psychological tension. While we were able to correct these cognitive biases by interacting with people in the past, today, we can choose our interaction area (McIntyre, 2019, pp. 51–69).

This situation, which is possible with new communication technologies, has led to more discussion of the concept of truth. First of all, new communication technologies that allow the user to produce content have caused deformation in the quality of the content. Digitization has also transformed the production and distribution processes of news, which is the raw material of the media. In other words, the form and functioning of traditional journalism practices have changed (Şen, 2021). Now, media professionals and every user with internet access can produce and publish content. This situation, which is possible with the emergence of Web 2.0 technology, has allowed being heard by the masses who cannot make their voices heard in the traditional media. There is no longer a need for media structuring as in traditional media. The user can transmit the message he wants to convey to the other end of the world with a smartphone or computer and internet connection, and everyone can see this message. This feature, which seems optimistic at first glance, has brought various problems. The spread of disinformation and misinformation has become easier with social media. In these environments, where control and content control are not very strict, people can quickly spread false or false information. The rapid nature of social media also has a share in this problem. In order to be clicked more on social media, it is essential to give the news or information first. This causes information to be shared without control. Information shared without checking its accuracy contributes to the post-truth period.

Another pillar of the new media on post-truth is algorithms, filter bubbles, and echo chambers. In new communication technologies, authenticity is replaced by the ability to appeal to emotions, and algorithms, echo chambers, and filter balloons make this situation familiar (Delal & Abanoz, 2021, p. 274).

Algorithms and artificial intelligence applications imprison people in filter bubbles with the information they provide. This situation, which is realized with the personalization feature of the new media, shapes the content that will appear in front of the user according to the search history. Thus, algorithms provide users with content they will like and hide content they will not be interested in (Delal & Abanoz, 2021, p. 274). Algorithms used by technology companies, especially Google and Facebook, were also on the agenda during the US Presidential elections. With the algorithms used, fake news was shown in the top positions in search engines, which enabled the news to be recirculated. The fact that the news at the top of Google search engines is accepted as correct by users has also caused this problem to grow (Kocabay Şener, 2019, p. 412).

Echo chambers also contribute to the post-truth period in this sense. People who follow thoughts, shares, and social media accounts that do not contradict their own thoughts are building a world where virtual reality is produced without criticism. On the one hand, the echo chamber effect strengthens one's current worldview; on the other hand, it causes the illusion of accepting this view as more accurate and universal. Users can easily limit the messages they want to be exposed to with a click in a way that supports their views (Narin, 2018, pp. 240–241).

Along with these developments, whether the news presented in the media, which has the mission of conveying the correct information and the truth to people, contains truth or not, has formed the media leg of the discussions about post-truth (Kocabay Şener, 2019, p. 384). In this sense, the post-truth trend is new because of the diffusing power of social media. The hostility to the truth that we encounter in every period of history has gained great opportunities with new technologies (Özçelik, 2021b, p. 191). This situation caused the post-truth problem to be discussed in the media.

Populism

Populism, a concept that emerged towards the end of the 19th century, takes its name from the word "Populus," that is, people. Populism, which has a structure that includes everything like the people (Belge, 2018), is a form of a regime that tends to establish a general relationship between the charismatic leader and the masses. Populism is a method that envisages appealing to fixed thoughts or prejudices rooted in the brains of the masses (Eco, 2012, pp. 161–162). The search for truth and solutions in political debates and conflicts is no longer critical. The tendencies and polarizing policies that reveal their truth and impose it as truth have gained strength (Bulut, 2021, p. 191).

Populism is in harmony with the era of the trivialization of truth. Both concepts are against rational reasoning, feeding on factual data, elites, and truth. Both draw their strength from perception management and the under-educated and low-income masses of the society. Rather than following what is actually going on or what the truth is, they follow what this crowd thinks is right. However, they do not do this directly from the audience's thoughts, and they catch the audience with emotional messages and fraudulent reasoning that will feed and support their stereotypical prejudices. Then they make them accept the ideas they want, and then they draw their politics on these ideas that they have placed in the masses. Both concepts try to appear democratic and undermine democracy. Its legitimator in every matter is the crowd it makes believe. In other words, their references are not reason, science, or art, but the opinions, prejudices, and beliefs of the most unequipped mass of the society. Moreover, they do this not secretly but openly by glorifying the people, vilifying the elite, keeping the traditions above reason, and fueling the prejudices that work for them, no matter how baseless (Alpay, 2017, pp. 57–58).

Populist movements have scattered belief systems; they are inherently difficult to control and organize; they lack consistency, and their effectiveness is in the form of tides of significantly varying frequency. Populism is a slippery and challenging concept. It lacks the qualities that could make it more tangible. It has embedded features that make it inherently variable. It is challenging to construct a generalized expression of populism as an idea or political movement, let alone a universal and comprehensive definition (Taggart, 2004, p. 2).

In every corner of the world, populism and radicalism increase fear and anger while reducing rational discussion environments. This situation, which harms democratic institutions, brings the voice of the crowd to the fore instead of the voice of experts (Kakutani, 2018, p. 15). In recent years, some of the world's most stable parliamentary democracies have seen so-called populist political movements and leaders come to the fore. The election of President Trump in the United States and the United Kingdom's referendum to withdraw from the European Union (Brexit) have both been interpreted as a populist backlash against the political elite and a challenge to the traditional institutions of liberal democracies (Speed & Mannion, 2017, p. 249).

Decreased Trust in Democracy

Another source of the post-truth era is the decline of faith in democratic institutions and the deliberate, conscious interventions of non-democratic actors. The idea of the welfare state, which was built after the Second World War, collapsed with the transition to the neoliberal order. Many studies have shown that trust in democracies has been on a steady decline in the last 40 years (Alpay, 2017, p. 55).

The historical process that led to the current destruction of balances in liberal or social democracies by populist forces has deep structural roots conducive to the post-truth situation. As seen before, the technological, cultural, and social transformations experienced have eroded the stability of the institutions and categories of modernity. Such corrosive effects have accelerated since the early 1980s (Cosentino, 2020, p. 26).

The search for truth and solutions in political conflicts and debates is no longer necessary. The distrust of systems and the lack of a solution to humanity's problems have weakened the relationship with the truth. Now, polarizing political forces reveal and impose their truths as truth (Özçelik, 2021b, p. 189). Voters and consumers are vulnerable to covert persuasion techniques. Voter manipulation is the foundation of democratic politics. It is known that emotions and feelings always dominate the mood of people. Authoritarian leaders increase their appeal in this period when post-truth trends are undermining liberal democracy. These leaders spread a widespread distrust of expertise, making it difficult to make the right decision in the public sphere, increasing the possibility of social conflict by separating power from reality (Picciotto, 2019, pp. 94–95).

In short, the risks associated with the post-truth era often relate to initiating or maintaining bad policies. Politicians in the post-truth era aim to secure and use arbitrary power while trying to change the status quo for the better (Picciotto, 2019, p. 92). This situation, which harms democracies, is also associated with populism. Rising populism in the world increases fear and anger and reduces rational discussion environments. This situation, which harms democratic institutions, puts the crowd's voice at the forefront instead of the voice of experts. The false claims of the UK in the Brexit process and the disinformation efforts of Russia before the elections in many countries such as France, Germany, and the Netherlands have damaged democracy (Kakutani, 2018, p. 15). Trump has also taken steps that harm democracy in the post-truth era. Trump told 2,140 lies in the first year of his presidency. In the first six months of his second year, he doubled his lies to 4,230. Trump lied on Twitter, at rallies, at press conferences, and in official statements; He lied about NATO leaders, unemployment, sex relations, about relations with Russia (Cabas, 2019, p. 16). These lies told in the political field have caused the truth to become insignificant, and both those who lie and those who are lied to have jointly built a post-truth era. In this construction, the parties know that their communication is based on lies. However, since there are mutual material and moral interests, these lies have been presented and accepted as truth (Alpay, 2017, p. 77).

In this period, when politicians are prone to making statements independent of facts and voters are prone to make decisions beyond logic (Karadut, 2020, p. 137), democracy suffers. This issue, damaging to democracy, is also an essential foundation of the post-truth era. Authoritarian leaders increase their appeal and undermine democracy with post-truth tendencies (Picciotto, 2019, pp. 94–95).

FUTURE RESEARCH DIRECTIONS

Post-truth, a frequently discussed topic in recent years, is especially interaction with new media technologies. Fake news spreads more easily with new media tools. People encounter dozens of fake news every day. This leads to the normalization of lies and the trivialization of truth. Fact-checking platforms created to combat fake news are trying to solve this problem. In future studies, the relationship between fact-checking platforms and truth is an issue that needs to be examined.

In addition, studies on post-truth can also be done in the metaverse, which has recently entered our lives.

CONCLUSION

Today's era, where the concept of truth is questioned more than ever, is called the post-truth era. The real problem today, when lying is normal, and more importantly, lying has become the norm, is seen as the fact that the truth has become unimportant. Although there have been lies in every period of history, there are claims that lying has become normal today. Today, the important thing is not the truth but the power of appealing to people's feelings, beliefs and prejudices.

In short, with the definition of the post-truth era, the focus of truth debates has changed. It is no longer discussed what the truth is or how to reach the truth, but why the truth has become unimportant. In the light of these discussions, the study first focused on postmodernism. Postmodernism, which has an uncertain and slippery ground, argues that there is no single truth. According to postmodernism, different truths change according to situations. This is the most essential feature of the post-truth era.

Another factor that paved the way for the post-truth era has been shown as the new media order. With the development of the Internet and computer technologies, a period has entered the era where users can also produce content. Information is now rapidly produced and shared. And the control of information is not as tight as in traditional media. This situation affects the quality of information, increasing intentional or unintentional information pollution. In addition, big technology companies bring people to content that will overlap with their thoughts through algorithms and filter balloons in these environments. Thus, people see their thoughts as the truth and cannot be aware of different opinions.

Another factor that harms the truth is the wave of populism that has been on the rise recently. An increasing number of politicians appeal to the prejudices and traditional beliefs adopted by the masses, without any basis, instead of the truth. The important thing is not the truth but winning. There is no problem in damaging the truth in order to gain power. In addition, with the decrease in trust in democracies, we entered a period where truth became unimportant. In this period, when politicians who try to show people their truth as truth are accepted, the masses do not care about the lies told to them.

These developments have changed the definition and importance of truth. In this post-truth period, even scientific truths have become easily questioned by non-experts. Science lost its importance; beliefs gained strength.

REFERENCES

Alpay, Y. (2017). *The Politics of Lies: Legitimating Lies, Trivializing Truth, and Fraudulent Reasoning Techniques* [Yalanın Siyaseti: Yalanın Meşrulaştırılması, Hakikatin Önemsizleştirilmesi ve Hileli Akıl Yürütme Teknikleri]. Destek Yayınları.

Belge, M. (2018). *"If you want...": Essays on Populism* ["Siz isterseniz...": Popülizm Üzerine Yazılar]. İletişim Yayınları.

Bolat, N. (2019). The New Roadmap of Modernism: Post-Modernism [Modernizmin Yeni Yol Haritası: Post-Modernizm]. In M. N. Erdem & N. Kocabay Şener (Eds.), *Communication in the Age of Posts* [Postlar Çağında İletişim] (pp. 33–59). Literatürk Academia.

Bulut, Ö. (2021). Philosophy, Truth and Beyond [Felsefe, Hakikat ve Sonrası]. In B. Özçelik (Ed.), *Post-truth Politics, Philosophy, Media, International Relations* [Hakikat Sonrası Siyaset, Felsefe, Medya, Uluslararası İlişkiler] (pp. 97–118). Nika Yayınevi.

Cabas, M. (2019). Tell Me Sweet Little Lies [Bana Tatlı Küçük Yalanlar Söyle]. In L. Mcintyre (Ed.), *Post-Truth* [Hakikat Sonrası] (pp. 15–19). Tellekt.

Chandler, D., & Munday, R. (2018). *A Dictionary of Media and Communication* [Medya ve İletişim Sözlüğü] (B. Taşdemir, Trans.). İletişim Yayınları.

Cosentino, G. (2020). *Social Media and the Post-Truth World Order: The Global Dynamics of Disinformation*. Palgrave Macmillan. doi:10.1007/978-3-030-43005-4

Delal, Ö., & Abanoz, E. (2021). Information Sharing and Misinformation about Covid-19 on Social Media in the Context of New Media Literacy [Yeni Medya Okuryazarlığı Bağlamında Sosyal Medyada Covid-19 ile İlgili Bilgi Paylaşımı ve Misenformasyon]. In F. Ünal Çolak & O. Yıldırım (Eds.), *Pandemic, Research and Discussions in the Digital World* [Dijital Dünyada Pandemi, Araştırmalar ve Tartışmalar] (pp. 265–296). Literatürk Academia.

Demir, Ö. (2018). *Philosophy of Science* [Bilim Felsefesi]. Sentez Yayıncılık.

Eco, U. (2012). *Turning Back the Clock: Hot Wars and Media Populism* [Yengeç Adımlarıyla: Sıcak Savaşlar ve Medyatik Popülizm] (S. Gezgin, Trans.). Doğan Kitap.

Foucault, M. (2001). *Fearles Speech* [Doğruyu Söylemek] (K. Eksen, Trans.). Ayrıntı Yayınları.

Frolov, İ. (1991). *Dictionary of Philosophy* [Felsefe Sözlüğü] (A. Çalışlar, Trans.). Cem Yayınevi.

Harsin, J. (2018). Post-Truth and Critical Communication Studies. In Oxford Research Encyclopedia of Communication (pp. 1–32). Oxford University Press. doi:10.1093/acrefore/9780190228613.013.757

Kakutani, M. (2018). *The Death of Truth: Notes on Falsehood in the Age of Trump* [Hakikatin Ölümü: Trump Çağında Yalancılık Sanatı] (C. Mizrahi, Trans.). Doğan Kitap.

Karadut, İ. C. (2020). Telling the Truth in the Post-Truth Age: Two Cases of Parrhesia [Hakikat-Ötesi Çağda Hakikati Söylemek: İki Parrhesia Vakası]. *Pasajlar Sosyal Bilimler Dergisi*, *4*, 125–140.

Keyes, R. (2017). *The Post-Truth Era: Dishonesty and Deception in Contemporary Life* [Hakikat Sonrası Çağ: Günümüz Dünyasında Yalancılık ve Aldatma] (D. Özçetin, Trans.). Delidolu Yayınları.

Kocabay Şener, N. (2019). Post-Truth If You Want Lies, Let Me Lies [Post-Hakikat (Post-Truth) Yalanlar İstiyorsan Yalanlar Söyleyeyim]. In M. N. Erdem & N. Kocabay Şener (Eds.), *Communication in the Age of Posts* [Postlar Çağında İletişim] (pp. 383–416). Literatürk Academia.

McIntyre, L. (2019). *Post-truth* [Hakikat-Sonrası] (M. F. Biçici, Trans.). Tellekt.

Narin, B. (2018). The Examination Of Personalized News Feed in The Context Of Echo Chamber Effect, Filter Bubble And Cyberbalcanization Concepts [Kişiselleştirilmiş Çevrimiçi Haber Akışının Yankı Odası Etkisi, Filtre Balonu ve Siberbalkanizasyon Kavramları Çerçevesinde İncelenmesi]. *Selçuk İletişim, 11*(2), 232–251.

Oxford Advanced Learner's Dictionary. (2016). *Post* [Dictionary]. https://www.oxfordlearnersdictionaries.com/definition/english/post_2?q=post

Özçelik, B. (2021a). Religion in the Post-Truth and Public Space [Hakikat Sonrası ve Kamusal Alanda Din]. In B. Özçelik (Ed.), *Post-truth Politics, Philosophy, Media, International Relations* [Hakikat Sonrası Siyaset, Felsefe, Medya, Uluslararası İlişkiler] (pp. 185–198). Nika Yayınevi.

Özçelik, B. (2021b). Presentation: To Defend the Truth [Sunuş: Hakikati Savunmak İçin] In B. Özçelik (Ed.), *Post-truth Politics, Philosophy, Media, International Relations* [Hakikat Sonrası Siyaset, Felsefe, Medya, Uluslararası İlişkiler] (pp. 1–12). Nika Yayınevi.

Picciotto, R. (2019). Is Evaluation Obsolete in a Post-Truth World? *Evaluation and Program Planning, 73*, 88–96. doi:10.1016/j.evalprogplan.2018.12.006 PMID:30562668

Şen, O. (2021). Robot Journalism [Robot Gazetecilik]. In M. Şahin & E. İlhan (Eds.), *Specialization Areas in Journalism* [Gazetecilikte Uzmanlaşma Alanları] (pp. 57–76). Pelikan Yayınları.

Speed, E., & Mannion, R. (2017). The Rise of Post-truth Populism in Pluralist Liberal Democracies: Challenges for Health Policy. *International Journal of Health Policy and Management, 6*(5), 249–251. doi:10.15171/ijhpm.2017.19 PMID:28812811

Taggart, P. (2004). *Populism* [Popülizm] (B. Yıldırım, Trans.). Bilgi Üniversitesi Yayınları.

Taş, O., & Taş, T. (2018). Fake News in Social Media and Syrian Refugee Crisis in the Post-truth Era [Post-Hakikat Çağında Sosyal Medyada Yalan Haber ve Suriyeli Mülteciler Sorunu]. *Galatasaray Üniversitesi İletişim Dergisi, 29*, 183–208. doi:10.16878/gsuilet.500943

Zabcı, F. (2021). Truth, Rhetoric and Politics [Hakikat, Retorik ve Siyaset]. In B. Özçelik (Ed.), *Post-truth Politics, Philosophy, Media, International Relations* [Hakikat Sonrası Siyaset, Felsefe, Medya, Uluslararası İlişkiler] (pp. 13–29). Nika Yayınevi.

ADDITIONAL READING

Baggini, J. (2018). *A short history of truth: Consolations for a post-truth world.* Quercus.

Farkas, J., & Schou, J. (2019). *Post-truth, fake news and democracy: Mapping the politics of falsehood*. Routledge. doi:10.4324/9780429317347

Lewandowsky, S., Ecker, U. K. H., & Cook, J. (2017). Beyond misinformation: Understanding and coping with the "post-truth" era. *Journal of Applied Research in Memory and Cognition*, *6*(4), 353–369. doi:10.1016/j.jarmac.2017.07.008

Ott, B. L. (2017). The age of Twitter: Donald J. Trump and the politics of debasement. *Critical Studies in Media Communication*, *34*(1), 59–68. doi:10.1080/15295036.2016.1266686

KEY TERMS AND DEFINITIONS

Modernism: It is an opinion based on sense and science.

New Media: Internet and computer-based communication tools.

Populism: Trying to influence the masses by appealing to their emotions rather than their minds.

Post: It means after, next, later.

Post-Truth: It means that the truth loses importance, and people do not care about it.

Postmodernism: There is no single truth in postmodernism; there is more than one truth. Indicates an uncertain period.

Truth: It means the truthfulness of thought.

Chapter 2
Grandiose Mirrors of the Self: The Narcissistic Narrative in Ads

Sena Şahin
https://orcid.org/0000-0001-6769-8640
Ondokuz Mayıs University, Turkey

Recep Yılmaz
https://orcid.org/0000-0003-3406-2755
Ondokuz Mayıs University, Turkey

ABSTRACT

Advertising narratives mostly use narcissistic discourses while appealing to the self of today's people to provide identification and transfer between the consumer and the brand. The study focuses on advertisements that promise to complete the lack of spiritual structure that the consumer's ego needs and desires based on a narcissistic narrative. The article's main question is how the promise of completion in the advertisement is realized through the egocentric structure in the advertisement narrative and how it is included in the story. Another focal point of the work is how and within which themes the transference between the narcissistic narrative in the advertisement and the consumer affects the consumer and how this interaction will be evaluated from a psychoanalytic point of view. This chapter offers the reader an analytical discussion to open these issues.

INTRODUCTION

TV commercials try to influence the consumer and include the consumer in the primary narrative promised by the commercial with the description they construct with plot, character, time, and place elements. They emerge so that the advertising narrative, which the adverting professionals consciously create, has a meaning expressed by each component.

Advertisements both realize the identification and transfer between the consumer and the brand and establish a bond by giving place to the consumers' desires, wishes, and needs. However, when the advertisement aims to appeal directly to the consumer's self, narcissistic narrative factors come into play,

DOI: 10.4018/978-1-7998-9251-9.ch002

causing the consumer to reconstruct their self-image through advertising, brand, and product. Advertisements promise to complete the lack of spiritual structure that the consumer's ego needs and desires based on a narcissistic narrative.

The consumer society transforms self-culture into the essential culture and indicator of the modern age through advertisements. A person preoccupied with himself without borders in the self-culture defines his/herself through the consumption of objects and tries to find his/her deficiencies in the media. At this very point, advertisements turn into fantasies and daydreams in which the narcissist satisfies his grandiose self and exhibitionism. Advertising, which builds this function on the narcissistic person's desire for unlimited power, success, and admiration, invites the consumer to his unique pleasure. The marketing business, which has to act according to the changing consumer trends, places the consumer in the center by switching to a consumer-oriented understanding. Today, brands focus on analyzing the life and self of the consumer, thinking like him, acting like him, capturing similarities with the consumer, and having the same personality, culture, and lifestyle to influence the consumer and establish a bond with him. With the globalizing world, brands that want to keep all consumers in their hands concentrate on the consumer self and market a lifestyle to the consumer. These lifestyles and self-designs focused on consuming and changing become an object that the consumer can put on like armor, completing the lack of the consumer's self and returning him to the first years of his life, when he was perfect and omnipotent.

As it is known, in the first years of his life, a person who is constantly satisfied by his mother as a narcissist loses all his primitive idealization and primitive omnipotence when faced with reality. The illusion of getting rid of the reality principle offered to man by the modern age invites him to break away from the fact of life and return to the fantasies of omnipotence and infinity and a break in reality. Advertising, one of these resting places, realizes this call through narratives. The people of the modern age no longer focus on tales and stories that appeal to everyone with general content but only on obtaining satisfaction and pleasure from narratives with a unique appeal. While the narcissistic narrative in the advertisement's content occurs between the brand and the consumer, it is built on individuality. The primary purpose of this study is to analyze how the narcissistic transformation in the consumption culture is pervaded via the advertising narrative and to take a glance at a psychoanalytic view of the narcissistic tendencies in advertising.

WHAT IS NARCISSISM?

The origin of the concept of narcissism is based on the myth that the Greek mythological hero Narcissus saw his reflection in the water and fell in love with himself. There are many versions of the myth, but the most common and classic is the one in which the love between Narcissus and Echo is stuck with the impossibility of the idealized self.

Narcissus was an impeccably beautiful young man favored by the nymphs, but he paid no attention to the fairies. A fairy named Echo, who is very fond of him, approaches Narcissus one day and is harshly rejected. Destroyed by his shame and grief after the event, Echo vanishes, leaving only his echoing voice behind. In the face of this demand of the water nymphs, who want Echo's revenge, the Gods decide to punish Narcissus with having unrequited passion: One day, Narcissus, looking at a clear puddle on the mountain, sees his reflection there and thinks he has met a beautiful spirit living in the water. He cannot separate himself from this image that looks at him above the water but does not respond and disappears every time he touches the water to embrace it. He eventually drowns and dies by falling into the water (Gençtan, 2018, p. 257).

Narcissus, who has an impassable and inaccessible mirrored armor against the outside world, builds all his perception and expectation on himself by only seeing himself and hearing only himself. Deceived by his reflection, he prefers his authentic self to his idealized self - that is, his image - and concentrates on satisfying himself only by desiring it. Narcissus, who died by drowning in water because he could not find a way to help his desire for his reflection, changes shape and turns into a narcissus flower living in water in the continuation of the legend. Narcissus perceives the world in a self-centered way, creating a grandiose and exhibitionist self-image. When his pleasure in being admired increases to such an extent that it undermines his reality, he is deceived by his reflection. His personality becomes dependent on a particular object, as his object-hunger for the old sense of perfection is stuck in Narcissus' archaic self-object. Narcissus, who accidentally finds his search for his thing of self in his reflection on the water, becomes insensitive to the outside world by becoming dependent on his reflection with the excessive intensity of his object search. Since he constructs his self-image design only on himself and cannot find an object of identification, he falls into the error of his reflection by following the first thing that he perceives as like himself as if he were like him. The self-representation of the narcissistic person, like Narcissus, is directed only at himself. That's why seeking oneself in others is interrupted when he cannot find the perfect person to identify. So much so that when this situation turns into the idea that he is unique and superior to others, he thinks that everyone admires him, and he adopts a superficial and lacking empathy attitude in his relations with others.

In classical psychoanalysis, narcissism is defined as the "reversion of libido to ego" and treated as primary and secondary narcissism based on libido theory and object choice (Freud, 2000). The numerous debates on narcissism show that narcissism coordinates the border between life and ourselves, allowing us to find the strength in ourselves that will enable us to adapt to living conditions. Narcissism has two dimensions, normal and pathological narcissism. In both sizes, the focus is on maintaining existence without harming oneself. According to Kernberg, normal narcissism is based on the integrity of the self, external elements, and inner psychic structures and depends on the sustainability of the balance between them (2019, pp. 296-299). Suppose a narcissist cannot maintain that balance between all systems; in that case, an ideal self-image creates not to damage the self and maintain its integrity, and normal narcissism turns into pathological narcissism. On the other hand, Kohut emphasizes that narcissism develops due to pauses in a typical development line, and it underlines that narcissism has pathological and standard dimensions (2020-a).

The most acute clinical syndrome of narcissism is abnormal self-esteem. The individual perceives himself as superior to other people, cannot establish deep close relationships in his life, and lacks empathy. Narcissistic personality type with a grandiose self-image; s/he considers her/himself unique and special, with fantasies of unlimited success, unlimited power, and intense admiration for others. In narcissistic people, "There is a lifelong pattern of superiority (in behavior and fantasy), a constant need for appreciation, and a lack of empathy" (Morrison, 2016, p. 550).

ADVERTISING NARRATIVE AND SELF-STORIES

Advertising narratives are consumer stories prepared to influence consumers for the brands' products and services and the campaign's goals. These consumer stories, which develop around a plot, often have all the narrative elements. For something told to be considered a narrative, it must have a narrator, a sequential sequence, and a plot transformation based on a causal framework on a temporal and spatial plane. In addition to the concept of narrative, classical narrative theories, and approaches, "the use of inter-genre and inter-media approaches and narratological concepts is appropriate and expanded to include genres other than prose" (Dervişcemaloğlu, 2016, p. 39). Advertising texts consider "a type of narrative" because they contain narrative elements. The advent of narrative advertising marks a progression from print ads with story elements to radio ads. Brand-oriented creative content includes the narratives in question in television commercials and creates support visually and audibly for these. With digitalizing, the changing product and consumers make the advertisement completely narrative-oriented, and advertisement narratives create through new technologies used to connect with the consumer (Yılmaz, Çakır, and Resuloğlu, 2017, pp. 133-152).

The primary purpose of narrative advertisements is to convey the main message about the brand and product to the consumer through a plot. The narrative structure of the ad consists of two main elements: Chronology and causality. In the narrative, chronology shows the flow of the sequential series of events and provides the perceptibility of the narrative by offering the time of the story events. On the other hand, causality enables the elements in the narrative to be associated with each other and turn into an inference within the framework of the plot (Escalas, 1998; Escalas, 2004).

Chingching Chang emphasizes that narrative advertising is shaped around a plot in which the product is at the forefront and that "the variety of the narrative can be achieved by changing the plot" and discusses "strategies of narrative repetition" for the diversification of the narrative: (1) Same plot strategy: They are advertisement narratives in which users in different segments of the target audience are planned based on a familiar plot, with the consumption theme of the same product. For example, The success of a vitamin advertisement uses the central theme of success in different target audience segments (at school, work, sports). (2) Different plot strategies: They are advertisement narratives the consumption theme is composed of different plots suitable for the product's characteristics. The narrative structure emphasizes that the same product is ideal for more than one user. For example, different plots are designed to use a multi-purpose cleaning product in different situations and events. (3) Continuous plot strategy: These are advertisement narratives in which the exact product has a constant consumption theme over the same or a similar plot. For example, A chocolate brand's constant use of the same happiness theme with the same plot (Chang, 2009, p. 52).

Advertising narratives have an essential place in establishing the consumer and brand bond. They are used to position the brand, product, or service in the consumer's mind and differentiate it from other brands and products. In addition, such advertisements provide the audience with what and how they can consume, what image they can have, and models that they can take as examples. By making them a part of the consumption culture, they ensure the continuity of the act of consumption. Like brands, people today use symbols to position themselves in the minds of others. Consumers can position themselves in society by using the product or brand's characters and values to reshape themselves. In this positioning process, they tend to prefer brands that are compatible with their self-image or brands that are compatible with their ideal self-image (Odabaşı, 2019). This tendency is considered in the consumer behavior literature to match self-image and product-image and is called 'self-image congruence' (Sırgy, 1982).

While consumers turn to brands that they can identify with, brands enable a person to reconstruct, develop or strengthen their self-concept. In this respect, brands would allow consumers to gain status and prestige in social and social life.

Consumers who try to reshape themselves through advertisements create their narratives by transferring what they have gained through stories to themselves. Escalas and Bettman argue that the brand and consumers are created the "Self-Brand Connections" each other. Accordingly, the closer the consumers' self-perceptions and the evoked by the brand, the deeper the self-connections established between the consumer and the brand (Escalas & Bettman, 2003). Today, brands act as if they have a self by being personalized through advertisements: Brands or products have ideals, values , and purposes. The more the self-connotations of brands are compatible with the connotations of the consumer's authentic or ideal self, the consumer can act through brands; and it tends to include brand stories in their narratives, so advertisements appear as a one-sided narrative and as a two-sided interaction within a structure that allows the consumer to create their narratives depending on the story processing process (Taşkıran & Bolat, 2013).

Ad's Transfer Stories

Advertisements aim to establish consistent connections between the consumer and the brand by giving information about the brand to the consumer. The primary purpose of the double-sided interaction created by the advertising narrative is to influence the consumer through the narrative and ensure the consumer's brand loyalty by establishing a bond with the brand or product. When the consumer identifies with the advertising narrative or thinks that the advertisement will be compatible with his self-image, he can transfer the experience and information obtained from the advertising narrative to her/himself, and the self-narrative can be formed through advertising.

Antonino Ferro emphasizes that the theme of interpretation in psychoanalysis is related to the narratological same theme and that narratives are also formed in psychoanalysis, even if it has a specific structure. Meaning is not created solely by the analyst's effort or the patient's behavior and discourse. This situation, he explains by putting forward the concept of "transformational common narrative" or "co-narrative transformation." The collaborative narrative is "how analyst and patient 'dance' along with Line C until they can move from C to D - where this is possible." According to Ferro, transference is the deciphering of meaning or the production and construction of meaning from interpretations and occurs as the "interaction of the here and now" (Ferro, 2006, pp. 1-7). The emergence of narratives is also revealed by transference experience; "The transference experience is communicated and understood by the analyst partly through projective identifications and partly through characters developed in the patient's narrative" (Goldberg, 2015, p. 497).

Like the reader-text in literary narratives, and the analyst-analyst relationship in psychoanalytic therapy, advertising has a narrative and plot based on the desires of an audience. As in the relationship between the analyst and the analysand, a transfer occurs between the advertisement and its audience. While watching the advertisement, the viewer "enacts" the personal story and conflicts in a special presentation and evaluates the product as a unique space. He symbolically redefines himself through the advertisement. When appropriate conditions are met, it affects the buying and consuming behavior. The "transferential" area in advertising narratives is realized through the consumer's interpretation of the advertisement by adding his personal history and reshaping his own past story. This remodeling proceeds based on the consumer's desires and expectations. Transference allows the past and its wish-based scenarios to come to life in signs with such a vivid reality that the configurations create the effect of fact. In a sense, although the history of the constructions has not changed, it can be said that rewriting it in the discourse of the present, it is preparing for a different future (Brooks, 2016, p. 82). Advertising promises to enable the consumer to become the person they want to be in the future, through a discourse of the present, as in the transference of the consumer's "past and its aspirational scenarios."

Like stories, advertisements aim to gain a place in the consumer's mind. However, this purpose is based on a commercial concern. Advertising aims to create information about the product or change opinions to favor the product. Just as the analyst, structuring stories and transferring them to the analysand, hopes to construct a new narrative that evolves into a new ending to produce a "solid belief" that allows for new confirming memories or a fiction that has the potential to replace what has happened in the past (Brooks, 2016, p. 81), the advertisement also presents a fiction to the consumer as if it will belong to him, and expects the consumer to construct a new narrative on the product itself. In advertising, the transfer enables the reproduction of fiction with interpretation and structuring. When the consumer adopts the story told in the advertisement by integrating it with his personal history as a new narrative, he can define himself based on the product's functionality and the brand. At this point, advertisements should be evaluated as narratives that can affect the consumer self and their "transference" quality.

Possible Scenarios and Self Stories in Advertising

Advertising constantly gives consumers "imagination guides," asking them to think about what they will become or gain when using the product or brand. It enters the consumer's mind, just like a daydream, and presents the possible scenarios in which they use brands and products. The more the consumer can identify the dream with the product, the more he believes in the reality of the dream and is satisfied, and the more the bond between them increases. Thus, the target audience becomes inclined towards purchasing behavior by choosing the way of realizing the dream to achieve the satisfaction they feel from the dream.

The concept of "mental simulation," which is essential in terms of social psychology and consumer research, emphasizes the cognitive connection of consumers between the product and the brand. Mental simulation involves creating possible scenarios against the stimulus that the individual encounters. These potential scenarios often take the form of stories and narratives. Mental simulations usually appear as a narrative consisting of three parts: introduction, development, and conclusion. Considering a possible scenario, a behavioral action plan needs to be prepared. Advertising narratives create a simulation by presenting possible scenarios we may encounter in daily life, on an action plan, to the consumer. The action plan in advertising takes place through the positioning of the brand or product, and the possible scenario ends with the use of the product. When the advertisement imitates a possible scenario, the consumer transforms the possible scenario of the ad into a mental simulation by being cognitively stimulated and creating a mental simulation in which the main character is her/himself by interpreting and changing the possible scenario based on her/himself, in other words by creating a new and own narrative. According to Escalas, the mechanism by which mental simulation and stories persuade is the same. When the narrative of the mental simulation is transferred to the person's self, the simulation stimulated by the advertisement is adopted, and the advertising arguments are evaluated less critically, causing more positive and stronger emotional reactions. Suppose the action plan presented by the advertising arguments saves the consumer from negative scenarios, and the product solves the problems. In that case, the consumer can be persuaded to use the product through the narrative transfer of mental simulation. The more the possible scenarios in the advertising narrative are close to the mental simulation narrative of the consumer and the more the action plan can save the consumer from negative experiences, the more the target audience can identify with the brand and product by transferring them, and they can show the buying behavior. The consumer tends to identify with brands with a shared history, values , and experiences and establish a loyalty bond (Escalas, 2004).

Brands must go beyond just identifying the consumer's needs and developing products for the needs of the consumption culture. Consumers no longer only focus on the functional benefit of the product but also on purchasing behavior for the value and experiences offered by the product. The consumer no longer consumes the purely functional use of the product but consumes the story it presents to the consumer. Consumers create their own stories by turning to brands with shared values and experiences and transferring their stories to themselves. Modern consumers have become inclined to define themselves through the consumption of goods they own, create their desires, create their values, and expand their selves through consumption (McColl & Legorburu, 2019, p. 194).

The consumer, who clings to the act of consuming to identify himself with the consumption society, embarks on a journey to collect his "self-stories." It's a similar but shorter journey to Campbell's template. Ads offer a "call to adventure" that facilitates the audience's transformation into "heroes." At this point, the sage that the hero encounters on his journey appears in the advertisement itself and presents the magical truth to us. The template of the possible scenarios of the trip for "self-stories" in the journey of the consumer in story design is as follows:

Our hero -------------------- (write consumer need) sets out to satisfy his need; we give him a gift as his teacher, --------- -----------(insert product/service) we provide. This gift magically provides ------------------- (type statement of value, unique selling proposition, etc.); in this way, our hero ------------------ (write your advantage) can (McColl & Legorburu, 2019, p. 118).

NARCISSISTIC NARRATIVE IN AD

Background

Advertising narratives create areas of narcissistic exploration by appealing to the consumer's self and transforming his secret desires into needs that need to be satisfied, glorifying the consumer's individuality. The promise of the consumer to create a new self-narrative based on common past and values with advertising feeds the narcissistic side of the consumer and makes the consumer dependent on the narcissistic one. Whereas advertising was aimed at products and sales in the past, today, advertising has a "lifestyle" marketing purpose (Lasch, 2006, p. 125). However, thanks to the "self-culture" that dominates the current era, advertisement for the bored and insatiable consumer who becomes alienated from his own life as he becomes an individual; this lifestyle creates behavioral patterns and ready-made representations and markets them with the promise of a grandiose self-image. Product orientation evolves into consumer orientation, and the mere features are not crucial to the modern consumer. The consumer, who does not care about the maximum benefit from the product, is ready to pay for the experience and pleasure that the product will provide, not the product.

When the person, who is insufficient to satisfy his narcissistic grandiosity and exhibitionism, tries to be happy through fantasies, which are the most distinctive feature of narcissism when he is not satisfied with the reality offered by modern life. The narcissistic narrative creates an opportunity for the consumer to realize the omnipotent fantasies of the narcissistic personality; unlimited power, unlimited success, unexpected attention from others, and more become experienced through the product or brand presented in the advertisement. While the advertising narrative promises to complete the void created by the narcissistic age of modern people, it turns the plot from a product orientation to the person using the product. The product's person has a different and unique appearance from other characters and is considered superior to others. The feeling using the product in the plot is omnipotent; He is the one who is constantly successful, robust, perfect, and never under challenging situations and does not ask for help from anyone even if he is left. The other character, who does not use the product or brand, is described as inadequate and worthless. From the narrative and plot to the slogan and music, it's all designed to be part of a unique experience. Slogans are not sales-oriented but in a form that directly appeals to the consumer. While narcissistic tendencies blend into advertising narratives and echo in consumer trends, the new egocentric structure of society turns into an adapted version of all the diagnostic criteria defined by psychiatry. Ultimately, each epoch develops its forms of pathology that exaggerate the basic character structure. In an individualist era, the consumer, who has to deal with himself with all his self-centeredness, obtains the experience of the self-object he needs in the form of a ready-made pattern through advertisements (Lasch, 2006, p. 81).

Increasing narcissistic values in the cultural field are turning the central theme of the advertising narrative into "self-admiration." While modern man strives to arrange his ordinary life by his constant search for self-admiration, approval, and attention, with alienation from everything that the age brings, he tends to follow the popular and the watch, distinguishing him from the others, to maintain this order. Today, the source of the desire for physical beauty is the fountain of self-admiration. Looking beautiful is just another way of gaining attention, status, and popularity for narcissists. Having perfect white teeth, gorgeous hair, a brand-new sports car, or an attractive girlfriend always serves the same psychological function—making others believe we are relaxed, unique, famous, or influential. The ego language of the advertising narrative causes the consumer to reinforce self-admiration, causing him to develop his "obsession with self-promotion." The consumer tends to show himself "as the best" while continuing his ordinary life in advertising narratives that claim to be special and unique. Advertising and marketing practices prepare a program that shows how to strengthen the "me" that the consumer has and gives the consumer "introductory lessons in self-admiration" and improves their self-promotion skills. Modern man does not want to introduce themselves with their gender, age, name, and social roles; They tend to present themselves through the consumption of goods they own. By transferring the power, attractiveness, uniqueness, and uniqueness in the advertising narrative and offering as the fundamental premise of the advertisement, it uses it as an extension of itself and tends to define itself through consumption (Twenge & Campbell, 2015, p. 218).

Advertising and marketing practices facilitate the consumer's positioning in social relations and life. They exhibit all the alternatives that will allow the consumer to create their "self-story" as they wish. The consumer, who is constantly emphasized to be unique and privileged in the advertising narrative, gets the illusion that using the product or brand is enough to make him unique. With a grandiose attitude, he tries to transform his life into a dream universe where he is omnipotent and unique.

Another narcissistic theme in advertising narratives is "claiming." Advertising narratives show how the consumer will strengthen the "me" he has to focus on the theme of "claiming rights" to provide the selfish motivation to activate the consumer. Advertising narratives impress the consumer, who acts with pleasure-oriented impulsivity, with advertising slogans and music, and encourages him to get what he deserves; L'Oréal Paris "Because you are worth it," because "you deserve the best," Doritos "Life is yours!

You make the rules!" etc. Advertising slogans such as "make your own rules" and "you should live your own life according to your desires" call the consumer in the imperative mood. Narcissistic narratives reinforce the pleasure-oriented images acquired by the consumer through advertisements and exploit the consumer's relationship with reality; by presenting the ideal selves in consumer fantasies and dreams with an embodied product, they are putting the perfect self into the illusion that they have achieved it.

When brands' promises are built on everyday experience and shared values through advertising narratives, they contain narcissistic discourses and narratives to form a bond between consumers and brands. Since individuals tend to establish and maintain close relationships with similar people, brands also use narratives to identify with the consumer and give them personality. Advertisers construct the advertisement language, slogan, and advertisement characters in a way that can provide similarity with the consumer to serve this purpose. Today, advertising narratives have a function not only to promote the product but also to the brand's narratives that people use to describe themselves; it conveys all the details to the consumer through narcissistic discourses, including who the brand is, what it cares about, what status it belongs to, who its close friends and social group are. Identification includes material elements as well as personal elements. A person who owns a Cadillac is more likely to identify with other people who own a Cadillac than someone who owns a Ford. This type of identification is called narcissistic identification. In the case of narcissistic identification, the person not only identifies the qualities of an external object with his personality but also desires the object even though he has it and wants to expand his relations with the thing. Such persons desire an object that fulfills a function lacking that can satisfy it. Unlike object choice, the person does not only want to have the thing but tries to help his blocked or unfulfilled desires through narcissistic identification. Suppose advertising narratives can match the consumer's desired object with possible satisfaction scenarios in the consumer's mind. In that case, they can establish a link between the consumer and the brand by realizing a narcissistic identification. In the advertising narrative, the object of identification occurs through the protagonist. The characters in the advertising narrative contain narcissistic personality traits with which the consumer can make a narcissistic identification (Hall, 2010, p. 90; Yılmaz & Çakın, 2017).

Narcissistic Personality in Advertising Narrative

According to Twenge and Campbell, narcissism is the plague of the century, and this epidemic is spreading vigorously in culture. While the authors describe celebrities and the media as "super spreaders," they emphasize that they cause the epidemic to escalate rapidly. They discuss the transmission of narcissistic tendencies of consumer culture to consumers through the media and celebrities, and the prevalence of narcissistic pathologies in the following example:

An advertisement for Kohl's has a band singing "Because I'm amazing." As the band members' clothes change every second, the song says, "I'm the leader / I'm the winner / I don't need you / I'll beat you / Because I'm extraordinary." The rest of the song features phrases like "I'm going to make a lot of money / I'm going to buy a self-tanner." Those calculating the score of the characters in this song in the list of narcissistic personality traits at home may mark next to them: a curiosity for leadership and power; competitiveness; don't tell others you don't need it; exaggerated sense of self; materialism; smugness. A psychologist couldn't have written a more perfect narcissistic song than this. (Twenge & Campbell, 2015, p. 148).

The unique pathological tendencies of the narcissistic culture have been internalized by a modern man so quickly and so well that; it has gathered all the grandiose, exhibitionist nature of narcissism (Lasch, 2006). For this reason, the narcissistic personality in the advertising narrative appears to have a structure that includes all the DSM-5 criteria.

In the advertising narrative, the narcissistic person becomes so arrogant with his achievements that the product and brand he uses glorify him and act as if he has the authority to turn him into a God. He can find the power to eliminate all conflicts and extraordinary situations that he encounters in the advertising narrative. The narrative hero articulates the product and brand to himself; he bends reality in the narrative by having unlimited success, unlimited power, superior talent, and power. The selfish character, which crosses the threshold of a unique and unique world with the advertising narrative, never meets the ordinary in the narrative; only the characters suitable for their strength and uniqueness interact.

The state of entitlement, the most crucial feature of narcissism, also appears in the narrative. This situation is glorified with positioning and support in the narrative; the consumer deserves the best, the most perfect, and the most beautiful of everything. When the consumer builds his expectation on unlimitedness, he believes that he can get whatever he wants. All characters and people in the advertisement narrative have functions and features according to the interest of the narrative hero. All characters serve their interests (American Psychiatric Association, 2014).

Another essential feature of the narcissistic personality in the advertising narrative is that; it frequently resorts to defense processes. In the culture of narcissism, the only time the individual relaxes is through fantasies and daydreams, so the areas in which he actively uses defense processes are limited. Therefore, in the narrative, advertising allows the consumer to be swept away by the flood of desire. The most frequently used defense processes of the narcissistic personality in the narrative; are processes such as idealization, denial, and dreaming. In the narcissistic narrative, idealization is often handled with the methods of identification and sublimation, as it transitions to the product and brand through transference. (Lasch, 2006, p. 34)

Reconstructing the Self in Advertising

While concluding our study, it will be helpful to deal with the concepts of self-object needs, idealization, twinning, and mirroring in Kohut's theory of narcissism.

Kohut argues that there is a pause, a disruption in the development line of narcissistic injury, and emphasizes that identification and transference must occur for pathological narcissism to show normal development of the personality. If the child cannot achieve the necessary internalization regarding developmental and even self-object and image, they stay stuck in the archaic self-object, and their character needs objects throughout their life and creates a dependency on them. The person who wants to complete their self-image and prevent self-injury feels the need for the self-object and suffers from object-hunger (Kohut, 2020-b, p. 56).

Advertising promises to complete the object hunger and spiritual deficiency revealed by Kohut. The brand, service, and product in the advertisement; With the narcissistic narrative, it is presented as an object through that modern man can convey his need for self-object and reconstruct himself. The narcissistic narrative allows the consumer to regain the perfection he had in the primary narcissism stage with his fantasies of unlimited power and success, where he can achieve everything, he is omnipotent and perfect. The consumer, who yearns for the archaic self-object, can reconstruct a grandiose and exhibitionist self-image through the object in the advertisement. He idealizes his former perfectionism by transferring it to a self-object that is a transitional object over the product in the ad. This idealization enables the revival of the narcissistic self-image and positions the product or brand as a self-object. To ensure the sustainability of the selfish balance, advertising allows the self-image to be reconstructed omnipotent, with the promise of fulfillment. The human being, who lives between time and space in an accelerated way in modern life, satisfies his need for self and object hunger through a ready-to-consume representation or an image. The idealized and all-powerful self-object, in which the transfer takes place through advertising, also offers a solution to the problem of emptiness and fragility that occurs when the transference is separated or detached from the object during the analysis. If the consumer has an experience in which the bond between the brand is damaged or bruised, he gains the flexibility to re-construct his grandiose self-image with a different brand and product without experiencing emptiness and vulnerability (Kohut, 2020-b).

The self-object, which gains flexibility through advertising, is the same as the self-object; experiences as an extension are part of it. By identifying himself with the product and brand in the advertisement, he accepts the status, values , and perceptions represented by the product and brand as an extension of himself and integrates with it. Developing and renewed consumer trends have caused what brands mean to become an identity, a personality. The consumer no longer uses only a product but transfers the personal characteristics of the product to himself; For example, by using one product, he internalizes the courage of the brand, and by using another brand, the brand's nature-loving, attractiveness, courage, and creativity, just like an extension of himself, tries to compensate for what is lacking in himself from external sources.

When we consider Kohut's theory of 'Self-Resolving' in Narcissism in advertising, another point we should mention is what self-object needs are and how they emerge in advertising. Self-object needs, according to Kohut, are the need for idealization, twin, and mirroring. Whether or not the advertising narrative has a narcissistic narrative, it ideally presents the product or brand in all circumstances. The transfer of idealization constitutes the basic premise on which it is built in the advertising narrative. The individual who wants to regain his archaic strength and perfection reconstructs his self-image in a grandiose and exhibitionist way through advertising; it places and transfers the desire and ideal of omnipotence to the product or brand. It integrates the narcissistic ideals in the advertising narrative about the product and brand itself. It satisfies the needs of the self with the promises of the product or brand. Mirroring involves responding to the approval, admiration, and exhibitionism of the narcissistic person's grandiose self. Kohut expresses mirror transference as the mother's eyes shining like a mirror to the child's exhibitionist show, the child's response to his narcissistic-exhibitionist pleasure, and emphasizes that the child should internalize the response received as a value to himself. The lack of mirroring and the child's approval by the parent causes self-image damage and inadequacy. The child needs an object that will enable him to perform the mirror transfer, provide visual satisfaction, and reach pleasure. Advertising cannot provide the interaction that may meet the need for mirroring directly, but it can enable the person to satisfy the need for mirroring through indirect ways. The first of these, mirror transfer or the need to be mirrored, starts with the person seeing the advertisement narrative since it is provided by the visual sense, and it occurs through the identification of the grandiose self that the person has with the advertisement. Secondly, when the person uses the product and brand in the ad, the narcissistic experience occurs when the individual sees the pleasure, interest, and admiration that will meet the individual's need for mirroring (Kohut, 2020-a, p. 111).

CONCLUSION

Consumption culture in modern life; directs the consumer to their own to get away from the daily worries and problems of individuals and uses the narcissistic tendencies of the consumer as a trump card against the consumer. The changing and developing culture decomposes everything according to its symbols and values and can turn everything into an object of desire. Consumers can recreate their selves through characters. In a narcissistic period, the media, a world where the consumer can quickly reveal their blocked selfish investment, prepare idealized images, signs, and messages through advertising narratives, and even offers ready and fast consumable idealized object images without the consumer ever having to attempt the image upload process. For the picture presented by the advertisement, it is sufficient for the consumer to only engage in an identification process, but the objects created are not personalized objects, even though they are presented with the label of "personalized" in the advertising narrative; They are stereotyped images that combine quickly consumable, unsustainable, and even non-permanent pleasures that are common to the whole world. But the consumer has such an intense object hunger that he immediately consumes the images and focuses on searching for a new one.

In the advertising narratives that people are exposed to, every element, from the plot to the slogan and music, is designed to be a part of a unique experience and presented to the consumer with ready-made images and representations that can be consumed. All that remains for the consumer is to cross the reality threshold together through advertising, to realize an identification attachment with the idealized object, ready for narcissistic investment. When the consumer exposes himself through the product and brand because he uses the product or brand, the narcissistic experience occurs when the individual sees the pleasure, interest, and admiration that will meet the need for mirroring. When we look at the theme of idealization from self-object conditions in the advertising narrative, it is seen that the central promise of the narcissistic narrative in the advertisement is an idealization. The theme of idealization is used to establish or strengthen the bond between the consumer and the brand. It can enable the consumer to identify the narcissistic ideals in the advertising narrative with himself, allowing him to satisfy the need for the perfect through the product and the brand. The person's exit from this circle depends on creating suitable conditions for him to reach self-awareness. The sociological dynamics of the subject show that the circle is getting narrower and tighter for ordinary people, including their culture.

REFERENCES

Amerikan Psikiyatri Birliği (APA) (2014). *Diagnostic and Census Manual of Mental Disorders 5* [Ruhsal Bozuklukların Tanısal ve Sayımsal Elkitabı 5]. Hekimler Yayın Birliği.

Brooks, P. (2016). *Psychoanalysis and Storytelling* [Psikanaliz ve Hikâye Anlatıcılığı] (H. Demir Atay & H. Atayt, Trans.). Boğaziçi Üniversitesi Yayınları.

Campbell, J. (2013). *Hero's Eternal Journey* [Kahramanın Sonsuz Yolculuğu] (S. Gürses, Trans.). Kabalcı Yayıncılık.

Chang, C. (2009). Repetıtıon Varıatıon Strategıes For Narrative Advertising. *Journal of Advertising, 38*(3), 51–65. doi:10.2753/JOA0091-3367380304

Dervişcemaloğlu, B. (2016). *Introduction to Narrative Science* [Anlatıbilime Giriş]. Dergah.

Escalas, J. E. (1998). Advertising narratives: What are they, and how do they work? *Journal of Consumer Psychology*, 267–289.

Escalas, J. E. (2004). Narrative Processing: Building Consumer Connections to Brands. *Journal of Consumer*, *12*(1&2), 168–180. doi:10.120715327663jcp1401&2_19

Escalas, J. E., & Bettman, J. (2003). You Are What The Eat: The Influence of Reference Groups on Consumers' Connections to Brands. *Journal of Consumer Psychology*, *13*(3), 339–348. doi:10.1207/S15327663JCP1303_14

Ferro, A. (2006). *Psychoanalysis as Therapy and Storytelling*. Routledge Taylor & Francis Group.

Freud, S. (2000). *Metapsychology* [Metapsikoloji] (B. Büyükkal & M. Tura, Trans.). İdea Yayınevi.

Gençtan, E. (2011). *Psychodynamic Psychiatry and Abnormal Behavior* [Psikodinamik Psikiyatri ve Normaldışı Davranışlar]. Metis Yayınları.

Goldberg, S. H. (2015). Transference, the Interpersonal Field, and Psychological Transformation in the Work of Antonino Ferro. *Psychoanalytic Inquiry*, *35*(5), 495–511. doi:10.1080/07351690.2015.1044407

Hall, C. S. (2010). *Introduction to Freudian Psychology* [Freudyen Psikolojiye Giriş] (E. De1vrim, Trans.). Kaknüs Yayınları.

Jahn, M. (2015). *Narrative Theory Handbook* [AnlatıBilim Anlatı Teorisi El Kitabı] (B. Dervişcemaloğlu, Trans.). Dergah.

Kernberg, O. F. (2019). *Border Situations and Pathological Narcissism* [Sınır Durumlar ve Patolojik Narsisizm]. Metis Yayınları.

Kohut, H. (2020-a). *Self-Resolution* [Kendiliğin Çözümlenmesi] (O. Cebeci, Trans.). Metis Yayınları.

Kohut, H. (2020-b). *Self-Restructuring* [Kendiliğin Yeniden Yapılanması] (O. Cebeci, Trans.). Metis Yayınları.

Lasch, C. (2006). *Narcissism Culture* [Narsisizm Kültürü] (S. Öztürk & Ü. H. Yolsal, Trans.). Bilim ve Sanat.

McColl, D., & Legorburu, G. (2019). *Story Design* [Hikâye Tasarımı] (M. Benveniste, Trans.). Kapital Medya.

McCracken, G. (1986). Culture and Consumption: A Theoretical Account of the Structure and Movement of the Cultural Meaning of Consumer Goods. *The Journal of Consumer Research*, *13*(1), 71–84. doi:10.1086/209048

Morrison, J. (2016). *Diagnostic Guide for Clinicians Facilitating DSM-5* [DSM-5'i Kolaylaştıran Klinisyenler için Tanı Rehberi]. Nobel Akademik.

Odabaşı, Y. (2019). *Consumption Culture From Content society to consuming society* [Tüketim Kültürü Yetinen Toplumdan Tüketen Topluma]. Agora Kitaplığı.

Sırgy, M. J. (1982). Self-Concept in Consumer Behavior: A Critical Review. *The Journal of Consumer Research*, *9*(3), 287–300. doi:10.1086/208924

Taşkıran, N. Ö., & Bolat, N. (2013). Ad and Perception Relationship: A Review of the Functions of Sensory Organs in The Acquisition of Advertising Texts [Reklam ve Algı İlişkisi: Reklam Metinlerinin Alımlanmasında Duyu Organlarının İşlevleri Üzerine Bir İnceleme]. *Beykent University Journal of Social Sciences*, *6*(1), 49–69.

Twenge, J. M., & Campbell, W. K. (2015). *Plague of the Century: The Plague of Narcissism* [Asrın Vebası: Narsisizm İlleti] (Ö. Korkmaz, Trans.). Kaknüs.

Yılmaz, R. (2017). *Narrative Advertising Models and Conceptualization in the Digital Age*. IGI-Global. doi:10.4018/978-1-5225-2373-4

Yılmaz, R., & Çakın, Ö. (2017). A Review of Sulphur Coding in Advertising [Reklamda Süblatif Kodlama Üzerine Bir İnceleme]. *MANAS Journal of Social Studies*, *6*(4), 531–539.

Yılmaz, R., Çakır, A., & Resuloğlu, F. (2017). Historical Transformation of the Advertising Narration in Turkey: From Stereotype to Digital Media. In R. Yılmaz (Ed.), *Narrative Advertising Models and Conceptualization in the Digital Age* (pp. 133–152). IGI-Global. doi:10.4018/978-1-5225-2373-4.ch008

ADDITIONAL READING

Alford, C. F. (1988). *Narcissism: Socrates, the Frankfurt School, and Psychoanalytic Theory*. Yale University Press. doi:10.2307/j.ctt211qz5x

Anlı, İ. (2010). *Psikanalizde Narsisizm*. Nobel Tıp Kitapevleri.

Behrendt, R. (2015). *Narcissism and the Self, Dynamics of Self-Preservation in Social Interaction, Personality Structure, Subjective Experience, and Psychopathology*. Palgrave Macmillan.

Jahn, M. (2015). *AnlatıBilim Anlatı Teorisi El Kitabı* (B. Dervişcemaloğlu, Trans.). Dergâh.

Mollon, P. (2020). *Pathologies of the Self: Exploring Narcissistic and Borderline States*. Confer Books.

Ogrodniczuk, J. S. (Ed.). (2013). *Understanding and Treating Pathological Narcissism*. American Psychological Association. doi:10.1037/14041-000

KEY TERMS AND DEFINITIONS

Grandiose Self: The omnipotent and perfect self-image that the narcissistic personality ideally determines through archaic objects and wants to create in himself (Kohut, 2020).

Narrative Advertising: A type of advertisement that conveys the message of interest to the consumer about the brand and product through a plot by using narrative elements such as narrative characters, temporality, and spatiality (Yılmaz, 2017).

Narcissistic Identification: The state of a person's desire for an object that will fulfill a function that is missing in himself that can satisfy him and to reach satisfaction by having it (Hall, 2010).

Omnipotence: The primary (primitive) defense mechanism in which a person assumes that his power is unlimited, can do anything, and has absolute control over the world (McWilliams, 2017).

Primitive Idealization: It is a primitive defense mechanism that can continue from early childhood to adulthood. The individual encodes idealized individuals as if they have superhuman strength and can achieve anything (McWilliams, 2017).

Self-Object: Objects that the person experiences as an extension of himself and invests narcissistically to maintain himself. They are persons or experiences that are called objects because they keep the functionality of the self rather than a real object (Kohut, 2020).

Self-Object Needs: These are the needs that the so-called self-objects must meet to prevent the self-injury of the individual. Kohut's self-object conditions consist of the need for idealization, other-self transference, or twinning, mirroring (Kohut, 2020).

ENDNOTE

1 This work is derived from the master's thesis named "An Examination on the Narcissistic Narrative in Ads" and supervised by Assoc. Prof. Dr. Recep Yılmaz.

Chapter 3
Archetypes of Otherness: An Investigation of the Narrative Structures of Posters in the Construction of Soviet Ideology

Ömer Çakın
https://orcid.org/0000-0001-7853-6460
Ondokuz Mayıs University, Turkey

Mehmet Akif Günay
Gümüşhane University, Turkey

ABSTRACT

The Bolsheviks seized power in Russia with the October Revolution of 1917 and began the process of establishing a new society. Propaganda is used to influence the public in this process, and posters were an important tool in the propaganda toolbox. The archetypes of "otherness" in Soviet propaganda posters are the subject of this research. The goal of this research is to discover how otherness archetypes are used in the narrative structure of Soviet propaganda posters. To accomplish this goal, the study will conduct a review of pertinent literature and examine the characteristics and transformation of the Soviet Union's marginalizing images on posters. Additionally, the study will identify marginalizing elements and the manner in which they are used.

INTRODUCTION

Vladimir Ilyich Ulianov (Lenin) led the Bolshevik Revolution that overthrew the tsarist Russian regime in 1917. The Bolsheviks actively disseminated propaganda in order to gain control of this multicultural and multilingual geography, which was home to a diverse range of ethnic groups. In Russia, this system change resulted in significant changes. As a result, a new societal-building process began in Soviet geography. The locomotive of this process was propaganda.

DOI: 10.4018/978-1-7998-9251-9.ch003

From the Bolshevik revolution to 1991, posters were a vital part of the Soviet Union's mass media. The posters were successful in influencing and changing society. Posters mirrored the regime's philosophy as a political propaganda tool. Other ideas, on the other hand, were censored on the posters (Kall, 2003, p. 90). Posters have played an important role in the social, economic, political, and cultural structuring of society as ideological weapons. The public was educated about the images and ideas of the time period through posters. Political, social, and economic issues were depicted on posters with visual messages by the Soviet administration, and this effort contributed significantly to public awareness.

Artists who had previously worked in a variety of fields and styles of artistic expression began to create posters that were bright, professional, persuasive, and, most importantly, psychologically effective (Afonskij, 2016, p. 161). The effectiveness and accessibility of poster language are enhanced by a large number of hidden symbols that operate in a person's collective unconscious. The challenger elements are visually present on the posters in the posters. From an artistic standpoint, the Bolsheviks attempted to impose these inner and outer challenger elements on the public through their policies.

The Bolsheviks did not hesitate to create new values or reinterpret old ones in order to shape the new Soviet people. They have persuaded the public to adopt their values rather than the values of marginalized groups through propaganda posters. The people were asked to accept the system by seeing a happy and judicious state image on propaganda posters. Posters became an educational tool for the Soviet Union at this point. Education and propaganda were complementary wholes for the Bolsheviks as well (Barghorn, 1964, p. 3).

In politics, every word spoken is transformed into the truth without any critical filtering, and beliefs, convictions, and prejudices have taken precedence over reason. The concept of 'post-truth' is born in politics in this way. The truth is trivialized in politics and reflected back to the public as a deception (Karadağ, 2019, p. 4). During the Soviet era, poster artists' work expanded beyond the artistic works of gifted masters to become a tool for agitation and propaganda. This dramatic, satirical, joyful evocative (Afonskij, 2016: p. 160) was the marginalizing element in the narrative pages during the difficult trials of the Russian people in the twentieth century.

While some propaganda posters in the Soviet Union revealed the new system's values, others stigmatized the marginalized. In this regard, the focus of the research will be on these marginalizing elements in posters.

IRRATIONALITY AND RATIONALITY IN THE CONSTRUCTION OF SOVIET IDEOLOGY

The Bolshevik revolution, sparked by the intolerable conditions on the Russian front during WWI, was a radical challenge to the global capitalist order. The Bolsheviks, led by Lenin, were inspired by Karl Marx's ideas and believed that this revolution was only the first stage. Later, a socialist revolution led by the working class would overthrow the capitalist system, in which private property owners exploited the vast majority of the population. Factories, land, and other production assets would be owned and managed collectively by the entire society. Borders between countries would be abolished. Equality between men and women, as well as between the peoples of developed industrial countries and the peoples of underdeveloped colonies, would be established (Carr, 2011, p. 18). Marxism-Leninism was an ideology that opposed all forms of exploitation and aimed for an egalitarian world order ruled by the working class with an internationalist perspective (Bekcan, 2019, p. 372; Solodovnik, 2012). Lenin was a Marxist, and Marxism was unquestionably the foundation of his worldview. However, Lenin adapted and applied Marxism's theoretical ideas and principles to Russian reality in a way that spread throughout the world (Stalin, 1978). Lenin's interpretive guide to action for the Bolsheviks was Marxism. Marxism-Leninism ideology served as a guide for moving society toward its objectives. Lenin and subsequent leaders developed the basic principles and unified framework of this guide. (2008, Zinoviev)

In the years leading up to World War II, the ideological machinery of Soviet society began to take shape. However, it peaked in the postwar years, particularly after Stalin's death (Zinoviev, 2008). In Soviet society, the origins and rise of the ideology factor are linked to the changing social reality under a new political regime. The ideological foundations of Soviet society appeared in the mid-1930s, at the 17th Party Congress in 1934, and were formally declared in the 1936 USSR Constitution (Solodovnik, 2012). Measures were taken in the following periods to maintain the ideological foundations of Soviet society.

In a non-communist society, the main goal of communist ideology was to figure out how to turn that society into a communist one. A number of practices were required to achieve this: the socialization of all means of production, the abolition of classes, the nationalization of private owners' and entrepreneurs' property, the communist party's seizure of political power, the centralization of all system power and control, and so on (Zinoviev, 2008). These and other similar practices were critical to the Soviet ideology's foundations. As a result, the communist society's existence was ensured. To develop ideological attitudes among the people, all of the major aspects of agitation and propaganda were used. The official media, the political education system in all enterprises and institutions, financial instruments, parties, trade unions, and other public institutions, schools, technical schools, and universities all played a role in spreading the Soviet ideology to all segments of the population (Solodovnik, 2012).

Although the decisions, changes, and practices made during the development of Soviet ideology were rational, they also had irrational aspects in many ways. It is reasonable to assume that the rational aspect of Soviet ideology predominates now that it has been declared a science. Because dialectical materialism, historical materialism, and the communist doctrine of society known as "scientific communism" are at the heart of Soviet ideology (Zinoviev, 2008). Soviet behavior, on the other hand, is irrational in many aspects of Soviet institutional life, as well as in domestic and foreign policies. The behavior of the Soviet Union as a whole is far from irrational. It has "rational aspects," particularly in terms of strategic and tactical methods, as well as the formation of political organizations. None of these procedures, however, overshadowed the fact that the entire Soviet operation was rife with conflicts spawned by an irrational doctrine capable of turning flexible tactics into inflexible dogmas (Fizer, 1957).

The Bolsheviks who took power had no choice but to use the state's ideological apparatus for their own ends (Althusser, 2016, pp.: 48-49). In order to maintain their power, the Bolsheviks had to send out a lot of messages to the people. The goal of these messages was to control the masses on the one hand, while also establishing hegemonic relationships on the other. All of these efforts were focused on changing people's perceptions (Bayrakcı, 2021, p. 93). For this, the government established an unrivaled hold on the state's ideological apparatuses, especially the mass media, which were effective in spreading the ideology (Cogandarjan, 2013, p. 182).

Taking control of the media creates a reality (post-truth) in which personal feelings and beliefs are more powerful than objective facts (Oxford Advanced Learner's Dictionaries 2021). The propaganda media of the Soviet Union demonstrated the irrationality of Soviet ideology. During the Soviet ideology construction process, truth was less effective than emotions and personal beliefs in forming public opinion (Conserva, 2009, p. 1). It was obvious that post-truth existed (Raptis 2020, p. 58). To summarize, Soviet ideology was constructed irrationally, particularly through the use of mass media as propaganda tools.

POST-TRUTH AND VISUAL PRODUCTION

A massive accumulation of spectacles characterizes modern production societies. Prepresentations takes the place of every direct experience (Debord, 1996, p. 1). According to Feuerbach, the appearance is the essence of the period, politics, and science (2008, p. 16). Whether it's information or propaganda, advertising or direct entertainment, the spectacle is the current model of socially dominant life in all of its forms. The desire for modernization and unification spawned by spectacle prompted the Russian bureaucracy to embrace democratic ideology (that is, the dictatorial ideology of market freedom, which became moderate by recognizing the rights of the audience) as a single body in 1989 (Debord, 1996, p. 7). Since 1917, the same shows or images, particularly visual propaganda tools, parades, and so on, have played a key role in the construction of Soviet ideology.

Visuality has always been more important than other senses for civilization. Berger emphasizes the significance of seeing by stating that seeing precedes speaking (2014, p. 7). Guenon emphasizes the importance of seeing by stating that the visual symbol's elements are also expressed verbally (Guenon, 2012). Looking is a deliberate act. The object becomes reachable as a result of this action (Berger, 2014, p. 8). By limiting one's thinking about things, the act of seeing allows one to focus more on the object. Today, the power of seeing has triumphed over the power of believing and has become life itself (Mirzoef, 1998). The visual environment of the world has changed as a result of rapid changes in communication technologies (photography, cinema, television, etc.) and the digital age. The ability to communicate has reached new heights thanks to visual language (Bolat, 2019, p. 1116).

The ability to distort the truth through visuality has increased due to the power of seeing, society's willingness to consume the visual, and advances in computer technology. However, this visual situation has paved the way for society and various authorities to have a strong preference for distorting the truth by concealing it.

Prior to the Bolshevik revolution in Russia, a struggle and polarization over the media erupted between the two sides. Polarization is one of the most important aspects of post-truth information. This polarization is achieved not only through written texts, but also through images selected or created with the post-truth goal in mind. Because, in most cases, photography as a visual communication tool has a much higher persuasive effect than written texts (Özdemir, 2019, p. 1056). As a result of advancements in communication and computer technologies, as well as the distorted structure of visual symbols, these images are now used for post-truth purposes.

Advances in digital technology have also accelerated the spread of misinformation about visual symbols. According to studies, people's ability to perceive both original and manipulated images is limited. People are unable to tell whether a real-world image has been manipulated or not. People are more likely to believe what they see as a result of this. If people can't tell the difference between real and fake details in photographs, manipulations can often change what they believe and remember (Nightingale, 2017, p. 1-2). Memories, beliefs, and behaviors are all influenced by images (Newman, Garry, Bernstein, Kantner, & Lindsay, 2012; Wade, Garry, Read, & Lindsay, 2002; Yılmaz, & Çakın, 2017). As a result, visuality played a crucial role in the adoption of Soviet ideology.

Context is a crucial component in the creation of post-truth reality through visual symbols. Some objects are represented by visual symbols. Images are not the same as reality in this context. Images are nothing more than extensions of reality. Photographs, in particular, and images in general, are captured in real-time. Original, internal, and external contexts are the three types of context. The original context refers to the unbroken reality, the person who created the image's psychological exposure, and his knowledge of other images. The external context refers to the location and presentation of the image. The internal context is about the self-evident (Barret, 2012). Changing the context of an image has a significant impact on its meaning.

Different external contexts, and especially adding text, can easily change the meaning of an image in most cases (Barret, 2012, p. 138). The image's potential as a representative tool is enhanced by a variety of tools that employ cultural and aesthetic conventions to produce a text (Fiske, 2011) that serves as the foundation for post-truth reality. The headlines or captions beneath the image influence the masses' perceptions of what is right and wrong. When Fiske looked at the "mirror of truth" photograph, he discovered that the newspaper's management surrounded the image with words to reduce ambiguity and increase repetition—in other words, to make the meaning fit our preconceived notions. Indeed, changes in the context of representative tools have a significant impact on what people think about and how they think about it.

PROPAGANDA IN THE SOVIETS

Propaganda is derived from the Latin word propagare, which means "planting shoots of a living plant into the ground to obtain new plants."(Geçikli, 1999, p. 266; Brown, 1963, p. 10). Propaganda, according to the Turkish Language Institution, is the use of words, writing, and other forms of communication to introduce, adopt, and spread a doctrine, thought, or belief to others. Propaganda has been a major topic among academic disciplines, especially in the first half of the twentieth century, as an important political communication tool (Satır, 2018, p. 568).

The foundation for creating and maintaining the communist individual is ideological indoctrination of the Russian people. This process starts with a person's birth, continues throughout their life, and only ends when they die. Ideological indoctrination affects every level of society and every aspect of people's lives (Zinoviev, 2008). Propaganda was used effectively in this way to indoctrinate Soviet ideology.

Lenin was a key figure in the Soviet Union's propaganda efforts. As a result, Lenin serves as a propaganda guide for the Soviet Union (Doğan, 2021, p. 422). Long before the revolution, Lenin's views on the importance of propaganda differed from the modern propaganda phenomenon. Starting with a quote from Plekhanov, he described how Russian revolutionaries need to use propaganda to reach and organize the masses (Yıldırım, 2014, p. 10). In this regard, Lenin states (2011, p. 86):

Today, We should define the difference between propaganda and agitation in a different way than Plekhanov did. "We must understand the revolutionary illumination of the current social order or its partial phenomena when we speak of propaganda, regardless of whether it is done in a way that is understandable to individuals or the general public." Agitation, in the narrow sense, refers to the mobilization of the masses to take specific actions, the proletariat to participate in social life. We need to learn how to support direct revolutionary intervention.

It's appropriate to say that the Soviet Union used propaganda to manipulate public opinion as well as to create a collective consciousness. The Bolsheviks used propaganda to try to change society's thought and behavior patterns. They also desired to manipulate society in their favor. Both internally and externally, propaganda was effective (Howell, 1975, p. 137). The goal was to announce the revolution to society and to protect and consolidate power on the inside, while fighting capitalism on the outside

(Reeves, 2004, p. 51). The Bolsheviks used propaganda to try to erase the social reality of the Tsarist regime from public memory and persuade the masses to adopt their own ideology (Satir, 2018, p. 572).

The Soviet regime placed a high value on literature and art. There were about 45 thousand writers, journalists, and editors in attendance, as well as over 100 thousand people from other cultural, educational, and political fields. The difficult and dangerous event for the spread of Soviet ideology drew tens of thousands of artists. The organization for agitation and propaganda was given a special place by the Soviet leaders. In the USSR, over 112 thousand people were constantly making verbal propaganda. "Every Bolshevik is an agitator," was one of the Bolshevik Party's first and most important slogans. The primary propagandist army was made up of party members, members of the Young Communist League, and non-party activists. These individuals were chosen for their ability to persuade the public through actions as well as words. The propagandist had to be well-versed in the needs, personal lives, and problems of all members of his cell, as well as their daily work in the factory or collective farm (Cogandarjan, 2013).

Before the October Revolution, the link between propaganda and the masses served as a functional principle in the Soviet Union as well. To convey the desired image of the Soviet paradigm, two major challenges had to be overcome. Furthermore, it was expected that the country would be completely encircled by the new socialist hegemony created by propaganda (Yıldırım, 2014, p. 11). In the case of the Soviet Union, propaganda was as important as the military or special services in the construction of the state. However, Soviet propaganda was "broken" when it came to the USSR's strong ritualization of life (Pocheptsov, 2015)

Throughout Soviet history, the Department of Agitation and Propaganda became the highest ideological governing body in the cultural sphere. The Narkompros, the Main Political Directorate of the Soviet Army and the Soviet Navy, the central committee of the Komsomol, and the sub-departments of agitation, propaganda, press, and national minorities formed the board formed by members of the central committee department, according to the Propaganda Department regulation approved in November 1921. (Chogandaryan, 2013, p. 181). As a result, the Soviet Union established a centralized, unified system of information and propaganda. This system was run by party organs and covered all channels for influencing public opinion both inside and outside the USSR. Figure 1 depicts the overall system in the Soviet Union (Bokerija and Dieva, 2015, p. 84).

The propaganda system was occupied by the ruling party controlled mass media from the beginning of Soviet power. The party's "ideological weapons" were the press and radio, and journalists were referred to as "officers of the ideological front." The press, it is widely assumed, served as a collective propagandist, agitator, and organizer. As a result, almost all of the media's content became propaganda, aimed squarely at bolstering the political system and the masses' ideological education. Individuals' consciousness and behavior were influenced by the press as a powerful ideological influence factor. "There is no better propaganda tool in the world than the press magazines, newspapers, pamphlets," Stalin stated flatly. The publishing was described by the Soviet state's leader as "large-scale machine production." The Bolsheviks' Central Committee of the All-Union Communist Party resolution of November 14, 1938 defined the press's leading role in Soviet propaganda. According to this definition, "the press should be the decisive weapon in propaganda" because it allows "almost everyone to succeed in telling the truth." This allowed complete control over the propaganda-sourced data (Chogandaryan, 2013, p. 182). Almost all media content became propaganda after the press was turned into a decisive weapon, and it was directly aimed at strengthening the political system and ideology education of the masses. The press acted as a powerful ideological influence factor on people's consciousness and behavior, steering their actions in a specific direction (Lucsev, 2016, p. 167).

Figure 1. Institutional background of the Informational Propaganda Mechanism in the USSR

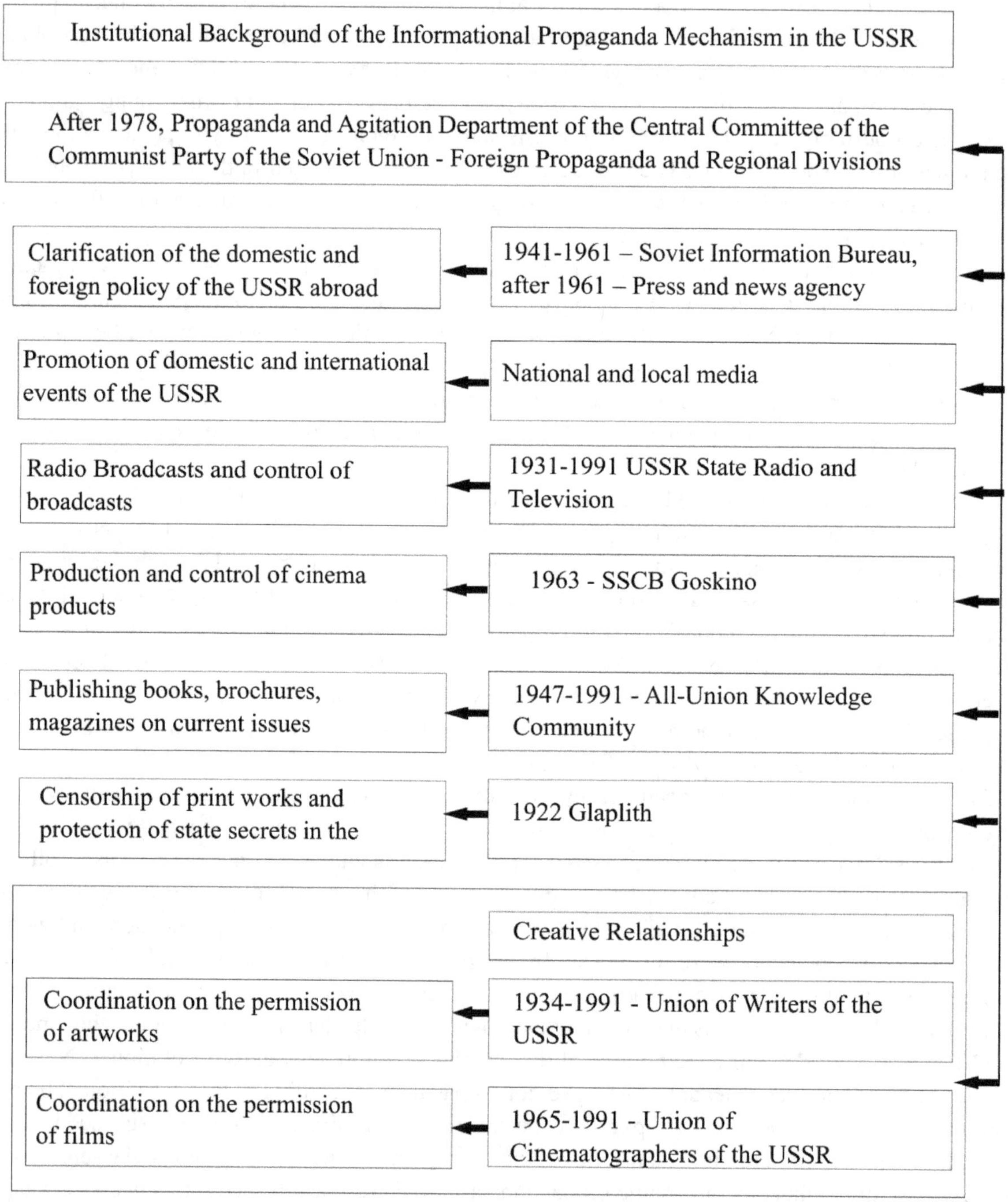

Posters in the Soviets

Posters were the primary visual tool of ideological propaganda in the Soviet Union, promoting a way of life, the eradication of ignorance, the preservation of health, the fight against the negative aspects of the existing system, and the "capitalist lifestyle.". Soviet posters covered topics such as anti-religion, agitation, anti-alcohol, military, and anti-imperialism. The posters highlighted communist construction, industrialization, aviation, rail transportation, and space exploration achievements. The movie poster advertised the upcoming release of a new film. The posters brought people together in times of crisis, helped them survive, inspired hope and confidence, inspired action, raised civic awareness, and emphasized the importance of duty to the motherland. In times of peace, posters served as both an ideological weapon and a powerful marketing tool for producers (Alekseeva & Vinickaja, 2018, p. 5).

In the early Soviet period, posters were the primary form of propaganda in the USSR, as they revealed the regime's developments and rules. Despite the fact that the posters date from earlier in Russian history, the Bolsheviks greatly expanded thei design and use of them. They were at the heart of the Soviet Union's propaganda efforts as a means of disseminating the government's policies and initiatives through the mass media (Pisch, 2016, p. 3). During the reconstruction and war periods, the Bolsheviks used posters to distribute brief news and government decrees to the public via the Russian Telegraph News Agency (Öksüz, 2017, p. 470).

Posters were the most effective form of mass media for spreading Soviet ideology. Propaganda posters in the Soviet Union, in particular (Rowley, 2006, p. 1320), emphasized that the Soviet people behaved in accordance with the ideology and that the people's minds were shaped in accordance with the goals. The printing press was used effectively in this process. "The communist revolution was won not with bayonets, but with the printing press," wrote V. Polonsky (1925, p. 14). The press was seized as a result of the confiscation of printing houses' assets, and the publication of apolitical popular prints was prohibited. The seizure of print media had the same connotation as the seizure of mail, telephones, and telegraphs. Poster art was once thought to be on par with the press, radio, and cinema because of its controllability (Nikolaeva, 2012, p. 129).

The Soviet poster, inextricably linked to the era, shaped the visual culture of Soviet society. The posters, which were produced and distributed as part of the USSR's cultural code, featured symbols and signs that were familiar to every citizen. The Soviet poster is traditionally viewed from three angles today (Jarskoj and Romanova, 2009, p. 444):

1. As a phenomenon in the history of Russian art,
2. As a historical resource for studying past sociopolitical discourse
3. As a system of visual codes of socialism, in line with visual anthropology.

During the Soviet era, there were four different types of posters. There are posters for propaganda, politics, education, science, and training. Each of these types serves a distinct purpose. The propaganda poster is remembered for its abrasive expressions. The posters' political purpose was to convey to the masses the meaning of a Soviet person's life. In schools, train stations, country clubs, and even the principal's office, such posters could be found. The educational posters were more specific than other types of posters because they included step-by-step instructions for performing specific agricultural tasks. The popularization of agricultural knowledge and various events in agricultural life were the subjects of scientific and educational posters (Esikova, 2009). Because of non-linguistic factors such as politics, ideology, and the country's social and economic situation, the theme of the Soviet poster has changed over time. With an ideological purpose, revolutionary zeal, and high artistic concern, the posters were transformed into a mass agitation, political, and educational tool (Danilova & Nurieva, 2015, p. 409).

MARGINALIZATION IN THE CONTEXT OF POST-TRUTH IN SOVIET POSTERS

Archetypes made it possible to reduce many of the actors in the Soviet myth to a limited number of main characters. The main characters can be classified as heroes, wise fathers, mothers, and enemy archetypes. Archetypes can be found in almost every aspect of Soviet culture, including the press, cinema, music, literature, architecture, fine arts, and posters. There are many different visual representations of heroes, such as war hero, politician, cultural hero, and self-sacrifice hero. Many symbols were replaced by the image of Stalin at the end of the 1920s. The mother archetype was born in the first half of the 1930s, with the ideal of returning to the public and the motherland (Gjunter, 1999).

The Soviet Union used mass media to erase images of the past from people's minds and replace them with its own values. Because the Soviet Union saw old values as impediments, they were trivialized and marginalized. In this context, elements from the past, as well as some current ones, that are seen as impediments to the new order, have been marginalized through the use of posters.

The old royal symbols were physically removed by the Soviet Union. Not only that, but the regime wanted to remove these symbols from people's minds and force them to adopt their own through propaganda (Alaniz, 2010, p. 31). Non-socialist views and values were restructured and marginalized in the past.

The Destruction of Religious Beliefs

For the Bolsheviks, religion was one of the most significant obstacles to the new order. As a result, they have declared open war on religion. Religion, according to Bolshevik leaders, is one of the most serious issues that saps the energy of those attempting to reach heaven in this world. In this context, the Bolsheviks believed that not only would the people be freed from the economic and political yoke, but that Marxism and Leninism would also serve as spiritual guides to them. The Soviet government was adamant in its opposition to religion and the church. They used marginalizing language to persuade the public and to harm the church's and clergy's reputations. (Saraç, 2019, p. 33-34). Because according to Lenin: '*Marxism has always regarded all modern religions and churches, and each and every religious organisation, as instruments of bourgeois reaction that serve to defend exploitation and to befuddle the working class.* (Lenin, 1909, p. 402).

The Soviet regime radically altered the people's Orthodox tradition. They made the church irrelevant in everyday life by forbidding religious dogmas in any form. The regimen also took drastic measures to erase the church from public memory (Şavlyutova, 2011, p. 192). The Bolshevik revolution resulted in the state seizing and destroying churches, as well as the execution of clergy (Shepler, 2008, p. 8).

The Soviet regime's anti-religious opposition was reflected in the posters. The clergy, the church, and religious elements are always depicted in a negative light in these posters. The images were presented in a straightforward manner in order to cause the general public to question religious values.

These posters claim that the clergy collaborate with capitalists to plot anti-Soviet schemes, that religious elements are anti-science, that religious holidays reduce worker productivity, that the church serves its own interests, and that the clergy oppose useful work. Religious values were generally trivialized in the posters and used as a marginalization element.

Clergy were depicted as thieves, alcoholics, fraudsters, immoral, society's exploiters, and the greatest obstacle to social development while attempting to keep society away from religion by humiliating and criticizing religious values. The public's perception of religion and clergy has shifted dramatically. The clergy's reputation among the people was ruined, and they were mocked as sycophants. As a result, the public regarded religious values as unimportant and unnecessary. Religious values and clergy were depicted in the posters, which accelerated the public's negative attitude toward religious values and increased their commitment to new values.

Anti-Alcoholism Movements

The Bolshevik regime tightened anti-alcoholism movements in the Soviet Union. The Bolsheviks banned the production of all types of alcoholic beverages in order to solve this problem, which had been unsolved during the Tsarist Russia period. While the prohibition lasted until 1921, some changes were made after that date, and only low-alcohol beverages were permitted (Solovev and Strasul, 1926, p. 243). The fight against alcohol has become mandatory due to the negative social, economic, and political consequences of excessive alcohol consumption (Paşin et al., 2011).

The anti-alcohol movement began with an uncontrollable volume of illegally produced liquor. Moonshine was produced by 8-10% of peasant households in the early 1920s. Police confiscated 75,296 illegal alcoholic beverages in 1923, and 295,003 people were prosecuted as a result (Solovev and Strasul, 1926, p. 244).

After 1930, the Soviet regime began to produce liquor on a regular basis. Alcohol sales to minors under the age of 16 are prohibited, and non-drinking zones are established across the country. Alcohol consumption was regulated differently at different times.

The Bolsheviks fought hard to eradicate the Tsarist period's drinking habits. The regulation was necessary for them because of the large number of Christian religious holidays. The heavy consumption of alcohol during these holidays was lowering the country's productivity. Due to the intensification of alcohol consumption and thus the disruption of production, the Bolsheviks opposed alcohol during these holidays, which lasted almost half of the year.

Alcohol abuse was depicted on Soviet posters as a social problem. The Soviet people were depicted as healthy in the posters created specifically for this purpose, and the posters urged people to abstain from drinking alcohol. The working class's struggle with alcohol was also extensively documented because it hampered production during this time period. In the posters, depressed members of the working class are depicted as exhausted, helpless, and marginalized. The message "no" was clearly stated that alcohol should not be consumed, especially during working hours.

The posters emphasize the negative effects of alcohol on the family unit. The message that alcohol destroys the family institution's peace and tranquility was brought to the forefront. As a form of marginalization, negative images of alcoholic mothers and fathers were used. On the posters, it is stated that parents who consume alcohol are unable to raise healthy children.

Additionally, the posters depict the accidents that employees will have while intoxicated, demonstrating their pitifulness.

Anti-alcohol posters, like all other posters in the Soviet Union on various subjects, were informative, educational, and stimulating, allowing people to choose their own path within the system.

The Image of the Enemy: Capitalism and Imperialism

One of the oldest archetypes that have appeared in all societies throughout human history is the enemy image. To stay strong, mankind required an enemy (Magomedov and Cogandaryan, 2013, p. 121). The Soviet regime had successfully implanted the enemy image at this point. 'The whole world is divided into two groups: we, the working people, and the colonial others,' Lenin said of capitalism's role as the enemy (Lenin, 1969, p. 323). The Soviet Union's stance against capitalist countries was also guided by Lenin's position. In addition, he clearly defined the Bolsheviks' anti-capitalist stance. The Bolshevik Revolutionaries made a radical break with both capitalist countries and past traditions (Sergeyeva, 2017, p. 223).

In propaganda posters, the distinction between the USSR and the capitalist West was frequently emphasized. "We and Them," in which the West is the Soviet Union's adversary, was compared to "East-West." The opposition to capitalism and imperialism was one of the most striking elements of the Soviet Union posters at this time. These two elements were constantly emphasized as threats as a result of a policy determined by the Soviet regime. The image of the capitalist was sharply and strikingly depicted on Soviet posters at the dawn of a new society and wars.

The posters contained a satirical narrative about capitalism and imperialism. The mockery of cartoons was used to depict the enemy. Furthermore, the quantitative superiority of socialism is depicted on posters as statistics. Imperialism was depicted as the enemy on posters as much as possible, with exaggerated negative features.

In the poster narratives, it was emphasized that the Soviet Union allocated more budget to education and industry as a social state, as well as the emphasis that capitalist countries' expenditures went to military needs. This idea implies that America's investment in military power has the potential to be offensive. Fedosov, 2016, p. 151).

CONCLUSION

In the Soviet Union, there was a close relationship between the visual arts and, as a result, posters and propaganda. In a society with a low literacy rate, the Bolsheviks recognized the poster's potential. Religious symbols are widely used in daily life in Russian society. The use of posters was motivated by a habit and sensitivity to visual elements (Taylor, 2003, p. 199). Sculpture, architecture, theater, cinema, painting, music, festivals, and posters were all used consciously to spread Soviet ideology. These tools cast a new light on Soviet symbols and images in the eyes of the public. Not only did the Bolsheviks seek to maintain power, but they also sought to redefine images, symbols, and discourses (Pisch, 2016, p.30). New ideology, vital norms, working orders, and holidays are explained to the public through visuality with these visual norms (Çaus, 2010, p. 220). The messages were easily understood by the target audience thanks to the posters. Posters with visuals and short texts were used in the Soviet Union's early years, much like they were in newspapers and radio. The posters depict a lot about the time period and play an important role in many of the events.

Soviet posters are agitation and propaganda tools, as well as visual tools that reflect the conditions of the time and clarify issues in the Soviet Union. Its functionality has also been enhanced by the ability to interpret the visuals and symbols that accompany the slogans without the use of commentary or text. It was one of the leading mass media of its time, addressing issues such as political propaganda, public education, and health care, according to its contents. Soviet posters now serve as a rich data archive about Soviet history, as well as raising awareness of the era through their flashy language.

In Soviet posters, the emphasis was on a symbolic narrative. The message was only obliquely revealed in the early Soviet posters' narratives, leaving it to the audience's interpretation. After 1930, the posters published underwent a significant transformation. The enemy is represented by a smaller figure, while the Soviet symbols are placed in the center (Nikolayeva, 2012, p. 376). In the poster narrative, traditional, national, and racial stereotypes were rarely used. On the foundations of the poster narrative, it is possible to see oppositional class, temporal and regional issues, and marginalized elements. In this way, the posters also reveal the Soviet Union's cognitive map. The subjects described in the posters are evaluated in two basic frameworks, as can be seen. While the Soviet Union is referred to as "us," the rest of the world is referred to as "them" and is depicted as marginalized on the posters.

It was the goal of the poster narratives during the Soviet establishment to change people's habits from the Tsarist Russia period to the new period's rules. By contrasting old and new norms, the posters emphasize the past and future. The past is demonized, but the future is idealized. Despite the fact that they are vastly different, the two periods are evaluated separately. While the past is shown in a dark light, the future is shown in bright light. While the previous regime and its elements were vilified in the poster narratives, the new regime's elements were highlighted and praised.

Posters were at the heart of propaganda in the Soviet Union, and an attempt was made to change people's minds by using visual and linguistic strategies to form Soviet-friendly thought and behavior patterns. During this process, an attempt was made on the manipulation axis. The public was informed about the new symbols and rituals created, the roles assigned to people, the destruction of religious beliefs, the anti-capitalist stance, and new behavioral patterns through posters. Everything associated with the Tsarist period has been visualized, trivialized, and marginalized, including opposing viewpoints. While negative elements such as trivialization and marginalization were depicted on posters in colorless or black, Soviet images and symbols, as well as the proletariat and factories, were depicted in red and became symbols of the new system's power.

As a result, the posters played an important role in mass re-education, mass consciousness communion, and Bolshevik culture ideologization. It has aided the people in their efforts to break free from their cultural traditions and heritage. In the Soviet Union, posters attempted to explain these concepts to the masses through visual expression in the creation of Marxist class ideology, communist education, and proletarian culture, which is a mass culture for society's lower layers. The main goal of marginalization posters for the Soviet Union was to keep class peace, reveal the USSR's new norms, respond to imperialism, and re-plan everything that was opposed to the new system.

REFERENCES

Afiş. (n.d.). https://www.britannica.com/dictionary/poster

Afonskij, S. A. (2016). Naličie i harakter arhetipov v iskusstve russkogo plakata, sozdannogo v period Velikoj Otečestvennoj vojny 1941-1945 gg [The presence and nature of archetypes in the art of Russian posters created during the Great Patriotic War of 1941-1945]. *Vestnik Rossijskogo èkonomičeskogo universiteta im GV Plehanova*, *3*(87), 159–169.

Alaniz, J. (2010). *Komiks: Comic Art in Russia*. University Press of Mississippi. doi:10.14325/mississippi/9781604733662.001.0001

Alekseeva, T. P., & Vinickaja, N. V. (2018). Fol'klornye tendencii sovetskogo ideologičeskogo plakata [Folklornye tendencies of the Soviet ideological poster]. *Vestnik Tomskogo gosudarstvennogo universiteta. Kul'turologija i iskusstvovedenie*, (29), 5-22.

Althusser, L. (2016). İdeoloji ve Devletin İdeolojik Aygıtları [Ideology and State Ideological Devices]. İthaki Yayınları.

Bayrakcı, O. (2021). İktidar-Hegemonya İlişkisinde Algı Yönetimi [Perception Management in the Power-Hegemony Relationship]. *Yüzüncü Yıl Üniversitesi Sosyal Bilimler Enstitüsü Dergisi*, (52), 93–108.

Bekcan, U. (2019). Stalin Döneminde Sovyet Dış Politikası İdeolojiden Saptı mı? [Did Soviet Foreign Policy Under Stalin Deviate From Ideology?]. *Pamukkale Üniversitesi Sosyal Bilimler Enstitüsü Dergisi*, (36), 371–382.

Bokerija, S. A., & Dieva, A. A. (2015). Opyt informacionnoj propagandy v SSSR kak instrument mjagkoj sily [The experience of information propaganda in the USSR as a tool of soft power]. *Vestnik Rossijskogo universiteta družby narodov Serija: Istorija Rossii*, (3), 81–89.

Bolat, N. (2018). Erkek Egemen Bir Dünyada Kadının Medyada Temsiliyeti Üzerine Bir İnceleme: Eşkiya Dünyaya Hükümdar Olmaz Dizisi Örneği [An Analysis on the Representation of Women in the Media in a Male-Dominated World: The Example of the TV Series Bandit Does Not Rule the World]. *Gümüşhane Üniversitesi İletişim Fakültesi Dergisi*, *6*(2), 1676–1703.

Bolat, N. (2019). Görsel Okuryazarlık Bağlamında Televizyon Dizilerindegeleneksel Mekânlar Üzerine Bir Çalışma [A Study On Tradıtıonal Spaces In Televısıon Serıes In The Context Of Vısual Lıteracy]. Uluslararası İletişim ve Yönetim Bilimleri Kongresi.

Brown, J. A. C. (1963). *Techniques of Persuasion: From Propaganda to Brainwashing*. Penguin.

Carr, E. H. (2011). Lenin'den Stalin'e Rus Devrimi 1917-1929 [Russian Revolution from Lenin to Stalin 1917-1929]. Yordam Kitap.

Çaus, N. (2010). Sovetskiye plakatı1917-1922 gg. Osnovnoye sredstvo propagandı sotsialistiçeskaya ideologii [Soviet Posters 1917-1922 Basic Propaganda and Social Ideology]. *Sotsial'no -ekonomçeskiye yavleniya i protsesı*, *6*(22).

Chogandaryan, M. G. (2013). Methods, methods and techniques of Soviet propaganda in the 1920-30s. XX century. *Theory and Practice of Social Development*, (4), 181-183.

Clegg, S. (1978). *Power, Rule and Domination*. Routledge & Kegan Paul.

Čogandarjan, M. G. (2013). Metody, sposoby i priemy sovetskoj propagandy v 1920-30-e gg. XX v [Methods, methods and techniques of Soviet propaganda in the 1920-30s. twentieth century]. *Teorija i praktika obŝestvennogo razvitija*, (4), 181-183.

Conserva, H. (2009). *Propaganda: A Question and Answer Approach*. AuthorHouse.

Cottingham, J. (1995). Akılcılık [Rationalism]. Sarmal Yayınevi.

Danilova, J. J., & Nurieva, D. R. (2015). Sovetskie plakaty kak sredstvo vizual′no-verbal′noj političeskoj agitacii [Soviet posters as a means of vizual′no-verbal political agitation]. *Mir nauki, kul'tury, obrazovanija, 2*(51), 408-411.

Debord, G. (1996). *Gösteri Toplumu* [Spectacle society]. Ayrıntı Yayınları.

Degot, E. (2000). *Russkoe iskusstvo XX. Veka* [Russian Art in the 20th Century]. M. Trilistnik.

Doğan, İ. (2021). Sovyetler Birliği'nde Din Karşıtı Propaganda: 1917-1960 Dönemi Üzerine Bir Değerlendirme [Anti-Religious Propaganda in the Soviet Union: An Evaluation of the Period 1917-1960.]. *Selçuk İletişim, 14*(1), 408–431.

Eagleton, T. (1996). *İdeoloji* [Ideology]. Ayrıntı Yayınları.

Esikova, M. M. (2009). Rasprostranenie agronomičeskih znanij i povyšenie èffektivnosti sel′skohozjajstvennogo proizvodstva v gody nèpa. Istoričeskie, filosofskie, političeskie i juridičeskie nauki, kul′turologija i iskusstvovedenie [Dissemination of agronomic knowledge and increasing the efficiency of agricultural production during the NEP years. Historical, philosophical, political and legal sciences, cultural studies and art history. Questions of theory and practice]. *Voprosy teorii i praktiki*, (2), 41-43.

Fedosov, E. A. (2016). S Sovetskim Soyuzom Navsegda Lozungi i obrazı vostoçnoevropeyskogo plakata 1948-1956 gg [İn With the Soviet Union forever, the slogans and images of the Eastern European poster of 1948-1956.gilizce başlık]. *Vestnik Tomskogo Gosudarstvennogo Universiteta*, (411), 171–176. doi:10.17223/15617793/411/23

Feuerbach, L. (2008). Hıristiyanlığın Özü [Essence of Christianity]. Say Yayınları.

Fiske, J. (2011). İletişim Çalışmalarına Giriş [Introduction to Communication Studies]. Pharmakon.

Fizer, J. (1957). The Irrationality of Soviet Behavior-* Gerhart Niemeyer with the assistance of John S. ReshetarJr.: An Inquiry into Soviet Mentality.(New York: Frederick A. Praeger, 1956. Pp. 113. $2.75.). *The Review of Politics, 19*(3), 399–400. doi:10.1017/S0034670500012110

Geçikli, F. (1999). Geçmişten Günümüze Propaganda Kavramı [The Concept of Propaganda from the Past to the Present]. *İstanbul Üniversitesi İletişim Fakültesi, 9*, 265-276.

Gjunter, H. (1999). *Sčastlivaja Moskva" i arhetip materi v sovetskoj kul'ture 30-h godov." Strana filosofov" Andreja Platonova: problemy tvorčestva* [Happy Moscow" and the mother archetype in Soviet culture of the 1930s. Country of Philosophers" by Andrey Platonov: problems of creativity]. https://lit.wikireading.ru/45173

Guenon, R. (2012). Niceliğin Egemenliği ve Çağın Alametleri [The Sovereignty of Quantity and the Signs of the Age]. İz Yayıncılık.

Hloponina, O. O. (2017). Censkiy mir v sovetskom plakate 1910-1930-x godov: evolutsiya mifologiçeskix konstrujtov [The World of Women in Soviet Posters 1910-1930]. *Znanie, Ponimanie, Umenie, 4*(25), 287-295.

Howell, R. (1975). The USSR: Sport and Politics Intertwined. *Comparative Education, 11*(2), 137–145. doi:10.1080/0305006750110204

Jarskoj-Smirnovoj, E. R., & Romanova, P. V. (2009). *Vizual'naja antropologija: režimy vidimosti pri socializme* [Visual anthropology: visibility regimes in socialism]. Moskva: BBK 60.5 V 76.

Karadağ, Ç. (2019). *Post-truth kavramı üzerinden medya ve siyaset ilişkisinin The Post, Spotlight ve Truth filmleri çerçevesinde incelenmesi* [Examining the relationship between media and politics through the concept of post-truth within the framework of The Post, Spotlight and Truth films] [Master's thesis]. İstanbul Gelişim Üniversitesi Sosyal Bilimler Enstitüsü.

Keyes, R. (2017). *Hakikat Sonrası Çağ: Günümüz Dünyasında Yalancılık ve Aldatma* [The Post-Truth Age: Lying and Deception in Today's World]. Tudem Yayın Grubu.

KurumuT. D.SözlükG. T. (n.d.). *Propaganda* [Propaganda]. https://sozluk.gov.tr/

Lenin, V. (1969). Polnoye sobraniye soçineniy [Complete collection of compositions]. T. 26, Gospolitizdat.

Lenin, V. (2011). Ne Yapmalı? [What to do?]. Evrensel Basım Yayın.

Lučšev, E. M. (2016). Antireligioznaja propaganda v SSSR: 1917-1941 gg [Anti-religious propaganda in the USSR: 1917-1941]. *Informatsionno-tekhnicheskoe agentstvo Ritm, 2*(20), 167-172.

Magomedov, R., & Çogandaryan, M. (2013). İstoriko-psihologiçeskiye osnovaniya obraza vneşnogo vraga SSSR v Pervoy Polovine 1930 godov [Historical and psychological foundations of the image of the external enemy of the USSR in the first half of the 1930s]. *Vestnik OGU, 3*(152).

Mirzoeff, N. (1998). *The Visual Culture Reader*. Routledge.

Newman, E. J., Garry, M., Bernstein, D. M., Kantner, J., & Lindsay, D. S. (2012). Nonprobative photographs (or words) inflate truthiness. *Psychonomic Bulletin & Review, 19*(5), 969–974. doi:10.375813423-012-0292-0 PMID:22869334

Nightingale, S. J., Wade, K. A., & Watson, D. G. (2017). Can people identify original and manipulated photos of real-world scenes? *Cognitive Research: Principles and Implications*, *2*(1), 1–21. doi:10.118641235-017-0067-2 PMID:28776002

Nikolaeva, M. F. (2012). Dinamika Obraza Vraga V Sovetskom Plakate (1917-1941) İ Modeli İdentifikatsii Sovetskogo Çeloveka [Dynamics of the image of the enemy in the Soviet poster (1917-1942) and models of identification of the Soviet person]. *Jurnal Dialog so vremenem*, (39), 372-386.

Nikolaeva, M. F. (2012). Sovetskij plakat (1917-1941): Meždu iskusstvom i medijnoj tehnologiej. Obŝestvo [Soviet Posters with Art and Technology (1917-1941)]. *Razvitie*, (3), 129–132.

Öksüz, G. Sovyet Rusya'da Bir Propaganda Aracı Olarak Din Karşıtı Alfabe [The Anti-Religious Alphabet as a Propaganda Tool in Soviet Russia]. *International Science Technology Conference*.

Oxford Advanced Learner's Dictionaries. (2021a). *Oxford Advanced Learner's Dictionaries*. https://www.oxfordlearnersdictionaries.com/definition/english/posttruth? q=post+truth

Özdemir, F. (2019). Post-Truth Çağda Görsel İletişim Aracı Olarak Fotoğraf [Photography as a Visual Communication Tool in the Post-Truth Age]. *Uluslararası İletişim ve Yönetim Bilimleri Kongresi*, 1056-1068.

Paşin, V. P., Bogdanov, S. V., & Bogdanova, Y. S. (2011). Antialkogolhaya Kampaniya 1985-1987 gg. V. SSCP [Anti-Alcohol Campaign 1985-1987 V. SSCP]. *Po Sovetskim Arhivnım Dokumentam i Rassekreçennım Materialam TSRU.*

Pısch, A. (2016). *Stalın in Sovıet posters, 1929–1953 archetypes, inventıons & fabrıcatıons*. Anu Press.

Pocheptsov, G. (2015). *Fenomen Sovetskoy Propagandi* [The Phenomenon of Soviet Propaganda]. https://ms.detector.media/manipulyatsii/post/13750/2015-07-19-fenomen-sovetskoy-propagandy/

Polonskij, V. (1925). *Russkij revoljucionnyj plakat* [Russia Regime posters]. Gosudarstvennoe izdatel′stvo.

Reeves, N. (2004). *Power of Film Propaganda: Myth of Reality?* Continuum.

Rowley, A. (2006). Sport in the Service of The State: Images of Physical Culture and Soviet Women, 1917–1941. *The International Journal of the History of Sport, 23*(8), 1314–1340. doi:10.1080/09523360600922246

Saraç, H. (2019). *Sovyet Propaganda Dili* [Soviet Propaganda Language]. Değişim Yay.

Satir, M. (2018). İdeoloji ve Sanat İlişkisi Bağlamında Sovyet Anıtsal Propagandası [Soviet Monumental Propaganda in the Context of the Relationship between Ideology and Art]. *Manas Sosyal Araştırmalar Dergisi, 7*(3), 565–583.

Şavlyutova, Z. (2011). Bor'ba sovetskoy vlasti s religioznım soznaniyem naseleniya Zaural'ya v 1920-e gg [The struggle of Soviet power with the religious consciousness of the population of the Trans-Urals in the 1920 ss]. *Vestnik Arheologii, antropologii i etnografii, 1*(14).

Sergeyeva, O. (2017). Vizual'nyy yazyk «krasnykh» i «belykh» plakatov perioda Grazhdanskaya voyny v Rossii [The visual language of the "red" and "white" posters of the period of the Civil War in Russi]. *Zhurnal sotsiologii i sotsialnoy antropologii, 20*(4), 210–229.

Shepler, R. (2008). *The Bolshevik campaign against religion in Soviet Russia: 1917-1932* (Unpublished Doctoral Dissertation). The Ohio State University.

Solodovnik, L.V. (2012). *Faktor ideologii v sovetskom obschestve: retrospektivnyi analiz v koordinatah ideologicheskoi bezopasnosti gosudarstva i obschestva* [The Ideological Factor in Soviet Society: A Retrospective Analysis in the Coordinates of the Ideological Security of the State and Society]. UDK 323.

Solovev, Z., Strasul, İ. (1926). *Alkogolizm* [Alcoholism]. BSE, T.2.

Stalin, J., (1978). *Leninizmin İlkeleri* [Principles of Leninism]. Ankara: Sol yayınları.

Taylor, R. M. (2003). *Munitions of the Mind: A History of Propaganda.* Manchester University Press.

Tolstaya, T. (2006). *Russkiy plakat: kniga -albom* [Russia poster Album]. Kontakt- Kultura.

Wade, K. A., Garry, M., Read, J. D., & Lindsay, D. S. (2002). A picture is worth a thousand lies: Using false photographs to create false childhood memories. *Psychonomic Bulletin & Review, 9*(3), 597–603. doi:10.3758/BF03196318 PMID:12412902

Yıldırım, E. (2014). Sovyetler Birliği'nde Propaganda ve Proleter Hegemonik İdeolojinin Kurulumu Üzerine [On Propaganda and the Establishment of Proletarian Hegemonic Ideology in the Soviet Union]. *Doğu-Batı Dergisi, 69*, 271-293.

Yılmaz, R., & Çakın, Ö. (2017). Reklamda Süblatif Kodlama Üzerine Bir İnceleme [A Study on Sublative Coding in Advertising]. *MANAS Journal of Social Studies*, *6*(4), 531–539.

Zinoviev, A. (2008). İdeologija Partii Buduŝego [Party ideology in the future]. Moskva: Litres.

KEY TERMS AND DEFINITIONS

Ideology: Ideology refers to thoughts (true or false) that represent a socially relevant group or class's circumstances and life experiences.

Poster: A usually large printed notice often having a picture on it that is put in a public place to advertise something.

Chapter 4
The Narrative of Violence in the Framework of the Post-Truth Concept in Television Series

Nursel Bolat
Ondokuz Mayıs University, Turkey

ABSTRACT

Violence shown in the media, and especially in television programs, manifests itself as an alarming narrative element. Establishing a narrative through violence is an important marketing tool for the television industry with its language that appeals to the general public. In television broadcasts, and especially in television dramas, violence is treated as a profitable theme for the broadcaster. Since violent programs are a subject that attracts viewers, television organizations also increase the dose of violence in their broadcasts. Along with the increase in violence in society, the role of the media's narrative of violence in directing the audience is starting to be discussed. At this point, the presentation of violence within the framework of the post-truth approach of the violence narrative presented in television series gains importance. In this context, the chapter examines how the presentation of violence through television series is blurred and affects the public opinion by highlighting emotions and various interests within the framework of the post-truth approach.

INTRODUCTION

People prefer mass media to have information about the world they live in and to get to know their surroundings. In addition, these tools are used as a means of entertainment and leisure. The media, which people and societies use for entertainment purposes as well as gaining information, also conveys certain narratives to the audience through images. Television, which meets the need for information and entertainment, also directs how people perceive the world and how they shape their behaviors. It is thought that television is effective in the emergence of aggression and violence with its visual and linguistic content, and also has a role in the increase of violence. However, the opinion of how much effect television has in increasing violence is controversial. Despite the view that television has a great effect on increasing

DOI: 10.4018/978-1-7998-9251-9.ch004

violence in society, a significant connection cannot be revealed. In addition, it is noted that there is a consensus on television directing and influencing violence.

Violence inflicted on people by people, for various reasons and with different dimensions, takes place in every society in some form as a social phenomenon. While violence is seen in different forms and dimensions in every age, it is also reflected in the dramatic narratives of the society in which it takes place. Although violence varies according to societies, television, which reflects the characteristics of the society, also reflects the violence narrative of the same society. As an important narrative element in television programs and especially television dramas, people become desensitized when violence is presented as a normal, ordinary phenomenon and as a part of life. The viewer, who becomes insensitive to violence, can watch the images of violence unresponsive after a while. With the normalization of violence with visual and auditory narratives, it is accepted and used as a phenomenon that is easily applied when necessary.

The audience, who is exposed to violence intensely through television programs, has a more pessimistic view of the world they live in and thinks that the world is woven with evil. The viewers, who live intertwined with all kinds of visual narratives of violence, feel insecure about the world they live in. The narratives of visual violence used in television series highlight the concept of post-truth by revealing the personal feelings and various interests of the audience in the face of objective reality, fading the objective reality and influencing the public. In this study, it is aimed to examine the violent narrative in television series according to the desensitization theory within the framework of the post-truth concept. In this framework, it is tried to be explained with examples from randomly chosen knees that deal intensively with violence both in terms of visual narrative and content narrative.

THE DEVELOPMENT OF VIOLENCE NARRATIVE AND ITS PLACE IN VISUAL NARRATIVES

Television viewers are constantly faced with different types of violence in their daily lives. At the same time, the audience relaxes with the fictional violence presentation on the screens full of fear and horror, and television is used as a means of purification. As a result of this situation, the adoption and approval of violence and crime and the tendency towards violence are increasing day by day (Çakır, 2008, p. 167). The audience, who is constantly exposed to the narrative of visual violence, confuses the real and fictional narrative after a while and experiences the illusion of reality. After a while, the narrative of violence is either quickly forgotten or accepted as normal. The violence narrative, which is fictionalized through television series, leads to the approval of violence through the use of bad characters after a while.

"Aggression is a strong, violent, effective action, act, action with the aim of dominating, defeating, directing: a behavior that has a hostile, injuring, abusive or destructive purpose against disrupting, hindering, nullifying a business." (Erten & Ardalı, 1996, p. 143). Throughout the history of humanity, violence has never been absent from the agenda of humanity. While sometimes using violence as a means to solve problems, sometimes it is focused on ways to remove violence from society. It is a fact that developments at the global level have effects and reflections on our society as well. In addition, just like every human and social event, the causes and determinants of violence are numerous (Fromm, 1984). Despite all these processes, violence is destructive and harmful to societies. Raising healthy generations and establishing a good future is possible by staying away from violence and its effects.

Although violence basically has many features, it draws attention as a phenomenon that changes according to time and social structure. The event of violence can gain meaning in different ways in different societies, and different perceptions can be encountered in the same community at different times. Changes in societies over time cause changes in norms (Ünsal, 1996, p. 31). Violence covers such a wide scope that it cannot be considered as a one-sided concept that can be limited to certain issues in general. Violence is a social phenomenon that is shaped on different foundations, from economy to psychology, depending on the structure of society.

It is defined by the World Health Organization (WHO) as "the situation where physical force or power is applied to another person in the form of an intentional threat or reality, causing or likely to cause injury, death or psychological harm to the exposed person" (Yılmaz & Erdem, 2018, p. 342). The exposition of the violence, so to speak, committed by man against his own species can be traced back to the beginning of human history. The murder of Cain's brother Abel by the books of the monotheistic religions reflects the narrative of violence. In addition, the narration of the violent events conveyed after this, the Prophet in Christianity. An example of this is the fact that the suffering inflicted on Jesus is clearly included both in the holy texts, in the visuals in the holy places and even in the works of art (Erdem, 2002, p. 1208). Violence is always highlighted in religious books and narratives. While the art of painting deals with violence intensely, the use of visual violence through religious-based paintings draws attention. Violence is also seen as a reflection of the oppression applied over religion on visual arts.

Violence has always been an important element in storytelling. The subject of violence has been used in hunter-gatherer societies since the hunters began to engrave their adventures on the cave walls and emerges as the first visual narrative examples of the storytelling of violence. It is seen that violence takes place in storytelling, including the pictures drawn and the works written before Christ. In the medieval literary works of Western civilization, violent attacks and detailed depictions of death are handled as an important narrative theme. For example, Shakespeare's famous plays have included elements such as kinship, suicide, and murder to a large extent. With the invention of the printing press, violence continued to play an important role in storytelling in books as well. Nineteenth century media critics consider the violence in the books as a mental epidemic (Trend, 2008, pp. 21-24). Later, it transfers the legacy of violence narrative, which has an important place in theater narratives, to cinema narratives. Cinema effectively uses the element of violence in its visual and verbal narratives. In addition to drawing attention to the visual narrative of cinema, it carries many types of representations of violence to its narratives in order to ensure that its films are watched by the audience (İlerialkan & Yılmaz, 2015, pp. 15-17).

Television entered the world of people in the mid-1950s as a means of consumption and entertainment, emerging as a relatively new phenomenon. Society immediately began to be concerned about the possible negative effects of television. Concerns for novels, plays, films, radio and the like have been inherited by television. Television's heavy use of violence in storytelling shows that these concerns are justified. Concerns for novels, plays, films, radio and the like have been inherited by television. Television's heavy use of violence in storytelling shows that these concerns are justified (Trend, 2008, pp. 24-27). Because while television has the characteristics of representation of many arts in the narrative, it could not be expected to stay away from the violence narrative. However, the biggest effect of television is that it brings these violence narratives into people's homes visually and verbally. When television carries violence to the living room of the houses, it condemns the viewer to live intertwined with violence uninterruptedly. In addition, when it starts using this violence with entertainment, the audio-visual power and effect of violence increases exponentially.

It is possible to see all kinds of violence in social media, which has emerged in connection with technological developments, since it has a structure that includes traditional media. For this reason, the phenomenon of violence in social media is openly expressed by everyone today. Today, the increase in the number of social media users, the ease of accessing social media whenever and wherever they want, is a situation that paves the way for being exposed to violence or resorting to violence. This situation clearly shows that online violence is increasing day by day (Çakın & Bolat, 2018, p. 320). In particular, violence presented in an uncontrolled manner increases its size and severity compared to other media. The fact that social media is an area where it is not possible to reach violence according to preference and control violence reaches threatening dimensions in terms of its effects.

Therefore, the processing and display of violence themes started with cave and wall paintings in the first periods, when there was no writing, spread with literary works, and increased its visual power with theaters. After the printing press, it reached the majority of societies with newspapers and books. However, ensuring the spread of violence in a more dangerous way through visual narrative continues with photographs and cinema. Violence, which enters the listener's house verbally through the radio, one of the technological mass media, is positioned in the most special place of people's homes with television, both visually and verbally. In this development process, the most criticized mass media tool and the best storytelling tool regarding the use of violence as a theme is television. All this developmental stage shows that the theme of violence is one of the basic and indispensable elements of storytelling. It is seen that television cannot be transformed into an audio-visual narrative tool free from violence. In the narrative told by television as the narrator of technology, it is seen that violence cannot stay away from being one of the most important and intensely used content elements. Broadcasters have been making an exaggerated use of violence in narrative on television from past to present.

TYPES OF VIOLENCE IN ITS NARRATIVES AND TRANSFER TO TELEVISION

As an important storyteller, television presents violence with different approaches such as physical violence, psychological violence, sexual violence, verbal violence and economic violence in its presentations of visual and auditory violence. Expressing the types of violence to be encountered in the content of television broadcasts is important in terms of detecting the existence of violence and evaluating its results.

Physical Violence

When the definition of physical violence is considered, "In the narrow definition of violence, with its indisputable and measurable qualities, physical violence is unique and is a harsh and painful act directed from the outside against the physical integrity of people.". Harsh and painful acts against people's bodily integrity often reveal acts of physical violence. These behaviors are actions such as kicking, slapping, punching, hitting with a stick, stabbing, using a gun, burning, torture, which cause pain, injury or death to people. Apart from acts of violence against another person, there are also acts of physical violence, such as suicide and suicide attempts, directed at oneself and harming their bodily integrity (Ünsal, 1996, p. 31). In social events, it is seen that acts of physical violence are experienced a lot in the society. These actions seen in social life also transfer their reflections to television narratives. In television programs, physical violence is seen intensely and openly in many programs that start with news and continue with serials.

Psychological Violence

Any kind of attitude and behavior that negatively affects, upsets, hurts people and makes people feel under pressure and threat (Güz, 2007, p. 89). Psychological violence has a feature that harms the victim's sense of self-worth, self-esteem, intimidation, and makes her feel powerless and helpless. In addition, it is a type of violence that aims to make the person who resorts to violence feel that they are under control of the person affected by the violence. Psychological violence is a type of violence that generally includes verbal and emotional abuse behaviors such as name-calling, humiliation, belittling, shouting, threatening, jealousy, social isolation, emotional and/or physical distancing. Although all kinds of violence are common today, psychological violence has become quite common in recent years. Although psychological violence does not directly cause physical harm, it has an effect on people's mental health.

Economic Violence

It is possible to evaluate economic violence as a kind of economic violence due to high inflation rates, unemployment level and insufficient social security opportunities in the social structure. Very low wages and chronic inflation threaten human life. Since this situation makes people more problematic and tense, it also catalyzes ordinary violence and increases aggressive behavior (Ünsal, 1996, p. 33). In societies where economic violence is experienced intensely, it is seen that people who are overwhelmed by economic problems tend to watch the ostentatious lives in television narratives. Luxurious lives, rich places and rich people's lives give the chance to live the lives that cannot be reached through these narratives.

Sexual Violence

Sexual violence, generally covers a wide range of harassment and assault, starting with cursing, gesturing, and raping against children, young people, women and other individuals. Saying sexually explicit words, groping, harassing, pressing, pressing for sexual intercourse and rape can be counted as examples of sexual violence. An important part of sexual violence acts also includes physical violence (Köknel, 2000, p. 203). Sexual violence, which is encountered in many areas in daily life, is also seen in television narratives. Especially sexual violence against women is one of the most intense topics. In television series, sexual violence can also be considered as the main subject of the series, depending on the place.

Verbal Violence

A type of violence applied in the form of shouting, bad speech, swearing, insults, scolding, humiliation. In verbal violence, the element of fear is considered as an important phenomenon. In this case, the words and actions applied are used for the purpose of intimidation and getting what you want. Insult, contempt, humiliation, harsh words, utterances, practices that undermine trust and lead to psychological abuse are perceived as verbal violence. Verbal violence, which is used as a method for discipline and discipline in social life, causes psychological harm to individuals and increases the tendency to violent behaviors (Güz, 2007, p. 90). Although it is seen that verbal violence is applied in every part of the society, it is seen that it is mostly used by men against men or against women by men. It is seen that verbal violence is used less than other types of violence in television narratives. Because verbal violence encounters censorship in television programs or series.

NARRATIVE OF VIOLENCE IN TELEVISION PROGRAMS

The basic elements of television consist of image and sound. Television is a mass communication tool that conveys any thought, idea, news about a certain subject, events, everything about life to the masses through the programs it broadcasts, using its own unique expression styles. While creating the content, the message to be conveyed is created in a way that will meet the expectations of the audience and keep its interest alive, taking into account the expectations of the audience. While creating the content, it is designed by using audio-visual materials through programs suitable for the message to be conveyed (Kars, 2012, p. 123; Akmeşe, 2020, p. 211). In this content creation process, it is seen that the theme gains importance as well as the audio-visual elements that will attract the attention of the audience. Violence remains an important theme in attracting the attention of the audience in television programs. For this reason, violence is embedded in television programs in many different forms.

It is evaluated that the images of violence in television programs satisfy the viewer's tendency to violence by identifying herself with the hero. Despite the research suggesting that the media does not play a role in reducing violence as a result of the constantly seen violence narrative, it is revealed that television acts instructive by triggering violence (Palabiyikoğlu, 1997, p.124). The viewer is constantly exposed to images of violence such as rape, robbery, killing, bombing, suicide, torture, fighting, and threats through various television programs. Violent content shows itself in the rankings of the viewer's interest in the programs, which brings about the intense processing of violence and sexuality (Sim, 1996, p.130). Television programs with ratings anxiety lock the viewer on the screen by increasing the visibility of their programs with visual narratives in which violence is committed. While violence is the indispensable material of television programs, television series use violence intensely.

The intense processing of violence as a subject show that people witness many violent events such as fights, murders, assaults, extortion, torture and sexual harassment through various television programs, much different than in their real lives. Television presents a fictional world narrative rather than a reflection of the real world. Besides emphasizing that the violence in here is not the same since reality and fiction are quite different from each other, it is necessary to make the audience realize this (Uysal, 2006, p.123). Intensely confrontation with violence through television ensures the normalization of violence over time. In addition, violence becomes acceptable with the blurring of the real and fictional worlds.

Television regularly presents fictional violence with visual and auditory narratives. This violence narrative, which is presented as fiction, is evaluated as innocent violence. Because the narrative of violence presented as fiction is not real. Especially in television programs where entertainment is at the forefront, violence is presented together with humor, comedy and drama. These narratives give their messages to the audience with violent content. Therefore, violence becomes an important material of television programs with a narrative function that feeds the entertainment industry. However, when this fictional narrative of visual and auditory violence begins to reflect in the real world by being normalized and internalized, it presents an important social problem.

In dramatic violence rituals, the relative strength of people, ideas, and values is often displayed in the clash of personified forces. Being able to hit hard and strike fear into the hearts of their opponents makes one important. The battered hero finally triumphs over evil by subduing the villain. Suffering is a test of virtue and killing is the ultimate measure of man. Loss of life, limb, or mind, any reduction in freedom of movement, is the price for weakness or sin in the symbolic shortcut of ritual drama. What appears to be the solution to a problem is the art of staging the death of cursed powers and the downfall of unfortunate characters. The typical plot ends with a reassuring and often predictable conclusion about who is the better man (Gerbner, 1972, 44). Violence in television dramas is the most easily identified narrative by the audience, and in the fictional world, violence is used as an important element of representation in both visual and auditory narratives. Violence, which is found in a much more closed form in people's real life, is represented quite clearly in fictional narratives. In this representation, it functions as an important theme in terms of keeping the audience in front of the screen.

Violence seen on television is defined within the concept of "social violence", mostly anti-social behaviors that are effective in disrupting the social order. According to Türkdoğan; In the phenomenon of social violence, terrorism, suicide, murder, assassinations, kidnapping, ransom demand, hostage detention, burning - destruction, destruction, verbal and written protests, total conflict, riots, race - sectarian fights and privileged forms of action take place (Turkdogan, 1996, p. 341). Television dramas mostly use this socially based violence in their narratives. This violence creates not only the violent heroes that the audience will identify with but also the villains with the approach that they deserve violence.

According to Gerbner, values and powers also emerge through character building. While the good character is shown as an attractive type, the bad character is shown as a lack of character and the right one wins. In such a game, violence plays an important role. Violence is the simplest and cheapest dramatic act that poses a risk to human integrity and purpose in this game (Gerbner, 1972, p. 44).

Saying that it is obvious that television violence is communication, not violence, Gerbner said that fictional violence is a narrative space used to convey the desired message, rather than an act like in real life. In this world built on fiction, it tries to emphasize certain moral and social codes, the message it wants to convey, with representative violence based on exaggerated elements, unlike the real world. For this reason, the power relations in the fictional world revealed through television appear to be trying to describe the balance of power over the powerless, the weak, or the victim, according to their place.

Television programs are not broadcast solely for the purpose of informing and positively influencing and enriching the masses. In addition, it takes the form of areas that produce ideas that are contrary to society and sometimes affirm these ideas. Due to the fact that the general content of the programs is shaped for "interest and commercial" reasons while keeping the element of curiosity high, productions that are negative role models from time to time are also directed. It is seen that violence is one of the most used and important content in this regard (Ünsal, 1996, p. 29). While violence is seen in the form of force or pressure, coercion, attack and brute force, it sometimes takes the form of physical or psychological pain and torture.

Two social scientists, Freedman and Sears (1993), emphasize that acts of violence on television will be effective in stimulating thoughts towards aggression and will make those who observe violence more ready for action in terms of behavioral tendencies in this direction. It is observed that the approach to violence observed in society and violence on television is based on modeling or social learning process. As in all behaviors, learning principles such as identification, performing the behavior with the expectation of reinforcement, imitating the observed behavior emerge in violent behaviors. If something is learned from television, there is no doubt about it, it can be learned in aggressive behavior. However, more importantly, it is more important to learn when aggression is appropriate and when it is not in the socialization process. More importantly, hostile aggression and violence should not be allowed to be learned and not approved by the society (Palabıyıkoğlu, 1997, p. 124). In this learning process, besides the content and methods of violence applied by opposite sexes to each other, the violence applied by the same sexes to each other is spread to a large extent via television. Violence by men against men to be strong, show power, protect the family or fight injustice, which is typical of patriarchal societies, stands out as an important representational narrative in television series.

TELEVISION SERIES AND PRESENTATIONS OF MALE-BASED VIOLENCE

Among the program types of television, series/serials are the most emphasized dramatic productions as the most popular narrative (İnal, 1999, p. 263). In terms of the production process of television series, certain rules, temporal and material restrictions, a considerably wide division of labor, a good specialization and besides all these, a certain quantitative production process is required (Mutlu, 1991, p. 222). TV series, which attract attention as the main broadcasting element of television, which is encountered in many types, are beginning to be seen at the beginning of the most remarkable and popular television programs among the world television programs, especially in the 1980s.

After the start of private-commercial television broadcasting with a significant change in Turkey in the 1990s, research on the relationship between media and violence has determined that the area where violence takes place mostly in the media is in television. It is seen that bloody and abusive scenes fill the screens in all program types, from "reality shows" to news, which has become widespread in connection with the increase in private television broadcasting, especially since the 1990s (Palabiyikoğlu, 1997, pp. 123-124). These shows, which are held for the sake of ratings, are included in every program due to intense interest, and it is seen that the same type of programs is made in all similar channels.

The concepts of television and violence range from commercials to serials and in many broadcasts, especially violence against women is presented openly or covertly. Violence against women is presented and perceived as normal behavior by making the violence that is constantly placed in many programs ordinary. Almost every television content, especially fictional programs, can criticize violence on the one hand and turn it into a legitimation tool on the other. The television series, which attracts attention as the type of program most watched by the audience, shows violence against women as justified and necessary by basing it on traditional concepts. In addition, the intense desperation of women who have been exposed to violence in the news plays an important role in the ordinarization of violence and in the depersonalization of violence against women. While violence against women is legitimized and presented for different reasons in television programs, it leads to results such as resentment, submission, and acceptance of violence against women (Ünlü et al., 2009, pp. 95-97). Violence against women placed in television series is presented legitimately with concepts such as customs and traditions. This legitimation is constantly given to the audience, and after a while, those who do not abide by these rules are punished. While violence against women includes some of the violence shown in TV series, very different violent tendencies are also seen. The most used violence is violence by a male character against another male character.

The violence of men against men, which violence is seen intensely in television programs, is an important social problem. The characters who represent good chasing after the bad guy with weapons and punishing him are used extensively in television series. When the scenes of violence are evaluated in terms of reflecting the violence in real life, it is seen that these scenes are extremely unrealistic. In television broadcasts, it is treated that violence is a positive and approved behavior when applied by good people. Constructive approaches and behaviors that find a solution without violence are generally not preferred in television series. In real life, the police use their guns very little, while in television shows guns are used all the time. It is seen that weapons are frequently used in solving problems (Radecki, 1986, p. 17). Television, as a commercial enterprise, has audience concerns. For this reason, guns and violence through guns are used as an important narrative theme. In addition, the acceptance of the violence of the good character by the audience ensures that this type of narrative is used a lot. The positive reflection of violence through the characters in good roles brings with it many dangers.

Most of the studies on the violence relationship between television and television series have assumed that television has direct effects on the behavior of the audience (Geçer, 2013, p. 87). It is observed that the narrative of violence, which is fictionalized through serials, normalizes violence, and creates behavioral effects in the viewer, especially in children and youth, in the direction of imitating the perception of violence.

The effects of television do not end there, and its constant presentation of images of violence causes the audience to become accustomed to violence and to affirm it (Kara, 2011, p. 46). Violence, which is fictionalized especially on the main character in television series, distances her from real experience and reduces her personal reaction through the character it identifies with, while at the same time it makes her/his take violence for granted. Here, the reflection of violence as a struggle against a male-dominated power and injustice reveals the danger of accepting the violence of men against men.

In the programs presented with fictional narratives, the solution of the problem between good and bad characters is realized through violence and generally the good ones win. Man, unlike other living things, has the ability to solve problems through communication by using his mind and language. However, instead of using reason, tolerance and reconciliation, people seek a solution by using weapons, fights and wars. This was also the case in television broadcasts and violence emerged as the most basic problem-solving method (Öngören, Yanık, İşcan & Demirergi, 1994, p.81). The use of violence by the protagonists in movies or TV series and the solution of problems with this method encourages and encourages violence. The fact that the real results of the violence exhibited by the heroes are not shown in the television programs causes the heroes to be exalted in the eyes of the audience.

In the narratives of the television series, the subjects that focus on family and familial relations are discussed. In this context, the relationships that the characters establish with their parents, lovers, children, relatives, neighbors, and friends are seen in the foreground. The characters are presented with their home lives, families, and close circles in the series, in which the narratives that deal with work and working life as the subject are centered. While the TV series is about love in general, sometimes more than one love, the fact that couples cannot get together, as well as being unhappy, are obstacles in front of them. In this context, among the elements that create conflict between the characters in storytelling, elements such as traditions, customs, and family pressure come to the fore. In addition, hatred, jealousy, envy, and misunderstandings are also heavily processed in the elements that cause conflict (Çelik, 2000, p. 3). Conflict is an indispensable material for the programs to attract attention and gain viewers. In this context, the serials on violence in the narrative, in which he applies his own justice system with the concern of creating conflict and the audience, where human life is not important, and especially the mafia in which violence is experienced intensely, are the narratives in which the audience sees the content of violence intensely. Considering all these issues, it is seen that violence as a concept is the founding narrative element of the TV series discourse.

The widespread belief that the world is a violent place, that violence is a good way to solve problems, and that violent characters are people to be admired and emulated, results in the audience's perception of violence and aggression as legitimate, ordinary, and a fact of daily life (Trend, 2008, p. 79).

Despite this intensity of representations of violence, both visually and verbally, in the discourse and narrative of television series, "violence" as a concept shows itself mostly in representations of violence against men. In this respect, fights or armed attacks, in which both the perpetrator or the main character and the victim or the villain are male, resulting in serious injuries, are called violence. In television drama narratives, there are characters in which the victim is given as a male, but the audience does not identify with, and they are minor characters. These are male characters who are on the side of good or bad characters, who are responsible for protecting or supporting them, and who are seriously exposed to violence. The violence applied to these side characters, which the audience does not care about or in case of violence, also has an important place in the process of desensitization of violence.

THE CONCEPT OF POST-TRUTH AND TELEVISION

In 2016, "post-truth" was named word of the year by the Oxford Dictionary. 2016 is known as an eventful year for many people, full of surprises, controversial surprises and unexpected events. In the process after the political and social panorama of the period, even the desire to maintain the climatic feelings or beliefs, in which the objectivity and rationality to be marked with this post-truth, show the opposite of the facts (Llorente, 2017, p. 9). Post-truth, which left its mark on 2016, when unprecedented social and political events took place all over the world, literally tells the post-truth.

The concept of post-truth is defined as "the situation where objective truths/facts/facts are/are less effective than emotions and personal opinions/beliefs in determining/forming the opinion of the public/ public on a particular subject". In addition, it also emerges with definitions such as "post-truth, false reality, subjective realization, excess of truth, erosion of truth, trivialization of truth, bending of the truth" (Terzi, 2020, pp. 81-82).

The human in Plato's allegory of the cave has reached reality by moving from the shadows. In the state book, people who have been chained from their feet and necks since their childhood, who can only see the tip of their noses and who cannot even turn their heads, perceive the shadows reflected from the fire behind them and the reflections of the voices as real. Although the reality of the people in the cave has their shadows, the real reality, the real truth, is outside the cave (Plato, 2005, p. 138; Kaya, 2021, pp. 27-28). According to the famous philosopher Aristotle, Plato's most successful student and the teacher of Alexander the Great, the real thing is the changing universe; time is derived from regular changes and movements and is used to follow it (Bardon, 2019, p. 1; Sirer, 2020, p. 49). As Aristotle mentioned, time also has an important place in the change of perception of reality. In the process experienced, concepts are reshaped according to the conditions of the day. Today, the concept of trivialization of truth, which is put forward with the concept of post-truth, shows itself in many fields besides politics.

Beyond individual cases, postmodernism comes at the forefront of the factors that make possible the age when truth loses its importance. The lack of effort to reach the universal truth and the rejection of the universal truth caused meta-narratives to lose their importance, making the insignificance of truth possible (Alpay, 2019, p. 25). When it comes to the media, and in particular television programs and narratives, the use of "the trivialization of truth" in the Turkish language to be used in this research comes to the fore.

Postmodern media critic Jean-Francois Lyotard argues that metanarratives collapse because global communication and media technologies use information as a scholarly pursuit or a commodity traded in national and international markets. Another postmodern theorist Jean Baudrillard, with the concept of hyperreality, reality is reconstructed by the media; argues that there are real-world simulations in the minds of media consumers. Therefore, the media, and in particular television, are making significant progress in the trivialization of truth.

Television, as a means of entertainment and leisure, offers a simulation of reality rather than reality. In the simulation he has presented here, he rather exhibits a narrative structure in which the truth is trivialized. Violence, which is an important theme especially for television series, is trivialized and turned into an entertainment commodity. The post-truth emerges as unresponsiveness and insensitivity to the violence experienced on television. Therefore, post-truth, which is the most used concept of today and emerged after postmodernism, reflects the pacification of the audience by showing the way its reality is destroyed with a narrative that specifies how violence is trivialized.

VIOLENCE AND DESENSITIZATION THEORY

Some researchers questioned the assumptions of the excitation theory and stated that overloading the audience through television stimuli creates more anesthetic effects in humans, and especially in children, rather than the emergence of aggressive behaviors. The most important result of the anesthetic effect of the violence transmitted through television broadcasts is seen as "depersonalization". Researchers such as Cline, Craft, and Courrier emphasize that excessive exposure to violence, either directly or through the media, transforms into a psychological dullness and emptiness with normal emotional reactions to violent programs (Mutlu, 1999, p. 125-126; Bolat & Çakın, 2018, p. 305). Awareness of reality and fiction in the narrative or the blurring of the border between reality and fiction determines the response to violence. It manifests itself in the form of imitation according to its place and in the form of depersonalization according to its place. It manifests itself in the form of imitation according to its place and in the form of depersonalization according to its place.

The intense violence and constant exposure to this violence through television desensitize the natural emotional and physical reactions of the audience and renders it unresponsive. After a while, continuous scenes of violence warn the audience less and the violence watched on television reduces the physical reactions to violence in the real world over time. Especially when it comes to children, extraordinary images of violence, which are watched for the first time, become ordinary when they are presented with constant repetitions. Due to their nature, people give a negative emotional reaction when they see blood and violence. However, when exposure to violence is given repeatedly, the reactions become ordinary and people become desensitized (Bushman & Huesmann, 2006, p. 348-352). Children and viewers, who are constantly exposed to the same visual and verbal narratives, see the television narrative as an ordinary narrative and do not attach importance to the narrative without violence.

By visualizing and repetitively presenting violent events and themes, traumatic images create anxiety, fear, and tension in all people, primarily children, adolescents and young adults, and in parallel with all these, violence, horror, death, pain, blood and makes it insensitive to losses (Palabıyıkoğlu, 1997, p. 124). After a while, violence, pain, blood and death become an ordinary events for the audience, and especially the incident or violence perpetrated by the actor becomes positive. In addition, the violence applied to the villain provides relief rather than tension and fear. This unknowingly increases the tendency to violence.

The effects of television programs are not limited to this, but the images of violence that are constantly presented cause the audience to no longer react to violence. Because, with the presentation style that stands out in the size shown by the television, it distances the audience from the real experience, thus reducing the effect of the event, making it difficult to react, numbing the audience, and desensitizing it. In addition to the effects of violence being given only dramatically, its presentation by introducing the element of humor trivializes violence and increases the power of desensitization by disabling the reaction against violence. Teaching violence, which is embedded in laughter and entertainment, combines with the imitation method and increases its effect (Zorlu, 2016, p. 20). Violence, which is placed in the humor in an innocent image, places itself positively in the mind of the audience in this innocent phenomenon. Violence, which the audience affirms in humor, takes its place in a depersonalized manner when confronted later.

REFLECTION OF VIOLENCE OF MAN TO MAN IN TV SERIES IN THE FRAMEWORK OF THE CONCEPT OF POST-TRUTH

In television series created based on fiction, the solution to the problem between good and bad characters is generally realized by using violence and generally good characters win. Man, unlike other living things, can solve problems through communication by using his mind and language. However, instead of using reason, tolerance, and reconciliation, people seek a solution by using weapons, fights, and wars. This is also the case in television broadcasts and especially in television series, and violence emerges as the most basic problem-solving method (Radecki, 1986, p. 17). The television audience is in front of the screen to have fun. Violence in television series is turned into an entertaining element to meet this need. This expectation of entertainment has led to the fact that the pain and sadness caused by violence are not shown. In the entertainment world of television, violence has gained a symbolic meaning beyond reality. However, the fun, symbolic and unrealistic use of violence makes it fantastic but also has negative consequences. This situation desensitizes the audience to violence and at the same time changes the perception of truth. However, the fun, symbolic and unrealistic use of violence makes it fantastic but also has negative consequences. This situation desensitizes the audience to violence and at the same time changes the perception of truth. The relationship between the real world and the world presented by television as a communication tool has been the subject of many studies in terms of truth. Despite its supposedly realistic nature, television offers individuals an imaginary world. This world, as a post-truth world, renders violence trivial in the face of truth.

The display of violence in television series more intensely than violence experienced in the real world offers the audience the opportunity to experience and learn more violence than in daily life. This experience and learning process increases the tendency of individuals to engage in aggressive behavior. The fact that the presentation of violence takes place in television programs more intensely and more than the presentation of violence in the real world stands out in the process of trivializing the truth with its unrealistic approach within the framework of the concept of post-truth.

The mafia-themed series process, which started to come to the fore with the "Kurtlar Vadisi" series on Turkish television and continued with the series shot as a continuation, uses violence as the main theme. TV series such as "Kurtlar Vadisi", "Eşkıya Dünyaya Hükümdar Olmaz" and "Çukur", which attract attention, especially with their high ratings, base their narratives entirely on the violence of men against men. In addition to receiving high ratings, these serials stand out as leading and remarkable serials that deal with the theme of violence by men against men.

Kurtlar Vadisi

Among the main reasons why the TV series "Kurtlar Vadisi" has an important place among the television series broadcast in recent years; Factors such as the subject of the series, being a mafia series, containing more and open violence, and lasting longer can be listed. In the series, the pain and difficulties experienced by the heroes of the series are also discussed for the interests of the country with nationalist discourses. The general discourse is the epic stories of heroes who risk death for the survival and peace of the state.

According to Füsun Çuhadaroğlu, Kurtlar Vadisi is a serial that has been influential in the establishment of violence in society. Because in this series, the concept of violence is combined with the concept of power. People, and especially young people, cling to anything that makes them feel powerful, they want to be, and if television presents power as a phenomenon that can only be gained through violence, viewers learn that in order to be powerful, they need to use violence. Instead of the media message that violence is bad behavior, "Violence is power, it is necessary to resort to violence to be strong" (2007, p. 57-58) gives the message.

The nationalist discourse in the series is mainly based on acts of violence that justify dying and killing for the continuity of the state. This situation also legitimizes the violent scenes and arguments that can be developed over national values for the audience of the series. In the studies on this series, it has been emphasized that the series contains violence and may be a factor in the increase in the tendency of violence in the society. In the studies on this series, it has been emphasized that the series contains violence and may be a factor in the increase in the tendency of violence in the society. In the first years of the series, it is seen that the discussions mostly focused on violence and praising the mafia. It is also possible to see in newspaper reports that the TV series "Kurtlar Vadisi" has a negative impact on people and increases violence. Those who committed murder, injuring and extortion, saying that they were affected by the series, were reported in the newspapers.

The use of violence for entertainment purposes in television series is trivialized by associating violence and mafia rules with concepts such as the protection of the state, its continuity and nationalism. Here, the truth, whose main purpose is to attract the viewer to the screen with the theme of violence, is covered up and the truth is trivialized. Therefore, the fact that men use violence against men intensely, by putting forward different interests and covering them with the mask of these interests, the reality is changed and the importance of the concept of post-truth is revealed.

Çukur

Which stands out with its violent content, has been reaching a large audience since the first day with its cast and theme. The series is about the events that take place in a neighborhood where illegal activities are intense, and violence is treated as an ordinary situation. The characters of the TV series draw attention with their similarities to the famous bullies of a period who lived in Turkey before. The series deals with the struggle of criminal organizations in the environment where the events take place. The internalization of violence, messages that the public conscience can be relieved through illegal communities, and the perception that justice will be provided by punishment on the street are also intensely processed in this series. The tattoos that the actors of the TV series have made on their bodies, the rings they use, the pocketknife, etc. tools have entered the lives of viewers and especially young people. Violence is the main theme of the series' narrative. As in all other mafia and crime series, justice is carried out by these criminal organizations. The use of violence for entertainment purposes is also seen intensely in this series. The viewer identifies himself with good characters and the violence of the man against the man in the name of providing justice is approved. The audience, who will not accept the use of violence by certain forces in real life, accepts this through serials. Because violence contributes to the trivialization of reality by desensitizing the audience within the entertainment logic of television. The audience, who will not accept the use of violence by certain forces in real life, accepts this through serials. Because violence contributes to the trivialization of reality by desensitizing the audience within the entertainment logic of television. Thus, the audience affected by the TV series accepts the truth that the characters in the TV series try to build on their own laws rather than the laws of the state. Therefore, the truth changes from within the framework of the concept of post-truth. Thus, the audience affected by the TV series accepts the truth that the characters in the TV series try to build on their own laws rather than the laws of the state. Therefore, the truth changes from within the framework of the concept of post-truth.

Eşkıya Dünyaya Hükümdar Olmaz

This is another series that includes mafia and violence and has a high viewership. The series tells the story of Hızır Çakırbeyli and his family, who are climbing to the top of the underground world he entered at a young age. The Bandit Doesn't Rule the World is another series that includes mafia and violence and has a high viewership. The series tells the story of Hızır Çakırbeyli and his family, who are climbing to the top of the underground world he entered at a young age. Every man who enters the underworld swears to rebel against injustice. As he gets stronger and richer, he becomes the source of these injustices. No one speaks or expresses this but turns into a benevolent person as atonement for all the crimes he has committed and the violence he has committed. Hızır has a mission to take from the rich and give to the poor and protect the weak. When he gets angry, he loses himself and increases the extent of violence. He uses violence against all men, strong and weak.

In this world, power is in money and position. The power takes place in the common area of the mafia leaders gathered around a table. Violence revolves around this table again. As in other mafia series, violence is applied to those who deserve violence according to them. Even though arms smuggling is carried out, it is acted with national feelings. The interests of the state are above all. Violence is legitimized by this identity. Violence is thus trivialized, and the truth is trivialized by making it a necessary and mandatory identity. The affirmation of violence is masked through the narrative of national interests, and it is ensured that violence takes its place within the framework of the concept of post-truth. The affirmation of violence is masked through the narrative of national interests, and it is ensured that violence takes its place within the framework of the concept of post-truth.

CONCLUSION

The history of humanity has been using the tradition of storytelling from the first day and keeps it in its life for entertainment purposes. Storytelling, which started in the oral culture period, continues effectively in the written culture period. In the age of visual culture, which is the important cultural feature of today, it has been television that has taken on the role of storytelling and is a good storyteller. The basic mission of television is to entertain the audience. In the age of visual culture, which is the important cultural feature of today, it has been television that has taken on the role of storytelling and is a good storyteller. The basic mission of television is to entertain the audience. In the process of entertaining the audience, it uses the storytelling that has existed in human life since the first day. While setting up and editing television stories, it chooses themes that will attract the attention of the audience and keep him on the screen. From past to present, both verbal and visual narratives use violence as a theme in order to maintain interest, create excitement and support tension. It uses violence in different forms in serials, which are important storytelling programs for television. Television adds many elements of violence to its narratives, such as physical violence, psychological violence, economic violence, and sexual violence.

In addition to violence against women, children and elderly people in television series, an important theme is seen as violence by men against men.

Violence by men against men in television series is mostly seen in crime series and mafia series. The representations of violence, especially in mafia serials, are given through good characters and bad characters. In the television series narratives, the violence of the good character over the bad character is presented positively, but the violence of the bad character is not accepted. In the television series narratives, the violence of the good character over the bad character is presented positively, but the violence of the bad character is not accepted. Violence is shown as legitimate in terms of preserving the established order and authority by the good character of the existing order in television series. Mafia serials encourage violence as well as illegal behaviors with the violence they contain and their explicit and covert messages. The violence used in the TV series is given in a much more exaggerated way than the violence that is possible to encounter in daily life.

Violence is an indispensable theme in television programs and especially television series. The fact that violent programs on television not only normalize violence but also present it as ordinary and a part of life, causes the audience to react less to violence in real life. After a while, this situation manifests itself with the insensitivity of the television audience to violence. The viewer, who has become desensitized to violence, becomes more demanding of the violence narrative fictionalized on television. After a while, the audience begins to believe that the solution to evil will come through violence.

The fact that the media presents the truth in line with their own truths and that television establishes its own reality while telling its stories reveals the trivialization of truth within the framework of the concept of post-truth. The fictionalized violence presented through television series brings with it the depersonalization of the audience and the trivialization of truth. The TV series "Kurtlar Vadisi", "Çukur" and "Eşkıya Dünyaya Hükümdar Olmaz", which are mentioned in the study, are TV series that build their narratives on the mafia and violence. In these serials, while the violence of men against men is affirmed as the violence of the good character against the bad character, the truth is trivialized by hiding the violence among different narrative forms. Violence, which is bad and is avoided behavior, is presented as an acceptable form of violence that confirms the structure of the post-truth concept, which has gained importance today.

REFERENCES

Akbulut, T. N. (2004). Women's Discourse on Turkish Television [Türk Televizyonunda Kadın Söylemi]. *Kadın Çalışmalarında Disiplinlerarası Buluşma, Vol, 2*, 157–162.

Akmeşe, Z. (2020). *The Effect of Framing on the Production of Content and Meaning in Television [Televizyonda Çerçevelemenin İçerik ve Anlam Üretimine Etkisi]* (E. Sirer, Ed.). Literatürk Publication.

Alpay, Y. (2019). *The Politics of Lies [Yalanın Siyaseti]*. Destek Publication.

Bardon, A. (2019). *A Brief History of the Philosophy of Time [Zaman Felsefesinin Kısa Tarihi]* (Ö. Yalçın, Trans.). Türkiye İş Bankası Kültür Publication.

Bolat, N., & Çakın, Ö. (2018). In N. Sargın (Ed.), *"Violence" as a Marketing Motif in Television Series: The Example of the Sen Anlat Karadeniz, Virtual Realm / Media Violence [Televizyon Dizilerinde Bir Pazarlama Motifi Olarak "Şiddet": Sen Anlat Karadeniz Dizisi Örneği, Sanal Alem / Medya Şiddeti]*. Hegem Publication.

Bushman, B. J., & Huesmann, L. R. (2006). Short Termand Long-term Effects of Violent Media on Aggression in Children and Adults. *Arch Pediatr Adolesc Med, Vol, 160*(4), 348–352. doi:10.1001/archpedi.160.4.348 PMID:16585478

Çakın, Ö., & Bolat, N. (2018). *An Analysis of Violence and Violent Posts on Social Media, Virtual World /Media Violence [Sosyal Medyada Şiddet Ve Şiddet İçerikli Paylaşımlara Yönelik Bir Çözümleme, Sanal Alem / Medya Şiddeti]*. Hegem Publication.

Çakır, S. (2008). Media and Violence [Medya ve Şiddet]. *Doğu Batı Düşünce Dergisi*, (43), 161–180.

Çelik, N. B. (2000). Introduction: Television, Women, and Violence. In Television, Women and Violence [Televizyon, Kadın ve Şiddet]. KİV Publication.

Çuhadaroğlu, F. (2007). Psychological Dimension of Violence: Youth and Violence Studies. In *Symposium on Preventing Violence Against Children and Adolescents*. Aem Kitap.

Dursun, Ç. (2010). News Ethics Against Violence Against Women [Kadına Yönelik Şiddet Karşısında Haber Etiği]. *Fe Dergi, 2*(1), 19–32.

Erdem, M. N. (2020). An Argumentative Study on the Presentation of Violence in Media Content [Medya İçeriğinde Şiddetin Sunumu Üzerine Argümantatif Bir Çalışma]. *MANAS Journal of Social Studies, 9*(2), 1198–1217.

Erten, Y., & Ardalı, C. (1996). *Psychosocial Structures of Aggression, Violence and Terrorism* [Saldırganlık, Şiddet ve Terörün Psikososyal Yapıları]. YKY Publication.

Fromm, E. (1984). *The Origins of Human Destructive [İnsandaki Yıkıcılığın Kökenleri]* (Ş. Alpagut, Trans.). Payel Publication.

Geçer, E. (2013). *Media and Popular Culture–TV Series, Television and Society [Medya ve Popüler Kültür–Diziler, Televizyon ve Toplum]*. Metamorfoz Publication.

Gerbner, G. (1972). Violence in Television Drama: Trends and Symbolic Function, Television and Social Behavior: Media Content and Control. National Institute of Mental Health.

Gültekin, Z. (2006). Before Iraq: The Valley of the Wolves [Irak'dan önce: Kurtlar Vadisi Dizisi]. *İletişim Kuram ve Araştırma, 22*, 9-36.

Güz, H. (2007). Violence and Youth Perception of Violence. In *Prevention of Violence Against Children and Adolescents Symposium*. Aem Kitap.

Güz, N. (2007). The Role of the Media in Preventing Violence. In *Child and Adolescent Symposium on the Prevention of Violence Against*. Aem Kitap.

İlerialkan, D., & Yılmaz, R. (2015). Script: How to Write? How They Write [Senaryo: Nasıl Yazılır? Nasıl Yazıyorlar?]. *Alfa*.

İnal, A. (1999). *Television, Genre and Representation [Televizyon, Tür ve Temsil].* Mahmut Tali Öngören'e Armağan.

Kars, N. (2012). *Let's Make a TV Program for Everyone to Watch [Televizyon Programı Yapalım Herkes İzlesin].* Derin Publication.

Kaya, R. (2021). An Old Truth A New Concept: The Trivialization of Truth or Post-Truth [Eski Bir Hakikat Yeni Bir Kavram: Hakikatin Önemsizleşmesi ya da Post-Truth]. *Isparta Okulu Dergisi, 1*(1), 25–35.

Köknel, Ö. (2000). *Individual and Community Violence [Bireysel ve Toplumsal Şiddet].* Altın Kitaplar Publication.

Llorente, J. A. (2017). *The post-truth era: Reality vs. perception.* UNO Developing Ideas.

Mutlu, E. (1991). *Understanding Television [Televizyonu Anlamak].* Gündoğan Publication.

Mutlu, E. (1999). *Television and Society [Televizyon ve Toplum].* Türkiye Radyo ve Televizyon Kurumu Publication.

Nalçaoğlu, H. (2003). A Framework for Understanding the Media and Society Relationship. In S. Alankuş (Ed.), *Media and Society* (pp. 43–57). İletişim Vakfı Publication.

Öngören, M. T., Yanık, F., İşcan, C., & Demirergi, N. (1994). *What Violence Is This [Bu Ne Şiddet].* Kitle Publication.

Palabıyıkoğlu, R. (1997). Media and Violence [Medya ve Şiddet]. *Kriz Dergisi, 5*(2), 123–126.

Platon. (2005). *State* [Devlet] (S. Eyüboğlu & M. A. Cimcoz, Trans.). Türkiye İş Bankası Publication.

Radecki, T. (1986). Violent Entertainment. In *Mass Media and Violence*. Hürriyet Vakfı Eğitim Publication.

Sim, Ş., (1996). Media and Violence [Medya ve Şiddet]. *İletişim Fakültesi, 3*, 127-131.

Sirer, E. (2020). *New Curriculum New Audience [Yeni İzlence Yeni İzlerkitle].* Literatürk Publication.

Sözen, E. (2008). *Icon Usage, Media Sensitivity to Violence Panel [Simge Kullanımı, Medyada Şiddete Duyarlılık Paneli].* RTÜK Publication.

Terzi, A. (2020). On the Concept of Post-Truth and Its Turkish Equivalents [Post-Truth Kavramı ve Türkçe Karşılıkları Üzerine]. *Türk dili, 69*(820), 80–86.

Trend, D. (2008). *The Myth of Violence in the Media [Medyada Şiddet Efsanesi]* (G. Bostancı, Trans.). YKY Publication.

Türkdoğan, O. (1996). *Social Violence and the Reality of Turkey [Sosyal Şiddet ve Türkiye Gerçeği].* Timaş Publication.

Türkoğlu, N. (2010). *Social Communication [Toplumsal İletişim].* Urban Publication.

Ünlü, S. B., Uluyağcı, N., Uzoğlu, C., & Bayçu, S. (2009). Violence Against Women: A Study on Violence Against Women in TV Series [Kadına Yönelik Şiddet: TV Dizilerinde Kadına Yönelik Şiddet Üzerine Bir Araştırma]. *Selçuk İletişim, 5*(4), 95–104.

Ünsal, A. (1996). An Extended Typology of Violence, Violence [Genişletilmiş Bir Şiddet Tipolojisi, Şiddet]. *Cotigo, 6-7*, 29–36.

Uysal, M. (2006). *Media and Violence, Violence as a Social Problem Symposium* [Medya ve Şiddet, Toplumsal Bir Sorun Olarak Şiddet Symposium. Ankara, Turkey: Academic Press.

Yılmaz, R., & Erdem, M. N. (2018). *An Analysis on Coding Violence in Advertising, Virtual Realm / Media Violence [Reklamda Şiddet Kodlamaları Üzerine Bir İnceleme, Sanal Alem / Medya Şiddeti].* Hegem Publication.

Zorlu, Y. (2016). Violence in the Media and Its Effects [Medyadaki Şiddet Ve Etkileri]. *Humanities Sciences, 11*(1), 13–32.

ADDITIONAL READING

Arendt, H. (2016). *Şiddet Üzerine* (B. Peker, Trans.). İletişim Publication.

Köknel, Ö. (2013). *Şiddet Dili*. Remzi Publication.

Şenbalkan, Ş. (2013). *Kadına Şiddet.! Madalyonun Öbür Yüzü*. IQ Kültür Sanat Publication.

KEY TERMS AND DEFINITIONS

Depersonalization: The most important effect of violence in television broadcasts that creates an anesthetic effect on individuals is "depersonalization". The intense display of violence in the media and the constant exposure to media violence cause depersonalization of individuals' natural emotional and physical reactions. In fact, scenes of violence warn individuals less over time, and in summary, the violence watched in the media reduces the physical reactions to violence in the real world.

Narrative: An all-encompassing meaning that tells or presents a story. Whether it is a picture, written text, moving image, or a combination of all these, the narrative is revealed. Television series are also known as storytelling tools with text and visuals.

Post-Truth: Post-truth, chosen as the word of the year in 2016, is defined as the determination of public opinion by personal feelings and beliefs rather than objective facts. Most of the academic studies are on the negativity of populist discourse overcoming "reality" and thus finding more supporters of the irrational than the rational.

TV Series: It presents people's emotions to the audience within the framework of curiosity, as a television version of the stories told by storytellers in traditional times. Dramas that reveal the modern interpretation of traditional stories by exaggerating and sometimes exploiting people's thousands of years of experience and their networks of relationships with each other are called television series.

Violence: Violence is defined as harsh and painful behavior directed from outside against the bodily integrity of people. Television fills people with hatred, grudge, and greed. News, reality shows, movies, TV series and even cartoons are marketing the biggest truth of life, death, to people. In order to increase interest and eliminate commercial concerns, television programs sometimes broadcast negative role models in which the element of curiosity takes place more. Violence is one of the most important areas in this regard.

Chapter 5
Informatics Truth:
News Media in the Post-Truth Era

Onur Şen
https://orcid.org/0000-0001-8054-5876
Ondokuz Mayıs University, Turkey

ABSTRACT

Today's technological developments have enabled the digitalization of communication and transform it into different forms. With the said digitalization, individuals have had the opportunity to communicate very quickly, exchange information, produce content, and access information about their environment much more. Besides many opportunities brought by digital transformation are reflected to individuals, it reflected to the field of news media, which provides information flow to individuals. The reflection of digitalization in the news media emerged as a result of especially distributing and producing information very quickly and reaching large masses. The acceleration of the flow of information has made it necessary to focus on the concept of truth. So that, as a result of the intense information flow in the 2016 US Presidential Elections and the Brexit referendum in England, the production and distribution of news in the post-truth era has become questionable. From this point of view, the truth of the information produced in the news media will be examined in this study.

INTRODUCTION

In today's world, people can access information anytime and anywhere. So that today, thanks to mobile internet technologies and intelligent cell phones, people can be aware of many issues such as health, finance, social environment, and politics with a few finger touches (Bartlett, 2020, p. 1). Although there are conveniences in accessing information and news today, this situation brings negativities. As a matter of fact, among the information and news that people can easily access in today's world compared to the past, there is also unreal, false, or false information. It can be stated that many news that people reach through information and communication technologies, whose source is not clear and which does not have proof statements, may be false. The emergence of fake news dates back to the 17th century. Fake news that existed in the past is now continuing in a different form. Compared to the past, the current

DOI: 10.4018/978-1-7998-9251-9.ch005

form of fake news stands out with the development of internet technologies and the rise of social media platforms worldwide and its spread to the masses (Bhaskaran, Mishra & Nair, 2017, p. 42).

Developments in information and communication technologies have rapidly integrated into people's lives. The mentioned integration has been realized with digital transformation (Balcı, Bekiroğlu & Karaman, 2019, p. 39; İnal & Şevik, 2019, p. 190). The transition to Web 2.0 in internet environments has transformed people into users who can produce and consume content. In other words, people can produce their information (Delal & Abanoz, 2021, p.265; Resuloğlu & Yılmaz, 2017). This information spreads quickly in countries where social media platforms are used at a high level. From this disseminated information, people accept what is suitable for them and do not accept what is not suitable for them (Şimşek, 2018, p. 12).

Many opportunities brought by digital transformation are also reflected in the field of news media, which provides information flow to people and people. The reflection of digitalization on the news media is especially evident in the distribution and production of information (Bekiroğlu, Kaya & Yaman, 2019, p. 153; Şen, 2021, p. 58). The news media performs the production and distribution of information digitally, rather than through traditional methods, and delivers it to large masses. Due to the transformation of information production and distribution with the digitalization process, the concept of post-truth has become questionable in today's ecosystem. In parallel with this discussion, in the last quarter of 2016, Oxford Dictionaries determined the word of the year as "Post-Truth". In the light of these discussions, the truth of the information produced in the news media will be examined in this study. The examination in the study will be made through how the news narrative is set up in the internet news media organizations operating in Turkey, which is about the tension between Russia and Ukraine that started in the past years and is now quite rising. Van Dijk's critical discourse analysis will be used as a method in the study. The texts to be analyzed in the axis of the determined method consist of the news about the tension between Russia and Ukraine on the news media sites ensonhaber.com, hurriyet.com.tr, and sozcu.com.tr dated February 12, 2022.

TRUTH, POST-TRUTH AND INFORMATION

Oxford Dictionaries defines the concept of "Post-Truth", which it chose as the word of the year 2016, as "the situation in which objective truths on a particular subject are less effective than emotions and personal thoughts in determining public opinion" (Oxford Dictionary, 2021). According to Oxford Dictionaries, the word "post", a prefix in the concept, does not reference an event or a later event. On the contrary, the prefix "post" refers to the trivialization and loss of meaning or shift of meaning of the concept (Carlson, 2018, p. 1881; Uluk, 2018, p. 90).

Although post-truth was chosen as the word of the year by Oxford Dictionaries in 2016, the concept started to be used in 1992 with its current meaning. Playwright Steve Tesich used the term in its current meaning in an article published in The Nation magazine in 1992. S. Tesich defined the concept as "Watergate Syndrome". In his article, Teisch mentions that the US Government made people believe in the war on groundless grounds (Kreitner, 2016).

It is known that the concept of "post-truth", which appeared on the political scene, spread to every area related to people's lives. In the post-truth age, "truth" is almost lost. In the face of the lost truth, the lie becomes normal. Non-truth information is becoming widespread in digitalized communication environments (Delal & Abanoz, 2021, p. 274).

The concept of post-truth; It can be said that refers to fabricated, reduced, or distorted situations that have no connection with the truth. Although post-truth was used in its current meaning in a theater play in 1992, the United States Presidential Elections in 2016 and the European Union referendum in the United Kingdom made the concept even more questionable in today's world. Moreover, the fact that information distribution has become relatively easy with the digitalization of communication makes the concept important (Salgado, 2018, pp. 317-318).

Post-truth age places people from "I think therefore I am" to "I believe therefore it is true" thought (Şimşek & Yalı, 2019, p. 50). For example, in the Brexit referendum in the UK, the breakaway Vote Leave coalition said, "We are sending £350 million a week to the European Union. Instead, let us fund our National Health System (NHS)". Although the claim in question was denied by official institutions, many people in the UK emotionally believed this claim and created their truths (Rose, 2017, p. 55). In a different example, it is known that the fake news that was served to the public during Donald Trump's campaign in the Presidential Elections held in the United States of America in 2016 was widely shared. It is known that, as with the people of the United Kingdom, a large part of the people of the United States create their reality with fake news (Uluk, 2018, p. 71). In this context, it can be stated that the main problem is that the layer between the truth and the lie becomes invisible in the post-truth eraIt is known that producing false or fake information in the post-truth era has become commonplace and even accepted by people. In the post-truth era, subjectivity and emotional intuition are superior to objectivity and rationality (Porgham, 2020).

In the post-truth era, truth has left its place in the ability to appeal to emotions. Especially with the digitalization of communication, this situation is becoming widespread with echo chambers and filter balloons on social media platforms. Today, people interact with people who share the same view and marginalize others. In other words, people are imprisoned in echo chambers with those with their own opinions. In these rooms, people are not exposed to any information other than the echoes of their views. People are firmly attached to information that does not contain truth, and because they do not encounter different ideas, they describe the information they receive as truth (Delal & Abanoz, 2021, pp. 274-275).

One of the essential instruments of the post-truth era is media platforms digitalized with information and communication technologies. People can communicate with each other quickly and without being tied to space and time, making the information flow unlimited. It is known that the firm idea that traditional media determined the agenda and public opinion of the society in the past has been questioned again with digitalized communication. On the other hand, traditional media has tended to converge in the face of digitalized communication and has moved itself to digital at many points. Based on these points, it is essential to examine the news media, which provides information flow to people in the post-truth era, as it was in the past.

NEWS MEDIA AND NEWS NARRATIVE IN THE POST-TRUTH ERA

With the rising developments in information and communication technologies at the beginning of the 21st century, computer and internet-based media tools, apart from traditional media tools and the digitalization of media tools, have enabled two-way communication instead of one-sided communication. In other words, people who are only consumers with traditional media tools have become both consumers and producers with computer and internet-based media tools. The fact that people are both producers and consumers takes place on their own or interactive network platforms. People can reproduce the information and information they see subjectively correct with these network platforms. In other words, people can use these networks to facilitate the creation of discourses of "truth" thanks to their platforms (Sawyer, 2018, p. 63).

As stated above, digitalized media tools have a different appearance compared to traditional media with the development of information and communication technologies. Although the instruments used by digitalized media tools are different from traditional media tools, they include digital media features (Yılmaz & Taşkıran, 2015, p. 13). There has been a transformation in news media practices with digitalization, and online journalism has emerged apart from traditional journalism (Şen, 2021, p. 58). Although this transformation has brought many positive situations, it is a fact that it also leads to immoral purposes. Media is accepted as the fourth power in democratic societies after the legislative, executive, and judicial powers. In a different way, in democratic societies, many tasks have been attributed to the news media, such as conveying the demands and wishes of the people to the elected, controlling the political and economic elites on behalf of the people, and providing information on current issues (Harjuniemi, 2021, p. 3). The existence of online news media alongside traditional news media, besides showing a democratic function; also allows the circulation of many publications that are not genuine, unrealistic, against the professional principles of the press, operational, sensational, and false broadcasting in which personal confrontations are at the center, and attacks on the rights and freedoms of individuals. Exposure of people to untruthful data in the face of a high level of information flow can adversely affect social, cultural, and economic perspectives (Porgham, 2020).

The concept of post-truth, which came to the fore in the Brexit referendum campaign in the United Kingdom in 2016, occurred with two different possibilities in the context of news. The first of these possibilities have emerged with the spread of the news or information by the masses without ensuring the accuracy of the spread with the digitalization of communication. In other words, while gatekeepers in traditional media can question the accuracy of information or news entering the public circulation, questioning is violated with the emergence of digitalization. In the second possibility, political people have turned to digital communication environments by taking advantage of the decrease in trust attributed to traditional media environments today. Along with this orientation, the news narrative specific to the post-truth era was emphasized by using digital communication media to influence the public (Marshall & Drieschova, 2018, p. 92).

Some opinions oppose the uploading of negative outputs (such as fake news and disinformation) brought about by the rapid spread of digital communication technologies to digital communication users. For example, Ünal and Taylan (2017: 82) state that the problem of fake news or fake/distorted/false information cannot be reduced to only digital communication users but traditional news media organizations, various companies, or trolls are among the parties to the problem. According to Ünal and Taylan (2017: 82); While digital communication environments are evolving into a medium where information and news flow accelerate, both with the shares produced by media professionals and the content produced by digital communication users, on the other hand, it is becoming an environment where fake news or fake/distorted/false information spreads rapidly.

The concepts of "disinformation and misinformation" and "fake news" are essential in investigating informatics truth. The first of the mentioned concepts, disinformation, can be defined as distorting information about an event or subject, unrealistic information flow, downplaying the importance of information, and biased information. The second concept is misinformation; information can be expressed as the information source's deliberate failure to provide incomplete information about an event or subject (Yüksel & Gürcan, 2005, pp. 86-87). Fake news, which has existed in the past but has turned into a different meaning in the post-truth era, is defined as news that does not reflect the truth and that is usually fictionalized at the desk to attract the attention of the public (Yüksel & Gürcan, 2005, p. 71).

There are debates about fake news and false information, especially in the West, in the post-truth age, about truth's news narrative and who determines it. Moreover, it is known that the distrust of the news narrative of the mainstream news media has increased (Doui, 2019, p. 132). In the post-truth era, concepts such as truth, reality, and truth have lost their importance. So much so that disinformation or misinformation can easily reach people in this age. Also, in this age, fake news or fake information is considered normal by people (Delal & Abanoz, 2021, p. 274).

In the light of these discussions, it can be stated that in the post-truth era, the truth questioning of the news or information received from the news media is made by people with emotions and subjective elements. People perceive untrue news or information served by the news media as "truth". In this context, it can be stated that the truth status of the information constructed by the news media in the post-truth era has become questionable.

ANALYSIS OF THE NEWS ON THE TENSION BETWEEN RUSSIA AND UKRAINE

Purpose and Subject

As in the past, the media plays a leading role in people's access to information today. Today, the digitalization of communication has deeply affected the production and distribution practices of the media. So much so that people can now access news and information within seconds. However, in the post-truth age, truth and lies are intertwined. Narrative constructs in media information in the post-truth era have become questionable in terms of truth. In this context, the study's aim is how the news media's narrative fiction is constructed. The subject of this study is the storytelling of the news about Russia-Ukraine tension in internet news media organizations operating in Turkey.

Universe, Sample and Limitations

The universe of the study is internet news media organizations operating in Turkey. Internet news media ensonhaber.com, hurriyet.com.tr and sozcu.com.tr were determined as samples in the study. The typical universe in the purposive sampling technique was used to determine the sample. Three conditions were considered in determining the typical sample. The first is that the news media, which is the sample, operate in the internet environment. Secondly, according to Alexa (2022) system data, they are in the top three among internet news media operating in Turkey. The third is that the subject of the study took place in the internet news media on February 12, 2022. In the selection of the aforementioned date, the statements that came from Europe and America that war would break out on February 12, 2022, were influential. The study's limitations are the news of the internet news media selected as the sample.

Method

Van Dijk's Critical Discourse Analysis (CDA) technique was used in the study with a qualitative research method design. Critical discourse analysis is expressed as an approach fed from various theoretical sources and contains various perspectives (Evre, 2009, p. 134). V. Dijk (2003, pp. 13-14) states that discourse analysis is vital in expressing thoughts and mutual communication. In this context, it can be stated that the artificial truth desired to be given in the news produced in the post-truth age will be revealed through discourse analysis.

The Critical Discourse Analysis developed by V. Dijk to analyze news texts consists of *macro* and *micro structures*. In critical discourse analysis, macro and microstructure are divided into sub-headings (Özer, 2011, p. 85):

Macro Structure

1. Thematic Structure
    a. Headline(s)
    b. News Entry, (Spot(s) if there is no spotlight, the first paragraph of the news should be taken. If the news consists of a single paragraph, the first sentence can be considered a news entry)
    c. Photograph(s)
2. Schematic Structure
    a. Situation (Presentation of main event, Results, Background, Context information)
    b. Comment (News sources, Comments brought by the parties)

Micro Structure

1. Syntactic Analysis (Active or passive sentence structures, simple or complex sentence structures)
2. Regional Cohesion (Causal Relationship, Functional Relationship, Referenceal Relationship)
3. Choices of Word
4. Rhetoric (Photo, Credible information, Eyewitness statements)

Background

In order to fully understand the tension between Russia and Ukraine, it is necessary to look at 2003. In 2003, with the election of V. Putin as the head of state in Russia, there was a diplomatic crisis with Ukraine. The crisis in question was experienced when Russia built a dam in the Kerch Strait, close to the Tuzla Island of Ukraine. A different crisis emerged when Russia supported Viktor Yanukovych in the 2004 presidential elections in Ukraine. In the election, Viktor Yanukovych, supported by Russia, and Viktor Yushchenko, who had Western ideas, came to the fore as strong candidates. According to the election results, Yanukovych, supported by Russia, won the election. As a result of the popular uprising, which started with the result that emerged shortly after the election and went down in history as the "Orange Revolution", Yushchenko, who had Western thinking, became the head of state. During Yushchenko's presidency, Russia cut off the natural gas it sent to Ukraine twice, in 2006 and 2009 (DW, 2022).

The tension between Russia and Ukraine, a former Soviet Union country, started to increase with the rapprochement of the Kyiv administration with the European Union (EU). The pro-Russian Viktor Yanukovych, who came to power in Kyiv, suspended the EU Association Agreement in 2013 to prevent the country from turning to the West. Upon this decision, many events took place in Ukraine in 2013, and in 2014 internal turmoil arose. Thousands of pro-Western people gathered in Ukraine for months to protest Yanukovych's decision. There were occasional clashes as the pro-Russians took to the squares. With the events becoming uncontrollable, Viktor Yanukovych fled to Russia. As a result of the events, the Ukrainian people were divided into pro-Russian and pro-Western (AA, 2021).

The recent reflection of the tension between Russia and Ukraine on the world agenda started with the annexation of Crimea, a part of Ukraine, by Russia in 2014. In addition, conflicts occurred between the pro-Russian separatists and the Ukrainian army in Donetsk, which received support from Russia in 2014. The conflicts ended with a ceasefire in 2015. However, it is known that there were occasional clashes until the ceasefire in July 2020. It is known that around 15 thousand people lost their lives in the conflicts. Pro-Russian separatists, who unilaterally declared independence in Donetsk and Lugansk (Donbas region), where conflicts take place, continue to exist (BBC, 2022). The tension between Russia and Ukraine, which has continued since 2014, has entered the world agenda again due to the death of 4 Ukrainian soldiers in the Donbas region on March 26, 2021 (AA, 2021).

Findings

The news to be discourse analyzed was selected from the news published on ensonhaber.com (2022), hurriyet.com.tr (2022) and sozcu.com.tr news media on February 12, 2022. The news selection was made by preliminary examination. In the news that was taken into pre-examination, attention was paid to whether there were narratives specific to the post-truth era. As a result of the selection process, one piece of news from each of three different internet news media was analyzed.

Internet News Media: ensonhaber.com

Macro Structure

Analyzing the news of internet news media ensonhaber.com (2022) within the framework of macro structure.

Thematic Structure

Headline: "Russia-Ukraine tension will be reflected in fuel prices"
News sub-headings: A1"Concerns that Fuel Prices Will Rise As Donbas Events Climb", A2"Increase in Oil Prices Passed 4 Percent", A3"Oil A Barrel At $95.13", A4"Global Oil Demand Will Increase", A5"Golden Ounce Price Increased"

When the main headline of the news is considered within the framework of discourse analysis, it is mentioned that the tension between Russia and Ukraine is reflected in fuel prices. In this sense, it is understood from the news headline that the tension experienced will cause an economic problem. The headline contains information hiding and generalization. When it is reflected in the prices is not stated in the title, and the verb is used with the future tense. In addition, it is not stated which fuels it will be reflected on. In this sense, there is a generalization. The headline title in question is far from giving precise information. When the sub-headings are considered, it is seen that the sub-headings A1, A2, and A3 support the main headline. However, it is noteworthy that the A4 and A5 sub-headings are separated from the context because they are fictionalized as new news. Information hiding is available in all sub-headings.

News entry: "Russia-Ukraine tension was reflected in oil prices. Stock markets were affected by this tension, and the ounce of gold rose as well."

When the introduction of the news is considered, it is seen that there are differences in meaning between the news headline and the entry of the news. While the headline mentions the reflection of tension on fuel prices, it is mentioned in the first sentence of the news entry that it is reflected in oil prices. In addition, it is mentioned in the introduction that the tension between Russia and Ukraine affects fuel prices and stock markets, and an ounce of gold. In this context, other information other than the information is given in the title is included in the news entry. In addition to all these, it is seen that there is an information reduction in the news entry. It can be stated that the said reduction fits the narrative plane in the post-truth era. The tension between Russia and Ukraine is also reflected in the world ecosystem given in the news.

Photograph: When the news photograph is considered, it is seen that a design image is used. The expressions "What happened when Donbas was heating up" and "New price hikes are on the way" draw attention to the designed image. The examined image shows that the fuel filling vehicle and the fuel oil image are used. In this sense, it supports the news title. In addition, the statement "...it happened to the pump" also supports the news headline. It has been observed that an information reduction has been made in the statement of new hikes on the way. It is unclear what and when the new hikes will come and what they will cover.

Schematic Structure

Situation: When the news is examined in the title of the situation, the presentation of the main event emerges at the entrance of the news. The event in the news is the increase in oil prices, and this hike may affect fuel prices. However, when the news text is examined in its entirety, it is seen that the presence of different events in which there are breaks from the main event. For example, it is seen that inflation in the United States of America (USA) is mentioned at the end of the news text. Considering the news results, it can be stated that there were price increases due to the tension between Russia and Ukraine, which is why the news was made. It has been observed that background information is not included in the news. In the news, it is seen that the context information is based on economy, conflict, and fossil resources. When the news situation is considered as a whole under the title, the existence of information hiding comes to the fore. In this sense, the truth situation is problematic. The absence of background information has made the reality situation questionable.

Comment: When the news is examined in the comment title, it is seen that the news source is the secondary source. The news is constructed on the information provided by an agency. It has been observed that the explanations of the parties or interests if the subject of the news are not included. However, it has been observed that the statements of different countries, unions, and authorities that are not parties are included. For example, the fact that various statements from the Western world are included in the news builds the truth that the West is powerful in the news.

Micro Structure

Analyzing the news of internet news media ensonhaber.com (2022) within the framework of micro structure.

Syntactic Analysis

When the news is analyzed within the framework of syntactic analysis, the sentence structures are the active and passive (Ex. "US National Security Advisor Jake Sullivan also said that Russia may start to invade Ukraine before the "Chinese Olympics" is over.", "International Energy Agency's (IEA) final In the report, it was pointed out that the oil markets are tight.") is used in the structure. Also, sentence structures are simple.

Regional Cohesion

When the news is handled within the framework of regional harmony, it is observed that there is a causal, functional, and referential relationship in the news text. For example, the news article mentions the causal relationship "Russia-Ukraine tension was reflected in oil prices." appears in the sentences. Its functional relationship can be seen in the following sentences in the news text: "Oil prices increased by more than 4 percent after the increasing tension between Russia and Ukraine. Gold prices also increased after rising inflation concerns."

When the news is considered within the frame of reference relationship, it is seen that there are many statements about the increase in tensions: "As the Donbas events escalate, especially from the increase in pump prices…", "Oil prices, after the increasing tension between Russia and Ukraine," "… enter Ukraine" The rumors that he will give the order to the world are worrying the global markets…" In addition, the use of many referential relations belonging to the Western world builds the truth that the West is powerful and has a say.

Choices of Word

It has been observed that the words chosen in the news are remarkable and exciting. For example, it can be stated that word choices were made in words "…the tension was reflected in the oil prices", "While the Donbas events were heating up…", "…after the increasing tension…", "…it caused concern..." to increase the interest in the news and make the reader curious. It should be noted that; reality is represented from a different point by the words used. Namely, words such as tension, escalation, tension, and anxiety appear in the human mind with their first meaning. With the news text, the meaning begins to bend. In this context, it can be stated that there are differences in the narrative of reality.

Rhetoric

When the news is handled within the framework of rhetoric, it is seen that the statements of different state officials and institutions are included to increase the news's credibility. No eyewitness or numerical data were used. The design photograph used in the news contributes to the rhetoric. However, trying to support the news with a different context in the first paragraph after the news entry leads to doubts about the truth. In addition, there is no objective evidence in the news text. In this sense, it can be stated that there are problems at the point of truth.

Internet News Media: hurriyet.com.tr

Macro Structure

Analyzing the news of internet news media hurriyet.com.tr (2022) within the framework of macro structure.

Thematic Structure

Headline: "The blood pressure is too high... Biden: If we enter Ukraine, there will be a world war"
News sub-headings: A1"War May Begin Before the End of the Olympics", A2"Negotiations Failed", A3"Naval Exercise with 20 Ships", A4"Western Shipment of Weapons to Kiev", A5"Giant Bombers in England", A6" US Staff Also Arrived in the UK", "NATO on Vigilance"

When the title is considered within the framework of discourse analysis, the word groups "the blood pressure is too high…" were evaluated as panic-inducing. It is noteworthy that in the headline, the statement of the President of the United States of America (USA), Joe Biden, is given with a direct quotation. When the statement in question is taken into consideration, a truth emerges that the USA has the right to have a say in the region and the world. It seems that there is no evidence for the proposition put forward in the title. In this sense, the proposition that there will be a war stands out as the construction of truth. The title also includes information hiding and generalization. When the sub-headings are considered, information hiding is striking in the sub-headings A1, A2, A3, A4, A5, and A6. On the other hand, the subtitles in the news support the narrative of the news. It can be stated that the discourse established with the information given in the headlines of the news has references to the post-truth era.

News entry: "While the successive negotiations with the search for a diplomatic solution to the Ukraine crisis were inconclusive, the ropes in the field were tense. After the Russian army started a large-scale exercise, a 'world war' warning came from US President Joe Biden."

Considering the introduction of the news, it is seen that there are differences in meaning between the news title and the news spot. The spot of the news is structured in two sentences. When the expressions in the first sentence are examined, a reference is made to a crisis in Ukraine. It is stated that diplomatic solutions to end this crisis are inconclusive. Considering the second sentence, the statements of the US President regarding an exercise by Russia are included. Including the statements of the US President suggests that it is biased information. The USA is not a party to the event. However, it is seen that the USA has a say in the region. In this sense, it is seen that the truth that the USA is strong is built on the news narrative.

5W and 1H questions should be questioned in news entries. However, it is stated in the first sentence that there is a crisis in Ukraine; why, when, and how this crisis happened is not explained. In the second sentence, there is an exercise that Russia will carry out, and the information about where, how, and why this exercise will be held is not included. In addition, information on why and when the statements of the US President regarding the exercise in question were made was not included. In this sense, it can be stated that information hiding is made in the news narrative. On the axis of all these explanations, it can be stated that the news complies with the narrative plane in the post-truth era.

Photograph: It is seen that more than one photograph is used in the article. The primary photograph used shows the presidents of the USA and Russia. The absence of a Ukrainian image in the main photo of the news shows that the truth that Ukraine is powerless and defenseless is being constructed. In other photographs, it is seen that there are soldiers, a warplane, war maps, and a soldier holding a gun. It is observed that the fact that there will be a war is built with the use of these images.

Schematic Structure

Situation: It is seen that the main event in the news consists of the statements of US President Biden due to the tension between Russia and Ukraine. When the results in the news are examined, it is seen that the emphasis of "war will break out" as a result of the tension is frequently expressed. It has been observed that background information is not included in the news. Contextual information in the news was based on the balance of power, war, and fear between the West and the East. In this context, it is seen that the news, which is examined as a whole in the title of the situation, has the characteristics of the post-truth era.

Comment: When the news is examined in the comment title, the primary source is used in the news. The news in question was prepared and served by two reporters. It was seen that the comments from Ukraine were not included in the news. It is striking that there are many interpretations of the Western world. It is seen that Russia, among the parties of the event, made comments in the news. It can be stated that the presentation of reality is problematic due to the high level of Western opinion in the news.

Micro Structure

Analyzing the news of internet news media hurriyet.com.tr (2022) within the framework of micro structure.

Syntactic Analysis

When the news is considered within the framework of syntactic analysis, it is seen that the sentence structures are in an active structure (Ex. "US Navy Spokesperson Arlo Abrahamson also announced that four destroyers were deployed to the sixth squadron responsible for the European region "to support NATO allies," "The so-called 'ship terminator' in the exercise. 'Bastin' missiles were also tested.") Also, the sentence structures are simple.

Regional Cohesion

When the news is handled within the framework of regional harmony, it is observed that there is a causal, functional, and referential relationship in the news text in general. It has been seen that there are sentences used in the news within the framework of causal relationships and functional relationships. Within the framework of the referential relationship, it is seen that the word groups such as "ship terminator" and

"NATO allies" are mentioned in the news, and references are given to concepts such as war, east-west, and power. Within the framework of regional harmony, it is seen that the Westside is depicted actively, and the parties of the event are passively depicted in the news narrative. In this context, the truth of the superiority of the West is emphasized.

Choices of Word

When the news is considered within the framework of word choices, it has been observed that the words chosen in the news are remarkable, interesting, intriguing, and cause panic. For example, the words "high blood pressure" in the title is not only attracting attention but can also cause panic in people. It can be stated that it is desired to create a reality with word choices. As a matter of fact, the words used make people believe. It can be stated that reality is not represented by the word choices used in the news.

Rhetoric

In order to increase the credibility of the news, it was seen that the statements of different state officials were included. No eyewitness or numerical data were used. It has been observed that most of the explanations used in the news are based on probabilities. In this sense, it can be said that the truth is not clear.

Internet News Media: sozcu.com.tr

Macro Structure

Analyzing the news of internet news media sozcu.com.tr (2022) within the framework of macro structure.

Thematic Structure

Headline: "Russia-Ukraine tension: Putin to invade on Wednesday"
News sub-headings: A1"Secret Briefing Given", A2"Avoid While There Is A Plane", A3"Message From The Mayor", A4"257 Pion Cannon Deployed", A5"Blinken: We Are Ready"

When the title is examined, the tension between Russia and Ukraine is mentioned, and the invasion of Russian President V. Putin on Wednesday is brought to the fore. The title contains information hiding and generalization. There are no explanations about where and when the invasion will occur. The concrete reality cannot be reached when the main title is examined. When the sub-headings are considered, information concealment is striking in all sub-headings A1, A2, A3, A4, and A5.

News entry: "While the tension between Russia and Ukraine has been escalating since 2014, critical developments have taken place in the last hours... The statements of intelligence sources that Putin will begin to invade Ukraine on February 16 emerged in the news in the German media."

When the introduction of the news is considered, it is seen that there are differences in meaning between the news title and the entry of the news. The news spot is structured in two sentences. When the expressions in the first sentence are examined, although reference is made to the background information, no details are given. It is said that the crisis is escalating. In the second sentence, it is understood that the news was made with the information obtained from the German media. 5W and 1H questions should be questioned first in news entries. Although it is stated in the first sentence that there is a crisis in Ukraine, why and how this crisis emerged is not mentioned. In the second sentence, it is stated that Russia will start the invasion. The reason for the occupation was not stated. In this sense, it can be stated that information hiding is made in the news narrative. It can be stated that this situation fits the narrative plane in the post-truth era.

Photograph: It is seen that the tank image is used as the primary photo in the article. In this context, it can be stated that it supports the narrative in the news. It was seen that more than one photograph was used in the news. It can be stated that the fictionalized reality narrative in the news is supported by soldiers, warships, aid equipment, and satellite images in other photographs.

Schematic Structure

Situation: The presentation of main event in the news is the tension between Russia and Ukraine. As a result of this tension, we come across in the news narrative that Russia will invade Ukraine. The event in the news was considered necessary within the framework of news value, and therefore it was reported. When the results in the news are examined, it is seen that the emphasis of "war will break out" as a result of the tension is frequently expressed. However, objective evidence was not included. The fact that different explanations from the West are included in the news builds a truth that tension affects the world. It has been seen that the background information is included in the news in general terms. Contextual information in the news was based on the balance of power, war, weapons, and turmoil between the West and the East. As a result, it can be stated that the news narrative has features of the post-truth age.

Comment: When the news is examined in the comment heading, it is striking that the news source is the secondary source. It was taken from a foreign media institution and served by the editors. It was seen that there were no comments by Russia in the news. However, it is striking that there are many interpretations of the Western world. It is seen that the mayor of Kyiv, the capital of Ukraine, made a comment in the news. The use of second-hand sources and the views of the West indicate that the presentation of reality in the news may be problematic.

Micro Structure

Analyzing the news of internet news media sozcu.com.tr (2022) within the framework of micro structure.

Syntactic Analysis

When the news is handled within the framework of syntactic analysis, it is seen that sentence structures are used in active and passive structures. Also, sentence structures are simple.

Regional Cohesion

When the news is considered within the framework of regional harmony, it is observed that there is a causal, functional, and referential relationship in the news text in general. For example, in the causal relationship news text, "While the tension between Russia and Ukraine has been escalating since 2014, critical developments took place in the last hours." appears in sentences. The functional relationship is in the news, "The USA, which announced that Putin might attack Kyiv this week, also wanted its citizens to move away from the region. US National Security Advisor Jake Sullivan said: "Washington believes Putin will invade Ukraine within days." sentences are also visible. The explanation of the first sentence is in the second sentence. In this sense, it can be stated that there is a functional relationship. Since the expressions such as "pro-Moscow separatists," "also called the Atomic Weapon of the Soviets," "allies and partners around the world" in the news text depict different meanings, it has been evaluated as a referential relationship.

Choices of Word

When the news is handled within the framework of word choices, it has been observed that the words are remarkable, engaging, and fear-inducing. For example, the title's words "will invade" are attention-grabbing and fear-inducing. When we look at the different words in the news text, it can be stated that words such as "tension is escalating," "critical developments," "he will bomb Kyiv," and "he will hit on February 16" also have remarkable features. It is seen that there is no objective evidence to support the words used in the news. In this sense, it can be said that the fact that is wanted to be given in the news is tried to be strengthened in the choice of words.

Rhetoric

When the related news is handled within the framework of rhetoric, it is observed that the statements of different state officials and institutions are included to increase the news's credibility. In addition, exact dates support the rhetoric of the news. There were no eye-witness statements about the incident described. In this sense, it can be said that the truth in the news narrative is built.

CONCLUSION

Although the digitalization of the communication process makes it easier for people to access information, it also causes problems in the accuracy of the information in question. With the digitalization of mass media, people have turned into users who both consume and produce information. Along with these developments, a period called the "post-truth" era, in which the truth disappeared. In the post-truth age, people define the information suitable for them among the information they reach without limits, with objective and emotional attitudes, as truth.

The news media plays a vital role in conveying information to people. This situation, which was valid before the digitalization of communication environments, still maintains its validity today. In the post-truth era, news media can construct information in a way that appeals to people's emotions and can serve people through digital media. In other words, the news that is served can be produced in a way that is not true.

In this study, the truth of the information produced in the news media has been examined. The analysis above was carried out on the news media sites ensonhaber.com, hurriyet.com.tr, and sozcu.com.tr about the tension between Russia and Ukraine. In the findings obtained in the news analysis, it was seen that the media organizations reconstructed the truth of the information. It has been seen that news is produced with interesting sentences specific to the post-truth era, which can appeal to people's feelings. With a different narrative, the truth is reproduced with news narratives that will affect people and appeal to their emotions.

The headlines and entries in the news are usually in people's memories. It has been observed that there are differences in meaning in the titles and introductory texts of the news of three different internet news media. In addition, there are information reductions and generalizations in news headlines and news texts. It has been concluded that the truth of the news is tried to be strengthened with many words and images used. People accept information that fits their thoughts and exclude others in the post-truth age. Internet news media also want to prevent people from questioning the truth with their rhetorical instruments. It can be said that the use of sensational sentences and images in the analyzed news is aimed at reducing the questioning of truth.

In the analyzed news texts, Russia; has been seen that it is reflected to people as an occupier, a country with high military power, a defeatist, and a country that disrupts the world system. As for Ukraine; It reflects the reality that it is a powerless country that needs to be protected. In addition, by giving many references to the West in news narratives, the truth of the West's strength is constructed. As a result, these findings; may indicate that disinformation is being made in the news media in the post-truth era.

REFERENCES

AA. (2022). *Russia-Ukraine crisis in 5 questions* [5 soruda Rusya-Ukrayna krizi]. Retrieved from https://www.aa.com.tr/tr/dunya/5-soruda-rusya-ukrayna-krizi/2203164

Alexa. (2022). *Top Sites in Turkey*. Retrieved from https://www.alexa.com/topsites/countries/TR

Balcı, Ş., Bekiroğlu, O., & Karaman, S. Y. (2019). Self-Esteem as a Determinant of Social Media Addiction: A Study in the Case of Konya [Sosyal Medya Bağımlılığının Bir Belirleyicisi Olarak Öz Saygı: Konya Örneğinde Bir Araştırma]. *İletişim Kuram ve Araştırma Dergisi*, (48), 36-64.

Bartlett, J. C. (2020). Information Literacy and Science Misinformation. In K. Dalkir & R. Katz (Eds.), Navigating Fake News, Alternative Facts, and Misinformation in a Post-Truth World (pp. 1-17). IGI Global. doi:10.4018/978-1-7998-2543-2.ch001

BBC. (2022). *Ukraine-Russia crisis: What is the latest situation at the border, how did the tension escalate?* [Ukrayna-Rusya krizi: Sınırda son durum ne, gerilim nasıl tırmandı?]. Retrieved from https://www.bbc.com/turkce/haberler-dunya-60047078

Bekiroğlu, O., Kaya, S. & Yaman, D. (2019). Accumulations and Leaps of Media and Journalism in The Period of Digital Transformation [Dijital Dönüşümün Periyotlarında Medya ve Gazetecilik Alanındaki Birikim ve Sıçramalar]. *Uluslararası Türk Dünyası Basın Sempozyumu*.

Bhaskaran, H., Mishra, H., & Nair, P. (2017). Contextualizing Fake News in Post-truth Era: Journalism Education in India. *Asia Pacific Media Educator*, *27*(1), 41–50. doi:10.1177/1326365X17702277

Carlson, M. (2018). The Information Politics of Journalism in a Post-truth Age. *Journalism Studies*, *19*(13), 1879–1888. doi:10.1080/1461670X.2018.1494513

Delal, Ö., & Abanoz, E. (2021). Information Sharing and Misinformation about Covid-19 on Social Media in the Context of New Media Literacy [Yeni Medya Okuryazarlığı Bağlamında Sosyal Medyada Covid-19 ile İlgili Bilgi Paylaşımı ve Misenformasyon]. In F. Ünal Çolak & O. Yıldırım (Eds.), *Pandemic, Research and Discussions in the Digital World* [Dijital Dünyada Pandemi, Araştırmalar ve Tartışmalar] (pp. 265–296). Literatürk Academia.

Doui, A. (2019). Global and Arab Media in The Post-Truth Era: Globalization, Authoritarianism and Fake News. *IEMed: Mediterranean Yearbook*, *2019*, 124–132.

DW. (2022). *How did Russia and Ukraine come to the brink of war?* [Rusya ile Ukrayna savaşın eşiğine nasıl geldi?]. Retrieved from https://www.dw.com/tr/rusya-ile-ukrayna-sava%C5%9F%C4%B1n-e%C5%9Fi%C4%9Fine-nas%C4%B1l-geldi/60522203.

Ensonhaber. (2022). *Russia-Ukraine Tension Will Reflect on Fuel Prices* [Rusya-Ukrayna Gerilimi Akaryakıt Fiyatlarına Yansıyacak]. Retrieved from https://www.ensonhaber.com/ekonomi/rusya-ukrayna-gerilimi-pompaya-yansiyacak

Evre, B. (2009). Different Approaches to Discourse Analysis: A Classification Attempt [Söylem Analizine Yönelik Farklı Yaklaşımlar: Bir Sınıflandırma Girişimi]. In İ. Parlak (Ed.), Construction of Truth in the Media [Medyada Gerçekliğin İnşası] (pp. 107-152). Konya: Çizgi Kitabevi.

Harjuniemi, T. (2021). Post-Truth, Fake News and The Liberal 'Regime of Truth' – The Double Movement Between Lippmann and Hayek. *European Journal of Communication*, 1–15. doi:10.1177/02673231211046784

Hurriyet. (2022). *The blood pressure is too high... Biden: If we enter Ukraine, there will be a world war* [Tansiyon çok yüksek... Biden: Ukrayna'ya girersek dünya savaşı çıkar]. Retrieved from https://www.hurriyet.com.tr/dunya/tansiyon-cok-yuksek-biden-ukraynaya-girersek-dunya-savasi-cikar-42002279

İnal, U., & Şevik, E. (2019). Survive in Rating Battles. In R. Yılmaz, M. N. Erdem, & F. Resuloglu (Eds.), *Handbook of Research on Transmedia Storytelling and Narrative Strategies* (pp. 190–208). IGI Global. doi:10.4018/978-1-5225-5357-1.ch010

Kreitner, R. (2016). *Post-Truth and Its Consequences: What a 25-Year-Old Essay Tells Us About the Current Moment*. Retrieved from https://www.thenation.com/article/archive/post-truth-and-its-consequences-what-a-25-year-old-essay-tells-us-about-the-current-moment/

Marshall, H., & Drieschova, A. (2018). Post-Truth Politics in the UK's Brexit Referendum. *New Perspectives*, *26*(3), 89–105. doi:10.1177/2336825X1802600305

Oxford Dictionary. (2021). *Post-Truth*. Retrieved from https://www.oxfordlearnersdictionaries.com/definition/english/posttruth?q=post-truth

Özer, Ö. (2011). *News Discourse Ideology* [Haber Söylem İdeoloji]. Literatürk.

Porgham, S. (2020). *Why Is the Truth of the News Worthless in the Era of Post-Truth?* [Post-Truth Çağında Haberin Gerçekliği Neden Değersiz?]. Retrieved from https://gergedan.press/abd-baskanlik-secimleri-yaklasirken-post-truth-caginda-haberin-gercekligi-neden-degersiz-8150/

Resuloğlu, F., & Yılmaz, R. (2017). A Model for Interactive Advertising Narration. In R. Yılmaz (Ed.), *Narrative Advertising Models and Conceptualization in The Digital Age* (pp. 1–20). IGI Global. doi:10.4018/978-1-5225-2373-4.ch001

Rose, J. (2017). Brexit, Trump, and Post-truth Politics. *Public Integrity*, *19*(6), 555–558. doi:10.1080/10999922.2017.1285540

Salgado, S. (2018). Online Media Impact on Politics. Views on Post-truth Politics and Post Postmodernism. *International Journal of Media and Cultural Politics*, *14*(3), 317–331. doi:10.1386/macp.14.3.317_1

Sawyer, M. E. (2018). Post-Truth, Social Media, and The "Teal" as Phantasm. In M. Stenmark, S. Fuller, & U. Zackariasson (Eds.), Relativism and Post-Truth in Contemporary Society (pp. 55-69). Palgrave Macmillan.

Şen, O. (2021). Robot Journalism [Robot Gazetecilik]. In M. Şahin & E. İlhan (Eds.), *Specialization Areas in Journalism* [Gazetecilikte Uzmanlaşma Alanları] (pp. 57–76). Pelikan Yayınları.

Şimşek, M., & Yalı, S. (2019). Did It Real (Really) Happen: Representation of History in Post-Truth Times [Gerçekte(N) Öyle Mi Olmuş: Post Truth Zamanlarda Tarihin Temsili]. İstanbul: Yeni İnsan Yayınevi.

Şimşek, V. (2018). Post-truth and New Media: A Study on Social Media Groups [Post-truth ve Yeni Medya: Sosyal Medya Grupları Üzerinden Bir İnceleme]. *Global Media Journal TR Edition*, *8*(16), 1–14.

Sozcu. (2022). *Russia-Ukraine tension: Putin to invade on Wednesday* [Rusya-Ukrayna gerilimi: Putin, Çarşamba günü işgal edecek]. Retrieved from https://www.sozcu.com.tr/2022/dunya/rusya-ukrayna-gerilimi-putin-carsamba-gunu-isgal-edecek-6947902/

Uluk, M. (2018). *New Media and Fake News in the Post-Truth Era* [Hakikat Sonrası Çağda Yeni Medya ve Yalan Haber]. Dorlion.

Ünal, R., & Taylan, A. (2017). *The Fake News-False Enformatıon Problem in Health Communıcatıon And The Verıfıcatıon Platforms* [Sağlık İletişiminde Yalan Haber-Yanlış Enformasyon Sorunu ve Doğrulama Platformları]. Atatürk İletişim Dergisi.

Van Dijk, T. (2003). Discourse and Ideology: A Multi-domain Approach [Söylem ve İdeoloji: Çok Alanlı Bir Yaklaşım]. In B. Çoban & Z. Özarslan (Eds.), *Mythology, Religion, Ideology* [Mitoloji, Din, İdeoloji] (AteşN., Trans., pp. 13–112). Su Yayınları.

Yılmaz, R., & Taskiran, N. O. (2015). A Model for Mind-Device Dialectic and The Future of Advertising in The Social Media Age. In M. N. Taskiran & R. Yılmaz (Eds.), *Handbook of Research on Effective Advertising Strategies in The Social Media Age* (pp. 1–16). IGI Global. doi:10.4018/978-1-4666-8125-5.ch001

Yüksel, E., & Gürcan, H. İ. (2005). *News Gathering and Writing* [Haber Toplama ve Yazma]. Tablet Kitabevi.

ADDITIONAL READING

Allcott, H., & Gentzkow, M. (2017). Social Media and Fake News in the 2016 Election. *The Journal of Economic Perspectives*, *31*(2), 211–236. doi:10.1257/jep.31.2.211

Damlapınar, Z. (2008). Medya ve Siyasete Güvenilirlik: Medya Siyasetinin Toplumsal Algılanmasına Bağlı Faktörler. In Z. Damlapınar (Ed.), *Medya ve Siyaset* (pp. 187–207). Eğitim Kitabevi Yayınları.

Delal, Ö. (2021). Breaking the Narrative on Global Fault Lines. In R. Yılmaz (Ed.), *Handbook Of Research On Narrative Interactions* (pp. 162–180). IGI Global. doi:10.4018/978-1-7998-4903-2.ch010

Güven, A. (2020). Hakikatin Yitimi Olarak Post-Truth: Bir Kavramsallaştırma Denemesi. *İnsan ve İnsan*, *7*(23), 20-36.

Sarıoğlu, E. B. (2020). Yalan Haber, "Post-Truth" Kavramı ve Medya Üçlemesi: Geçmişten Günümüze Gündem Belirleyen Örnekler. *İnsan ve Toplum Bilimleri Araştırmaları Dergisi*, *9*(1), 377-397.

KEY TERMS AND DEFINITIONS

Information: It is the sum of thought and reality outputs communicated, disseminated, informed, or broadcast.

Journalism: It is the dissemination of news or events, phenomenon, and truths that concern the society to the public.

Media: All of the tools provide information flow and a communication environment to the masses.

News: Summary information about an event, an existing phenomenon, or a situation.

Post-Truth: The loss of the reality of the event or information rather than a reference to the aftermath of an event or information.

Chapter 6
Representation of Violence Against Women in Television News:
The Case of Emriye Metegül

Sereney Cantimur
Ondokuz Mayıs University, Turkey

Nursel Bolat
Ondokuz Mayıs University, Turkey

ABSTRACT

There are many ethical violations in the news of violence against women, which is frequently encountered in television journalism. In these ethical violations in the news of violence against women, statements that especially women are shown as victims, marginalized, objectified, and legitimizing violence are frequently encountered. The use of violence in the news also makes the issue of the reality of the news and how the reality is reflected problematic. Reality in the news is a recreated reality. In this study, the way the media handles the news of violence against women is analyzed according to Teun Van Dijk's critical discourse analysis theory through the news of violence suffered by Emriye Metegül. The aim of the research is to examine the news of violence against women in television news through the violence suffered by Emriye Metegül, to see unethical acts through the news, to examine the news by explaining how the representation of women is presented.

INTRODUCTION

Most people today spend more time listening to the radio and watching television than they do at work. The effectiveness of mass media is increasing day by day, administrations are trying to control the content of these tools. The decrease in the time allocated to reading in the movement of daily life directs people to audio-visual tools that can be obtained more easily and cheaply (Uğurlu, 2007, p. 289). Television has

DOI: 10.4018/978-1-7998-9251-9.ch006

been an attractive instrument since it was invented. Rating has been high even during the time of New Media instruments. According to the results of the 'Study on Television Watching Orientations', the mean daily duration of watching television in Turkey was three hours and 34 minutes in 2018. Results of the afore-noted study also indicated that the durations of watching television are close in Turkey, Germany, France, United Kingdom and India (Sirer, 2020: p. 184). It guides the audience with its news content and presentation formats. Television is important for viewers who want to watch the news, especially since it is audio-visual in the concept of news. The news on television reaches a higher number of viewers as it is transmitted visually and with sound. In television news, the first images that come to mind and welcome us are the images. In addition to the concepts of news and reality, this also highlights the discourse approach in the news.

The role of televisions as appealing to the eye and ear is precisely to integrate the world into the flow of images, rendering it useless and empty. The viewer's mind is completely preoccupied with the fullness of visual images. These intense images do not allow people to rest. The news or speeches presented can be listened to and heard while dealing with different jobs. However, images bind people to themselves (Ellul, 1998, p. 178). Although many images in the news are watched carefully by the audience, they make the audience insensitive after a while. The audience can watch even a news where very bad events take place without reaction. Violence and violence against women, which are among the indispensable topics of news programs, are used extensively as important news topics.

The forms of representation in which women are predominantly trivialized, portrayed as victims, accused, negated and ignored in the media often appear as the subject of violence against women. The view that the media have a central influence on the increase in violence in society has been debated since the beginning of the twentieth century. Theories that deal with the relationship between display of violence and aggressive attitudes on the effects of the media draw attention to the direct or indirect effects on behavior (Boztepe, 2017, p. 40). One of the purposes of the media is to get yourself watched. As a result of this purpose, the media gives quite a place to violence in its content. The prevalence of violence and murders against women in the world has caused violence to become a social issue. The fact that violent events take place in a comprehensive manner, the way they are practiced and the degree of closeness of the perpetrator or people to the victim of violence ensure that these events take place on the agenda of the media" (Nisan and Tuncel, 2020, p. 105). It is known that one of the most emphasized areas in terms of representation among the products in the media is news. The news tends to increase the interest in the news by highlighting the woman in this representation feature.

The phenomenon of violence, especially when evaluated in the context of media content, is a problematic area that has been discussed for a long time (Erdem, 2020, p. 1199). In the research titled "Media, Violence and Women", in which the form of violence against women in the Turkish print media is evaluated, news about violence against women is described as a police-courthouse case in the newspapers, these events are tabloidized, and the news texts and photographs about the event are exaggerated. It has been revealed that the events and photographs do not reflect the truth''(Ulusal, 2007, p.64). The news of violence in the print media in Turkey is generally on the 3rd page. Looking at recent years, it is seen that the news about violence is in the headline. Therefore, this situation reveals the interest shown by the media in the news of violence. At the same time, the reason for the interest shown by the press to news of violence is the interest of the society in these news. This situation leads to an increase in violence in the society. This violence is generally in the form of violence by men against women. "Because in Turkey, where the patriarchal system is dominant, male-dominated power, the violence of men against women has always been the subject of more media coverage" (Ulusal, 2007, p.1). While the media deals with the issues in the society as a reflection of the society, it organizes a content structure in line with the expectations of the society as content. Therefore, violence and violence against women are shaped around the expectations of the audience or the reader (İlerialkan, & Yılmaz, 2015, pp. 15-17).

While the media shapes the phenomenon of violence against women, they generally reflect the image of women as weak and with negative character traits (Baker, 2012, p. 316-317). This causes the media to report violence against women by making it into a tabloid, and the aim is only to earn financial income. The media, which started to act according to the interests of the society, exaggerates the news of violence, exploits emotions, and uses images of violence (Ulusal, 2007, p. 24). In this context, a form of discourse towards women develops in the media and this discourse becomes an important element of the media. The media uses the discourse of violence against women by constructing and disseminating the discourse of violence against women in the media.

Within the scope of this study, the handling of the news of women exposed to violence in the media will be examined through the news of Emriye Metegül. The problem of the research is the representation of violence against women in television news. The aim of the research is to examine the news of violence against women in television news through the violence suffered by Emriye Metegül, to see unethical acts and the trivialization of reality in the news, to examine the news by explaining how the representation of women is presented. This study is important in terms of raising awareness about the representations of women presented in the media. The universe of the research, the sample of violence against women in the television news, consists of the news of the violence suffered by Emriye Metegül on Show TV, Star TV and A Haber, which are television channels in Turkey. The research questions of the study; How is the female identity represented in the news of violence against women? How is news of violence presented? Does the presentation of news on violence differ in channels with different broadcasting policies? An analysis is made within the framework of these research questions.

NEWS CONCEPT

Oya Tokgöz, who entered the news with the definition of "the story or summary of the event or events", actually used concepts such as event, story and summary when describing the event (Tokgöz, 1981, p. 51). The concept of news, which expresses the new, always means that the events brought together from every location are conveyed to the society quickly and accurately (Özmen, 2014, p. 57). Therefore, the need for people to learn about what is happening around them, as well as their need to get information, is important in the development of journalism. This desire and need has given birth to the concepts of news and news.

Although it is very difficult to use precise expressions to describe the news, events that are more rare and interesting than the events or phenomena that are common in life and that everyone can experience at any time are more newsworthy. In addition, facts that are thought to be of interest to the general public are included in the function of journalism (Kars, 2015, pp. 5-6). First definitions of news; 'Everything that happens is news, news that we didn't know yesterday, news is a report of an event, news is whatever time is appropriate'. While the concept of news is accepted as everything that we did not know yesterday, it is known that it should have certain characteristics in terms of being impartial, accurate, up-to-date and important. According to Wilbur Schramm, news occurs in people's minds. In other words, news has an intellectual dimension and a subjective structure. 'news is not an event itself, but the concept that emerges after the event, the reorganization of the event' According to this, news is not an event, but an attempt to re-establish the real framework of an event (Bayraktaroğlu and Uğur, 2011, p.10; Wilbur, 1949, p. 259). There are many definitions about the concept of news. For this reason, it is difficult to make a comprehensive news definition. News, as a communication phenomenon, provides information to people who are curious about what is going on around them. It is necessary to use a clear and understandable language because it speaks to large audiences.

The news covers such a wide area that it cannot be limited to the written press only. This is because television and radio are the most consumed mass media and they are important for news. Visual media is more attractive than print media. In a study, it was understood that news programs are the most consumed content among visual media types. It is thought that the low reading habits in Turkish society also affect this situation. Therefore, journalism on television channels has developed and become an important field of journalism (İnal, 1996, p. 19). News is a social phenomenon and responsibility. The main task of the journalist is to collect and research the news with all the details and transfer it to the society. However, while the prominent commercial concerns in the field of journalism direct journalism, the density in the news of violence causes representation problems in the news of violence against women.

Violent acts can be carried out by supporters individually or collectively. Freud's claim Internalized masochism often causes externalization. Externalized aggression reflects itself in the following ways: acts of violence. Violence can easily be demonstrated in an appropriate setting (Sirer. 2020, 177). In the news, these acts of violence are reported in different languages and discourses.This reveals the language and discourse problematic in the news.

LANGUAGE AND DISCOURSE IN THE NEWS

According to Postman, the language used in the telegraph in the past has also affected the content of the news today. Due to its intended use, the telegraph had a different language than the one used in daily life. This was more of a "title language". In this case, too, the contribution of the telegram to public discourse was to glorify indifference and multiply helplessness (Postman, 2003, pp. 80-82). The discourse used in television news today also follows the discourse of the telegraph. The news has also been effective in the formation of insensitive and indifferent audiences. The word choices used in the news may reflect a certain ideological attitude and choice. However, this can be handled as "representation problem of power/power relations in discourse" rather than the word ideology.

News is studied as a discourse, as a specific example of socially constructed meaning and language in its use. Accordingly, it is not possible to distinguish easily the factors that are in a decisive position in the news content. The news transforms these factors within itself. At the same time, the news is in relation with the institutions and discourses that undertake different functions at the same time in the structure in which they exist. Thus, news cannot be understood in isolation from this existing network of relations (Ergül, 2000, pp. 81-82). Thus, the news is structured in a complex network and they form their discourses accordingly. However, although they reveal a discourse specific to the power and dominant structure, it also reveals a discourse that reflects the society from which it emerged and its expectations. Television is the medium in which language and discourse are most effective and supported by images.

TELEVISION JOURNALISM

Journalism is no longer limited to the printed media, newspapers and magazines. Radio and television, which are mostly visual and auditory, take precedence over the written media. In a study conducted in Ankara in 1993, it is understood that news and news programs are the most consumed contents. It is said that the fact that the audience prefers audio-visual television and radio broadcasts rather than the printed media is related to the economic, cultural and social structure. This preference orientation can be associated with three reasons; 1) Consumption time. 2) The financial aspect of consumption. 3) It is listed as sufficient cultural equipment for consumption (İnal, 1996, p.19-20). Therefore, it is turned into an industrial product and commodity that can be bought and sold specific to the capitalist system. Especially with private broadcasting, the value of news is valued according to the number of viewers, making it an object of consumption culture. The fact that the subjects that attract the attention of the public are presented to the market highlights the transfer of violence, which is an important commodity, to the screens. Violence, which is seen in all program contents, is seen as an important theme in the news.

With the use of images in television news programs, the intellectual dimension of the news has disappeared. The viewer finds himself in the events. As a result of the new technologies that have emerged recently, the audience can be "eyewitnesses" to the writing of history. This has been an extremely exciting development for the news (Parsa, 1993, p. 43). People can instantly watch a war or event live from where they sit. Television has both sound and image elements together. This has brought television to an effective position as a mass communication tool. The evaluation of television among the mass media that does journalism is due to its news bulletins and programs (Bülbül, 2001, p. 50). Television has surpassed other means of communication in terms of reporting. Television programs and especially news that are concerned about ratings bring similar violent news to the screen due to the high ratings obtained with images of violence (Bolat and Çakın, 2018, p. 323). For this reason, although violence is important for all media, it is used more conspicuously in terms of television. The power of the image puts television ahead of other media.

The structural features of television news are examined with five main elements. The first is the approach in which the news is built. According to this approach, news is established by reporters based on certain influences and requirements. Dramatically presented events are embellished by editing and adding music. This situation is aimed at constructing a new structure. The second is the approach that news is a direction. According to this approach, he argues that the news is not an event, but a point of view. Products that aim to understand are created by collecting products that contain culture, ideological and technical factors. The third is the approach that news is projection. According to this approach, news is a tool that shows the world as well as forming an ideology. The fourth approach says that the news is imitation. According to this approach, the events in the news are symbolized on the television screen. The news is reproduced. Therefore, an imitation emerges as a result of analogy. The last approach argues that the news is a show business. In other words, according to this view, the news tries to make the audience watch itself and keep it on the screen. Meeting the expectations and demands of the society will help to achieve the goal by determining the content that they find entertaining. The news gets more dramatic over time. The increase in the use of dramatic and fictional elements is also noteworthy (Özmen, 2014, pp. 57-59). Therefore, the news moves away from its real context and narrative structure and turns into a form of entertainment. This narrative structure has brought news and reality discussions. Is the news real, or is it experiencing a structuring process that shows the reality that reality is reconstructed?

HIDING REALITY IN THE NEWS

In a strange way, television can do it by showing, by showing something other than what needs to be shown in order to do the job of informing the information, or by showing what needs to be shown, in a way that does not show or makes it meaningless. He moves towards things that are slightly less visible, showing how he can conceal events by constructing them in such a way that they acquire a meaning that is in no way compatible with reality (Bourdieu, 1997, p. 23). While doing this, television uses its own hiding and deception skills. While giving the image as real, it gives it by hiding it with fiction.

The real thing is that there is neither complete truth nor truth in the media. Television news seeks drama features in the selection of some interesting stories. While he makes the story of a child's abduction interesting, he's not completely lying. But it does not give the complete truth. If it could reach the truth, we would have to be content with only the news program (Burton, 1995, p.125). However, the television also plays a game here. This play on display also increases the interest in the news and the number of viewers. In doing so, he moves away from reality as much as possible and creates a fictional world.

Today, television news has similar features to serials. In the news, there are dramatic fiction, background music, slow motion images, animations, movie fragments during the presentation of the events. All these techniques allow television news to approach TV series. Complex events and processes are given in a personalized way. This ensures that the distance between them and the entertainment programs decreases (Long, 2002, p.17). The fictional world, which is experienced in all other programs on television and accepted by the audience, continues in the news. Television news is also approaching the format of entertainment programs in this way. The audience is interested in these light and tabloid news in order to relieve the stress of busy life.

Framing refers to a comprehensive holistic formation in essence, in which the visual and auditory materials of the image are used together (Akmeşe, 2020a, p. 218). In television, framing is done for a purpose. Nothing exists by itself in the reality of the events revealed by the frame, that reality is the point that the framer wants us to see (Akmeşe, 2020b, p. 39). With its framing, television creates a different language between the world it is in and the real world. There is a difference between the reality in the studio and the reality outside. A world framed by a square screen is created on television (Pösteki and Kaplan, 2005, p. 99). This square frame can be filled according to the opinions of the person and institution that prepared the news. The aspect of the news that this frame is filled with determines the degree of its authenticity. This draws attention to the news-fact relationship.

The news-truht relationship creates a problematic relationship. What causes this relationship to become problematic is the transformation of the news process into an election process. The selection process, on the other hand, constitutes a biased process. Which truhts will be selected for news reporting, how and in what order the selected facts will be presented, and in which aspects they will be presented are parts of the selection process. Many individuals and institutions, from news sources, reporters, cameramen, editors, editors, advertisers and sponsors to owners of news organizations, are effective in this selection process. As a result, the product that emerges as news ensures that reality is reconstructed through a selection process (Uzun, 2002, p. 11). In a way, the news is the reality or the deception of the people who prepared the news. The news turns into the reality of these people and institutions that interfere with the news. One of the main points that stand out in the context of news reality is in the context of gender. In the news where the gender structure is prominent, the truth is reconstructed or trivialized.

GENDER DISCRIMINATION

Animus and anima represent both biological and psychological aspects of masculinity and femininity, which are thought to exist together in both genders (Akmeşe, 2021, p. 333; Coreyi 2015, p. 78). In the archetypal system, the relationship established with the opposite sex is seen as the factor that ensures compliance with the most basic conditions of life. Anima and animus archetypes, as the combination of masculine and feminine aspects of opposite sexes, have the potential to significantly affect male and female relations (Akmeşe, 2021, p. 333; Stevens, 2014, p. 100). In the social structure, men and women are subject to important distinctions despite all these features. The concept of gender is a very important concept used in studies about women. The concept of gender is divided into two in the literature in the field of social sciences. The first of these is biological sex, and the second is the concept of gender. The concept of biological sex defines two different genders that people carry biologically, male and female. The concept of gender, on the other hand, defines the different behavior patterns and roles of men and women in society. The patriarchal understanding prefers to see the state of being a woman and a man as two different phenomena. Therefore, this understanding tries to separate gender roles from each other with a sharp line (Dündar, 2010, p. 92). Accordingly, "gender culture", which accepts that gender is a social and cultural phenomenon, offers a broad framework for the individual and social relations. Therefore, gender culture is a complex culture that includes the definitions of men and women in a society, their images, behavioral patterns, gender-determining identities, the relationship between the sexes, their attitudes, marriage customs, family types, understanding of beauty, and clothing. it is used to describe a large area (Türköne, 1995, p. 14). With these definitions, the gender culture created by the society and the patterns in which women and men will take place in the society are also shaped.

To men in the social structure; tough, dominant, strong, judgmental, determined, successful, independent, ambitious, determined, active, for a woman; being soft, compliant, powerless, accepting, indecisive, unsuccessful, dependent, helpless, passive. "The system has transformed us into half and limited humans, dividing the qualities that make each of us fully human in the name of designated sexual roles, giving half to women and half to men." All individuals go through the process of socialization in order to be a part of the society in which they live, to be in harmony, to find a place of their own in the society. People gain identity as a result of this process they go through. "The socialization process gives women and men different identities in terms of their sexual roles and imposes different roles. In this process, family, friends, environment, school and mass media play an important role" (Dündar, 2010, p. 92). Therefore, men and women are separated and presented with certain identities. This separation is more evident when it comes to the media.

Representation of Women in the Media

The concept of representation is the basic element of the process of establishment and change of meaning among the members of a culture. For the concept of representation, the authors generally state that it is multidimensional. The concept of representation is used extensively in research focusing on discursive analysis in media texts. The concept, which is used in two senses, is first used in the sense of resembling or resembling something, while in the other sense it is used to replace, hold or take something. Two meanings are encountered in the media. Media creates meanings about the world thanks to the concept of representation. Media representing the world makes the world meaningful for the audience. "The representations established in the media are important. Because they reflect the place of the represented person, institution or object in social life and give legitimacy to this place. They even determine and reproduce our view of the world, society and human beings by being articulated with each other. Among media products, one of the most emphasized areas regarding representation is news" (Boztepe, 2017, p. 41). When we move forward through the representation of women in the media, studies reveal that the concept of powerlessness is reproduced through women, the body of women is objectified and transformed into an area of exploitation, and the media has an important role. It is possible to say that there has been an improvement in the representation of female identity over the years. But despite this, the gender gap and distinction remains the same. Showing women individuals as worthless in the media also affects the perspective of readers and viewers on women in the same direction (Çelenk, 2010, pp. 230 - 232). The structure created in the media for the representation of women takes place in the general narrative of the media. Although the representation of women, especially in news programs, has improved, there has been no significant change.

Representation of Women in the News

The system that produces and reproduces gender in human life will always exist. Although gender is not a fully conscious identity in the media environment, it is constantly being reconstructed through media, work and home environments in relation to the message and meaning structures that are everywhere today. In this process, by using the widespread use of television, it has a voice in the media's gaining an important role because it fills a very important part of human life and entertainment and information environment that reaches wide audiences. The media conveys the image of men and women through gender. This transferred image reflects cultural values and expectations in shaping gender roles (Kaypakoğlu, 2004, p. 93). Therefore, the media generally places how to behave with the principle of what gender stereotypes should be in society. While doing this, he emphasizes traditionalism by building his thesis on whether it is approved by the society or not.

The principle of selection in television journalism is the search for sensational, show-like news. Television can resort to dramatization in both senses; first, it staged the event, visualized it and increased the importance, gravity, dramatic and tragic character of the event. When there is a news about the slums, the event that will attract attention is the uprising that took place here. The word insurrection is an exaggerated word on its own (Bourdieu, 1997, p. 24). The second one tries to attract attention with the choice of words used in journalism. Therefore, the media reconstructs and presents reality. While doing this, the most important program he uses is the news. While the news is being created, reality is seen as a reconstructed reality. In this reality, the dominant meanings are a reality that makes selections from the social reality that emerges in the context of the news production process.

While words are associated with truth, images are associated with reality (Ellul, 1998, p. 46). However, the authenticity of the images should also be discussed, as the media reconstructs reality while constructing images. Violence by the spouse is viewed more moderately, especially in the context of the legitimizing discourses of violence against women in the media, where the woman is visually presented as a mother and wife. With the violence it constantly presents, the media normalizes and accustoms it to violence. While doing this, the woman who is tied to her home and has a family order is presented as the subject of honor, while the violence done to her is approved by making the woman outside as bad.

The expression 'honor killing', which is frequently used in the news where women are exposed to violence, and 'woman returning from night entertainment', and being used in rape or rape cases in the news of assault, or 'young girl with alcohol' are the leading words, and these women almost judge it as their own fault. It is implied that they incite or deserve attacks. The reasons for violence against women are explained in the news, and the reasons for the violence against women are presented in order. Violence perpetrated by male individuals against female individuals is described as a personalized problem in the media, and even the third pages of the news of violence, in which female individuals are portrayed as victims, convey the news stating that the violence perpetrated by male individuals is not related to the patriarchal structure (Nisan & Tuncel, 2020, pp.107-109). The news builds its representations of violence against women through killing. Because violence other than the act of killing is not considered to be newsworthy. At the same time, it is seen that the reaction shown is lower in case of violence against women in Turkey through their husbands. This situation leads to a phenomenon in which the woman who is subjected to violence by her husband remains silent.

METHOD USED IN THE STUDY

Qualitative research method was used in the research. The reason for choosing the qualitative research method is that the interpretation and analysis of the news is not measurable and it is not appropriate to express it numerically. The universe of the research consists of news about violence against women in television news. The sample of the research is the news of violence recently experienced by Emirye Metegül. The sample of the study was determined by the easily accessible case sampling technique, which is one of the purposeful sampling methods. With this sampling method, the research is carried out quickly and practically. Therefore, this sampling method was chosen because the research was fast and practical. Within the scope of the study, the news of Emriye Metegül on Star Tv, Show Tv and A Haber channels broadcasting in Turkey on March 7, 2021 were examined.

A literature review was conducted within the scope of the research. Then, in order to obtain the news to be used in the research, the news of Emriye Metegül on Show Tv, Star Tv and A Haber from the "YouTube" platform was examined. The news to be used in the research were determined according to different publication policies. Accordingly, in the research, the news of violence suffered by Emriye Metegül in Show Tv, Star Tv and A Haber dated March 7, 2021 took place as data. Teun van Dijk's critical discourse analysis method was used in the analysis of Emriye Metegül's news published on Show Tv, Star Tv and A Haber dated March 7, 2021.

Findings and Analysis

Teun Van Dijk's Critical Discourse analysis of the news of violence experienced by Emriye Metegül broadcast on A Haber, Star Tv and Show TV.

Show TV News Review "Violence Against Women" dated 07.03.2021 https://www.youtube.com/watch?v=qR2wdLCyliY

Thematic Analysis Within the Scope of Macro Structure Analysis

1. **Titles:** The title of "Violence Against Women" was used in the news, which lasted 3 minutes and 37 seconds. This title, with the word 'again', indicates that violence against women occurs constantly. Therefore, it presents the impression of a familiar situation.

2. **News Entry and Spotlights:** The drama that took place in a street in Samsun last night disturbed Turkey's sleep. A man kicked his ex-wife in the street. Worst of all, she did it all in front of their five-year-old daughter. Now her mother is in the hospital, her father is in prison, and the little girl is at her relatives' house with memories that cannot be erased from her memory if all the psychologists of the world came together. Here are the gifts given to a woman and her daughter on the eve of March 8, International Women's Day...' News entry has been made. At the beginning of the news, it was emphasized that what happened on the street was a drama and the whole country was sleepy. In addition, in the introduction emphasizing that a man beat his wife, whom he met on the street, very badly on the street and that the worst part of this situation was in front of their five-year-old daughter, the degree of violence was supported by a striking expression, 'to death'. It is not correct to make such an entry in the news for the purpose of attracting attention and being watched. In the expression as the worst side, being with their children was presented and attention was drawn to the age and gender of the child. Later, it was said that his mother was in the hospital and his father was in prison, with memories that could not be erased from his memory if all the psychologists of the world came together for the child. These sentences make the child very victimized and at the same time, presenting the worst thing in violence against women, that this situation is in front of their children, puts the situation of violence in the background.
3. **News Images:** In addition to the sentences used in the news entry, a child with his back turned symbolically is presented with a teddy bear in his hand. Later, the news was presented using video footage in the news. In this video, the images of violence that Emirye Metegül has been exposed to are given half openly. Even the blurry and intermittent video of the violence suffered by Emriye Metegül is not enough to cover up the violence. Even if the news is correct in terms of attracting attention, these video images should not be used in the news in order not to legitimize violence and not to accustom the eyes and ears to this situation. Afterwards, the interview footage of Emriye Metegül in the hospital with a foggy face is included in the news. Although his face is misty, the consequences of the violence he suffered are clear. The statements made by Emirye Metegül's sister and a person who saw the incident were also used in the news as a video. Photos of the perpetrator and Emirye Metegül are located next to the video images. As a result of the violence that Emriye Metegül was subjected to, the people around watched the incident with their mobile phones, the footage of the perpetrator being caught and subjected to violence by the people around him, and finally the footage of the perpetrator being taken to the police station. It would not be correct to present these images, as the presentation of responding to violence with violence will be remembered as a way to prevent violence. At the same time, the fact that when a woman is subjected to violence, the people around her first record it on video, directs the viewers in a negative way about what to do in such a situation.

Situation Section With Schematic Analysis

1. **Presentation of the Main Event:** The news is presented as Emriye Metegül's violence, a helpless woman lying on the ground covered in blood, and a little girl screaming for mother on her head, will always remember her father with these kicks. In the presentation of the news, Emriye Metegül's helplessness was emphasized. Since this emphasis is a presentation that shows the representation of women as helpless, it is a presentation that can affect other women as well. At the same time,

the emphasis on violence in front of the girl's eyes is at a level that can affect children as well. Therefore, it should not be emphasized in the news that the violence suffered by the woman, her helplessness against it and the fact that it happened in front of her children should not be emphasized, it should be considered that the audience, the child and Emriye Metegül, who will watch the news, may be affected by this presentation. The emphasis in the presentation of the news that Emriye Metegül, who was subjected to violence, was lying on the ground in blood is also wrong. Violence makes this situation possible. Therefore, it is portrayed as extraordinary, again in order to draw attention to the news. Violence is violence, regardless of its consequences, large or small. Separating it can lead to caring about the great and considering the despised as normal. There is no correct emphasis.

2. **Results:** As a result of the news, Emriye Metegül, who was subjected to violence, was taken to the hospital for treatment, and the perpetrator was sent to the police station and arrested. In the news, which also includes the statements of the perpetrator, the statements that he committed the violence because he did not show his child and because he was very angry were included. Including these statements is not correct as it legitimizes violence. At the same time, assumptions were made in the direction of the child's feelings and thoughts, and the news of violence against women was made more remarkable through the child. In terms of the possibility of seeing these news for the child individual and Emriye Metegül, this presentation has the right negativities.

Comment Section

1. **News Sources:** The video images of the violence suffered by Emriye Metegül, the expressions of Emriye Metegül and her sister, as well as the expressions of a person who witnessed the event were used as a source in the news. Although the video was broadcast in the form of blurred and cut images, the violence is understood. At the same time, the fact that children's screams are included in the news makes the situation quite dramatic. Even if the source is counted, the fact that the event is violence against women and the child's involvement was not taken into account. These uses are not correct in terms of news ethics.
2. **Comment:** The comments of the citizen who witnessed the event, Emriye Metegül and her sister were used in the news. However, if the news consisted of these testimonies instead of the video images used as a source, the presentation of violence against women could have been a more ethical presentation. Because in order to dramatize the news and draw attention, it is not right to present the woman as a powerless being in a situation where violence is evident and to include the child in this situation as long as possible.

Microstructure

1. **Syntactic Analysis:** In the news, it was presented by describing the violence that Emriye Metegül suffered and by expressing that it was often experienced in front of her child. It is not appropriate for the main theme of the news to actively state that this violence took place in front of his child's eyes. The news is about violence against women. Therefore, in order to make this even more dramatic, it would not be right to put a small child in the foreground. While the news is being told, the

sequence of events is also conveyed as if it is being followed and narrated one by one. However, it is not correct to convey this situation to the audience with all its information. The information conveyed to the reader along with the news must be at a level that will not affect the life of Emirye Metegül. Therefore, information such as what happened before the violence, the moments of being exposed to violence, how he received the blow of violence, in which region he received the violence, and assumptions made on his child should not be used.

2. **Regional Harmony:** When the sections in the news are examined, it is seen that Emriye Metegül was exposed to violence in the middle of the street, the citizens in the vicinity videotaped this situation, the violence of the perpetrator by the people around, the images of Emriye Metegül in the hospital and the images of the perpetrator while being taken to the police station. It is often stated in the news that the violence against Emirye Metegül took place in front of her child. It would have been more appropriate for the regions in the news to consist of interviews with Emriye Metegül taken after the treatment and interviews of those around her, instead of being the moment of violence. If such a formation had occurred, the effect of the news on Emirye Metegül and her child might have decreased.

Word Choices

In the news, the city where Emriye Metegül was subjected to violence, the time period, the way she was subjected to violence, the consequences, her desperation and especially her child's experience of the incident in front of her eyes are included in the news text. In terms of word choice, it is not correct to use words in the news that will emphasize the situation that the woman is a victim of, that is, the process she goes through due to violence. The purpose of the news should not be to further victimize women. The duty of informing the public, which is the main purpose of the news, should be ensured by paying attention to the words used. It is not correct to specifically state that the woman was covered in blood. Such a situation is possible after violence. For this reason, it is wrong to give it as an extraordinary situation as a result of violence in terms of preventing violence. At the same time, statements such as "he learned the violence, cruelty, ruthlessness and helplessness that took place before his eyes so early that maybe he was no longer a child", which are frequently made about children, increase the victimization of women and children even more. The news should convey the event as it is, assumptions and such dramatic use of words to attract attention are not correct in terms of news ethics.

The Rhetoric of the News

In the news, the violence experienced was presented using video visuals in order to be credible. These images used to support the news are not ethically correct. It would be more accurate to use other elements to support the news instead of these images.

Dated 07.03.2021 'Turkey Stands' Star TV News Review "Violence Against Women In Samsun Aroused Indignation" https://www.youtube.com/watch?v=aXq_O7P2s3k

Thematic Analysis Within the Scope of Macro Structure Analysis

1. **Titles:** In the news consisting of 4 minutes and 47 seconds, "Turkey Stands! The title "Violence Against Women Aroused Indignation in Samsun" was used. The title used in the news is used to

summarize the event in a short and ethical way and to draw attention away. Such a title is not appropriate as it will make it harder for the woman who has been subjected to violence to recover from the effects of the event she has experienced.

2. **News Entry and Spotlights:** The news was introduced as "Tomorrow is March 8th, International Women's Day. While various social responsibility projects are being carried out to draw attention to the problems of women, on the other hand, violence and murder have not been missing." In the news entry, it is not correct to compare the social responsibility projects for women with the violence perpetrated against women. This emphasis may cause social responsibility projects for women to lose their importance and spread the thought that they are not effective. Therefore, these two information presented together in comparison is not an accurate presentation. At the same time, the incident of violence did not result in murder. However, in order to draw attention, the word murder was added next to violence. Such information is not correct. This entry by the relatives of the victimized woman may create a misunderstanding.
3. **News Image:** Video images were used in the news. These video images include video images of the moment Emriye Metegül was exposed to violence, the moment the perpetrator was taken to the police station, the interview footage of a person who witnessed the incident, the reporter's presentation in the area where the incident took place and in front of the hospital where Emriye Metegül was taken, the interview of Emriye Metegül in the hospital, The doctor's interview consists of the interview of Emirye Metegül's sister and father. Although the moment of violence is given in a hazy way, violence is understood. It is not right for him personally to use the images where the woman is exposed to violence. These video images are images that emphasize violence.

Situation Section With Schematic Analysis

1. **Presentation of the Main Event:** The incident of violence experienced in the news was presented as "He battered his ex-wife for minutes near her child, ignored her little daughter's cries and cries, kicked the unconscious woman's head, punched her face". The expression used in the presentation of the news that the violence took place next to Emirye Metegül's child is an expression used in the news to draw attention. This emphasis may have negative effects on Emirye Metegül's child due to the incident. At the same time, the use of expressions describing violence is also used to draw attention, and it is not correct. Violence is any form of violence. Trying to make this even more important by describing it does not comply with news ethics and women's rights.
2. **Results:** The result of the news is presented with statements stating that the perpetrator was arrested, that the child who suffered the violence was with his grandparents and that he would receive psychological support. In this section, mentioning the situation of the child who has witnessed violence and the information that he will receive psychological support again emphasizes the child. It is not correct to emphasize the news by using this information about the child. The possibility that Emirye Metegül, who experienced the incident, her child, and the viewers and young children who are the audience will also be affected by this situation should be taken into consideration.

Comment Section

1. **News Sources:** Video images, the statements of two people who witnessed the event, and the statements of Emriye Metegül, her doctor, her sister, her father and the person who perpetrated the violence were used as sources in the news. The name of the person who prepared the news is also given in the news. Although the images of violence used as a source in the news are cut and mosaiced, it is not true because it clearly shows violence. These uses can victimize the woman and her child, it would be more correct to use other images.
2. **Comment:** The news included the words of Emriye Metegül, her sister, father, doctor and the person who perpetrated the violence, as well as the two witnesses to the incident. "Do you regret it?" It is not correct to pose the question to the perpetrator and present the answer given in the article. Such a presentation can create a perception of mitigation in the face of remorse for violence.

Microstructure

1. **Syntactic Analysis:** Active sentence structures and indirect sentence structures are used in the news. With the active sentence structures used in the news, the feeling that the person making the news has collected one-to-one data from the crime scene is given, while the indirect sentence structures include the words of the doctor or the perpetrator. It is not correct to enter the privacy of the woman and her child in the sentences told with this style of expression. It is openly presented to the audience that they are victims in their private lives. At the same time, the use of statements in which the perpetrator explains the reasons for committing violence may also be one of the elements that will legitimize violence. It is not correct to tell the news with such clear sentence structures.
2. **Regional Harmony:** News Emriye Metegül is battered, hospitalized, the perpetrator is subjected to violence by the people around her, and she is taken to the police station. It can be said that there is regional harmony in the news. However, it is not correct to give the images of Emriye Metegül battered, even if they are cut and mosaicized, and the violence is clearly understood. At the same time, even if the child's face is not visible, it is inevitable that the event will attract more attention because there is a child in the middle. It is unethical to draw attention to the news through a child. The fact that the victimization of Emriye Metegül and her child further increased was not taken into account. Instead, the information provided by the reporter in the area where the incident took place and the information given by the doctor at the hospital could have been sufficient.

Word Choices

The news emphasized the injured areas on Emriye Metegül's body, the severity of the coup, and the fact that this event took place in front of her children. Word choices are formed to describe violence. This situation puts the woman in an even more difficult situation. There should be no need for such a description in news about violence against women. In addition, the choice of words stating that the incident happened in front of their children and that even the screams of the child did not stop this violence are not correct and ethical. It is normal for a child who has witnessed such a situation to react like this. Emphasizing this and saying that this situation is ineffective are words that dramatize the news and are used to draw attention. The possibility of affecting the mother and child in their life processes should be considered.

The Rhetoric of the News

In order to support the violence experienced in the news, video images of the moment of violence were used and interviews were included. It is not correct to give the incident of violence even if it is cut and steamy. This steamed and cut video is a video visual that clearly explains violence. This situation enters the privacy of the woman and her child and further victimizes the woman and the child in the face of the incident. Another image could have been used to support the story. At the same time, the interviews used should have been given in a more superficial way without entering the private area of the woman.

"A Haber" Review "He Kicked His Ex-Wife Many Times in Front of His Child" Dated 07.03.2021 https://www.youtube.com/watch?v=_GcZ0ggens8

Thematic Analysis Within the Scope of Macro Structure Analysis

1. **Titles:** In the news consisting of 3 minutes and 11 seconds, "He Kicked His Ex-Wife Repeatedly in Front of His Child! The title ' is used. The title used in the news is a title established to draw more attention to violence through children. At the same time, the discourse that he was kicked many times is a discourse that depicts violence, but it was also established to attract attention. The title used in the article is not appropriate within the scope of the news about violence against women. The woman was evaluated under the name of ex-wife. In this evaluation, it provides a transfer as if the ex-wife of the perpetrator of violence is somewhat more normal, which puts the woman in the background.
2. **News Entry and Spots:** The article was entered as "A person beat and punched his ex-wife for minutes in front of the little girl's eyes, and when he fell to the ground, he hit his head on the concrete and kicked it". This introduction to the news includes expressions describing violence. This entry, which was made to further emphasize the violence, is not suitable for women's privacy. At the same time, the woman was again under the concept of ex-wife and marginalized. Including the child in the violence is unethical as it is done to draw attention to the news. It may cause the woman and her child who have been subjected to violence to become more traumatized by the event in their later lives.
3. **News Image:** Video images and images of the people involved in the event were used visually in the news. The video image, which contains the moment of violence in the news, reveals the violence, even though it was steamed and cut. At the same time, despite the steaming in the image of Emriye Metegül with her daughter, the child's face is understandable. These uses may have a negative impact on both Emirye Metegül's family and news audiences. Therefore, in the selection of these images and video images in the news, it would be appropriate to use them in a way that would not victimize Emirye Metegül and her child.

Situation Section With Schematic Analysis

1. **Presentation of the Main Event:** The news was made in the form of a presentation stating that the woman who was subjected to violence was beaten in front of her daughter, that the woman

fainted in the face of the violence she suffered, but that she continued to be subjected to violence, the ministers' statements on the subject, and the sister of Emriye Metegül, who was subjected to violence, was shocked. In the presentation of the news, the detailed presentation of the violence suffered by Emriye Metegül increases her victimization against violence. These moments of victimization can further victimize the female individual. Such a presentation is unethical. The person who perpetrated violence against Emirye Metegül was his ex-wife. However, the word 'wife' is mentioned in the news presentation. Since this information is not correct, it misinforms the audience. At the same time, a remarkable statement stating that Emriye Metegül was shocked before her sister's statements is again unnecessary. It is normal to be shocked by such an event. In this context, the presentation of the news could have been made in a shorter and clearer way, for informational purposes only, and not to attract attention.

2. **Results:** As a result of the news, the statements of Emriye Metegül's sister and those who saw the incident were included. In her sister's statements, there is information that Emriye Metegül has filed a complaint before, that her husband has been removed from Metegül, that the suspension period has passed, and that there is a child who witnessed the incident. The explanations of those who saw the incident are that Emriye Metegül is in good health and that they will be involved in the event that the perpetrator of the violence is punished. Although the child's situation is curious, it would be more ethical not to give enough information. Too many details can harm the child. At the same time, it would have been more accurate to have an interview with Emriye Metegül after the event and to give a voice recording for a first-hand explanation. Although it is relevant to state that Metegül's husband was complained about before and that a decision was taken to suspend her from the court, it could not have been given because it was an information that especially frightened women.

Comment Section

1. **News Sources:** The news included the statements of Emirye Metegül's sister as a source. At the same time, video images of the moment of violence were used to support the news. Even if the video images used to support the news are steamed and cut, they are not enough to cover the violence. It is not correct to use this video image in the news. Emriye Metegül is a video image that can have a negative impact on her family and the audience. It would be more appropriate to use a different image in the news, which would not make the woman and her family suffer more, and would not reveal the private life in this way. At the same time, only the statements of Emirye Metegül's sister are not sufficient as a source.
2. **Comment:** The news included the statements of Emriye Metegül's sister. However, the comments of the citizens who witnessed the event in the surrounding area were not included. The comments of the citizens in the surrounding area or the health workers who intervened in the hospital regarding the incident could have been included by paying attention to the ethical rules, without leaving Emriye Metegül and her child in a disadvantaged position.

Microstructure

1. **Syntactic Analysis:** Active sentence structures and indirect sentence structures are used in the news. With the active sentence structure used in the news, the impression was created that information was collected from the crime scene. However, with this active sentence structure used, it is not correct to describe what kind of violence the woman who has been subjected to violence experiences moment by moment. Recounting the violence experienced by women in this way conveys the traumaticity of the event to all viewers. Therefore, there may be a traumatic effect on the audience as well. At the same time, when this information is found for Emriye Metegül and her child who witnessed the event, there will be a high probability of experiencing the same trauma again. Therefore, the news should not be presented to the audience with all the information in the news, taking these into consideration.
2. **Regional Harmony:** When the sections of the news are analyzed, the moments when Emriye Metegül was exposed to violence, the statements of the witnesses and the statements of Emriye Metegül's sister are given. Regarding the regional coherence of the news, instead of giving the beginning of the news about the moments when Emriye Metegül was exposed to violence, it would have been more accurate to receive treatment in the hospital after her recovery or to have an interview and a voice recording. This situation would have been appropriate in order not to reinforce the victimization and to prevent the woman from entering the privacy area. In the news, as in other news, the form of violence was described and it was pointed out that the child was in front of his eyes. It is not correct to specifically state these situations. It is unethical to describe violence in order to attract attention when there is violence. At the same time, drawing attention to the fact that there is a child makes the event even more dramatic. This information could be given superficially.

Word choices

Words are often used in the news to explain that Emriye Metegül was subjected to intense violence in front of her daughter, and that Emriye Metegül, who was described as unfortunate, lost consciousness after being beaten by her ex-husband. In the words used in the news, it is not correct to emphasize the form and extent of the violence that Emriye Metegül has suffered. At the same time, the word choices that indicate that it happened in front of their children dramatize the event and are used to attract more attention. As in other news, the words that show the woman as mother and wife, and the expressions explaining why the violence occurs again normalize the violence and give the image that it is natural to experience it against a reason.

The Rhetoric of the News

Video images and statements of Emirye Metegül's sister and witnesses were included in the news in order to support the violence. The presentation of these video images used in the news to support the event is not correct. Other images that would not reinforce this grievance should have been used in the news.

CONCLUSION

As seen in the literature review of the study, news and television journalism have some ethical rules and social responsibilities. However, although these rules are sometimes applied, it is seen that some rules are ignored in order to be remarkable, sometimes out of the responsibility of informing the public under the name of news watching anxiety. The main purpose of the news should be to convey and inform the public about important events that concern the society without entering the private sphere of the people. In the process of transferring the news, the media presents the events in their own way.

The representations established in the media are generally important. The main reason for this lies in the efforts to reflect the represented person's place in the life process, as well as to establish legitimacy for this place. In addition, media are added to each other and shape people's perspectives on the world. News is one of the most representative programs in the media. The representation of women in the media is generally reproduced through the concept of the powerlessness of blood, and at the same time, the body that belongs to the woman is objectified and drawn into the field of exploitation. Researches reveal that the media has an important role in the transmission and placement of this situation. The reasons for violence against women are explained in the news, and the reasons for violence against women are presented in order. Violence by male individuals against female individuals is described as a personalized problem in the media, and images of violence are presented by entering the private area of women in order to draw attention to the news, even if the images are misted. Therefore, women are represented as weak, helpless, exposed to violence, ex-wife, mother. As can be seen in the reviewed Emriye Metegül news, the use of images and words that will victimize women is quite common in the news. While the woman is already a victim of the violence she has experienced, making her even more victimized is presented in a way that will negatively affect the woman's family, the audience and herself.

It is seen that there are similar posts in Show Tv, Star Tv and A Haber, three news channels in Turkey that were taken as a sample for the study. The results of the evaluation of the news on the television channel with three different broadcasting policies show that the choice of words, emphasis and news visuals includes uses that push women into the background, make them seem weak and helpless, marginalize and legitimize violence. News are presented on similar grounds to draw attention to the news.

Considering the increase in violence against women, it should be one of the issues that require sensitivity. Considering the uses that do not comply with journalistic ethics, it may be healthy to have journalists interested in women's rights advocacy in the teams of media workers, to increase the number of female employees in these teams, and to engage in the profession of journalism for these groups. In general, the presentation of news on violence against women requires more attention.

REFERENCES

Akmeşe, E. (2021). An Archetypal Analysis on the Transformation of the Individual in Play with Fire [Ateşle Oyun Filminde Bireyin Dönüşümü Üzerine Arketipsel Bir Analiz]. *İNİF E-Dergi, 6*(2), 325-339.

Akmeşe, Z. (2020a). The Effect of Framing in Television on Content and Meaning Production. In *Television 4.0 Society 5.0 New Curriculum New Audience*. Literatürk Publication.

Akmeşe, Z. (2020b). Framing in Television Main Newsletters: Türk Telekom Advertising Film Example [Televizyon Ana Haber Bültenlerinde Çerçeveleme: Türk Telekom Reklam Filmi Örneği]. *Middle Black Sea Journal of Communication Studies*, *5*(1), 37–49.

Baker, Ç. (2012). *Culturel Studies, Theory and Practice*. Sage.

Bayraktaroğlu, A. M. & Uğur, U. (2011). The Case of Magazineization in Television Journalism [Televizyon Haberciliğinde Magazinleşme Olgusu]. *Süleyman Demirel Üniversitesi Güzel Sanatlar Fakültesi Hakemli Dergisi*, *4*(7), 1–47.

Bolat, N., & Çakın, Ö. (2018). Violence as a Marketing Motif in Television Series: You Tell Black Sea Series Example. In *Virtual Realm/Media Violence and Social Conflict Traumas*. Hegem Publication.

Bourdieu, P. (1997). *On Television [Televizyon Üzerine]* (T. Ilgaz, Trans.). Yapı Kredi Publication.

Boztepe, V. (2017). Representation of Violence Against Women in Television News: An Analysis on the Murder of Özgecan Aslan [Televizyon Haberlerinde Kadınlara Yönelik Şiddetin Temsili: Özgecan Aslan Cinayeti Üzerinden Bir İnceleme]. *İstanbul Üniversitesi İletişim Fakültesi Dergisi*, *1*, 39-66.

Bülbül, A. R. (2001). *Anatomy of the News and Basic Approaches [Haberin Anatomisi ve Temel Yaklaşımlar]*. Nobel Publication.

Burton, G. (1995). *More Than Looks [Görünenden Fazlası]* (N. Dinç, Trans.). Alan Publication.

Çelenk, S. (2010). Representation of Women in the Media and Ethical Issues [Kadınların Medyada Temsili ve Etik Sorunlar]. *Academia (Caracas)*, 229–236.

Corey, G. (2015). *Theory and practice of counseling and psychotherapy* (10th ed.). Cengage.

Dündar, S. (2010). Representation of Women in Television News [Televizyon Haberlerinde Kadının Temsili]. *Erciyes İletişim Dergisi*, *1*(4), 91–105.

Ellul, J. (1998). *The Fall of the Word [Sözün Düşüşü]* (H. Arslan, Trans.). Paradigma Publication.

Erdem, M. N. (2020). An Argumentative Study on the Presentation of Violence in Media Content [Medya İçeriğinde Şiddetin Sunumu Üzerine Argümantatif Bir Çalışma]. *MANAS Sosyal Araştırmalar Dergisi*, *9*(2), 1198–1217. doi:10.33206/mjss.526941

Ergül, H. (2000). *Magazineization of News on Television [Televizyonda Haberin Magazinleşmesi]*. İletişim Publication.

He Kicked His Ex-Wife Many Times In Front Of His Child! (2021). https://www.youtube.com/watch?v=_GcZ0ggens8

İlerialkan, D., & Yılmaz, R. (2015). Script: How to Write? How Do They Write? [Senaryo: Nasıl Yazılır? Nasıl Yazıyorlar?]. *Alfa*.

İnal, M. A. (1996). *Reading the News [Haberi Okumak]*. Temuçin Publication.

Kars, N. (2015). *History, Theories, Discourse and Radio-Television Journalism of the News, [Haberin Tarihi, Kuramları, Söylemi ve Radyo-Televizyon Haberciliği]*. Derin Publication.

Nisan, F., & Tuncel, I. (2020). Presentation of Violence Against Women in the News: Emine Cloud Example [Kadına Yönelik Şiddet Olgusunun Haberlerde Sunumu: Emine Bulut Örneği]. *International Journal of Cultural and Social Studies*, *6*(1), 104–123.

Özmen, S. (2014). *Radio and Television Readings [Radyo ve Televizyon Okumaları]*. Derin Publication.

Parsa, S. (1993). *Television Journalism and Theories [Televizyon Haberciliği ve Kuramları]*. Ege Üniversitesi İletişim Fakültesi Publication.

Pösteki, N., & Kaplan, N. (2005). Illusional Lives. In Media Reviews. Beta Publication.

Postman, N. (2003). *Amusing Ourselves to Death Public Discourse in The Age Of Show Business [Televizyon Öldüren Eğlence]* (O. Akınhay, Trans.). Ayrıntı Publication.

Sirer, E. (2020). Violence Aestheticized in Sports Publications and Broadcasts. In *Handbook of Research on Aestheticization of Violence, Horror, and Power*. IGI Global.

Stevens, A. (2014). *Jung* (N. Örge, Trans.). Dost Publication.

Tokgöz, O. (1981). *Basic Journalism [Temel Gazetecilik]*. Anakara Üniversitesi Siyasal Bilgiler Fakültesi Publication.

Turkey Stands! Violence Against Women Aroused Indignation in Samsun. (2021). https://www.youtube.com/watch?v=aXq_O7P2s3k

Türköne, M. (1995). *Gender Culture of the Old Turkish Society [Eski Türk Toplumunun Cinsiyet Kültürü]*. Ark Publication.

Uğurlu, S. (2007). *"Interaction of Social Fabric with TV Programs", on Media Studies ["Sosyal Dokunun TV Programlarıyla Karşılıklı Etkileşimi", Medya üzerine Çalışmalar]*. Beta Publication.

Ulusal, D. (2007). Women in Violence and Violent News Presentation in the Written Media positioning [Yazılı Basında Şiddet Ve Şiddet İçerikli Haber Sunumunda Kadının Konumlandırılışı] [Master Thesis]. *Erciyes Üniversitesi, Sosyal Bilimler Enstitüsü, Gazetecilik Anabilim Dalı.*

Uzun, R. (2002). Entertainment Industry and Television Journalism [Eğlence Endüstrisi ve Televizyon Haberciliği]. *Kocaeli*, *1*/*2*, 9–27.

Violence Against Women! (2021). https://www.youtube.com/watch?v=qR2wdLCyliY

Wilbur, S. (1949, Sept.). The Nature of News. *Journalizm Quarterly*, 259 – 269.

ADDITIONAL READING

Arendt, H. (2016). *Şiddet Üzerine* (B. Peker, Trans.). İletişim Publication.

Köknel, Ö. (2013). *Şiddet Dili*. Remzi Publication.

Şenbalkan, Ş. (2013). *Kadına Şiddet.! Madalyonun Öbür Yüzü*. IQ Kültür Sanat Publication.

KEY TERMS AND DEFINITIONS

News: It is the news that presents current and interesting events, obtained from every moment and everywhere, to the public in an accurate and fast manner, in an objective manner. The news must be impartial in accordance with its own ethical rules. The purpose of the news is to convey the information obtained to the public.

Representation of Women: The representation of women presents women in limited patterns in the patriarchal society, especially in the media. Women are represented in the media as a mother, wife, responsible, homemaker, sexual object or powerless.

Television News: After it has been decided that the information received is newsworthy, conveying this news to the society via television with sound and images creates the concept of television news.

Violence Against Women: All kinds of violence (physical, psychological, sexual) that women suffer due to their gender, all acts that cause them pain, threats, bullying and restriction of their freedom, such as all these types of violence, are all within the concept of violence against women.

Section 2

View of the Entertainment and Marketing Worlds

Chapter 7
Truth in Football From the "Hand of God" to VAR

Esennur Sirer
https://orcid.org/0000-0003-0345-4158
University of Usküdar, Turkey

ABSTRACT

Today, dozens of cameras are placed at various points on the football field, making sure that no detail is overlooked. The positions are reviewed using the video assistant system (VAR). However, despite the existence of live broadcast cameras and their technology-integrated structure, there is a position to be discussed after the match; the truth is reinterpreted. As Umberto Eco emphasizes, live-action, where television time and real-time are closest to each other, is not a mere repetition of an event, but an interpretation. In the chapter, the poetics of truth in football is discussed in the historical and technological process.

INTRODUCTION

On June 22, 1986, Argentina and England had faced each other in the World Cup quarterfinals at Mexico's Aztec Stadium, and Argentina had reached the semi-finals with a 2-1 victory. During the match, both goals of Argentina had been scored by the famous football player Diego Armando Maradona. After this match, Maradona's first goal in the 51st minute was discussed rather than the second goal that had brought the victory. It was thought that Maradona had scored the goal by hand, but within the framework of the technical possibilities at that time and from the point of view of the camera, a definite decision could not be reached. Regarding that position in the match, Maradona had commented as the "Hand of God" making a religious and political reference by citing the depiction of God extending his arm to Adam to wake him up from a deep sleep without even touching him in Michelangelo's famous "Creation of Adam" (Aydın, Aslıtürk, 2017, p. 724) (Habertürk, 25.11.2020).

Mankind has made rapid progress in the field of technology in the past quarter century. Technological developments triggered each other, and technological transformation took place in many areas. Technological tools are now considered as an extension of our body and indispensable for life. The

DOI: 10.4018/978-1-7998-9251-9.ch007

camera, which is accepted as an extension of our eye, is one of these tools. With the advancement and cheapening of technology, the camera has become something that can be afforded by everyone. Cameras integrated into mobile phones began to serve for personal use, and from this point on, personal realities were produced from the camera's point of view.

In this period when content is produced individually over the internet and social media is on the spot, the productions that are watched most on the television screen are match broadcasts. Football is suitable for television broadcasting due to its inherent nature. The ball and players are followed by cameras placed at different points on a football field, and the enthusiasm of the match is presented to the audience in the format of a television program without interruption. In line with technological developments, it is possible to put any number of cameras on the football field. The live broadcasts of the match, which are decorated with details, turn into a visual feast thanks to technology. Innovative cameras and Video Assistant Referee (VAR) applications, previously tried in large football organizations, are used to make the football game even more attractive. While it is paid attention to not overlook any details thanks to the dozens of cameras placed at various points on the football field, positions are reviewed with the Video Assistant System (VAR). However, despite the existence of live broadcast cameras and their technology-integrated structure, there are positions to be discussed about the matches played in the sports programs on television, and the reality is reinterpreted.

As pointed out by Mathias Roux points, increasing the number of cameras and resorting to the arbitration of the camera is a technological trick, and this is based on a philosophically incorrect assessment. This is because a perfect image combining all points of view is logically impossible (2013, p. 36-37). In this context, the presentation of a selection made by dozens of cameras placed at different points in football matches leaves a question mark about the images that are not displayed on the screen. This situation leads to the creation of productions on which possible scenarios are written in another time period, such as commentary programs made after the match. Therefore, the camera reproduces itself by reproducing its own reality through the television screen.

FOOTBALL: A SIMPLE GAME

When checked chronologically, the indicators show that football was started to be played in China between 5000-2500 BC and in Egypt on similar dates. It is important that football, which has been adopted and identified with life since these dates, is still a popular game regardless of when and under what conditions it emerged. "Competition, war, struggle, race, creating and keeping group or class difference, preparation for war, being successful in other activities through skill development through football activity, reproducing class difference and relations, reproducing on clergy/theological power's self and their power, the realization of the "circus and bread", the "divide, set against and rule" policies under the name of entertainment and football, and gaining commercial interests" can be listed as the requirements for the emergence of an activity like football (Erdoğan, 2008, p. 9-11). Although football, which has been loved for thousands of years, is described as a simple game, it is observed that it plays an intermediary role for many situations.

Football took its closest form to its current form in England in the 17th century (Serim, 2014, p.189), and with the industrial revolution in the 19th century, it turned into an entertainment activity and became the focus of attention. "The fact that sports are dragging large masses after them is closely related to the economic, social and political consequences of the industrial revolution" (Talimciler, 2009, p. 50).

Starting from the second half of the 19th century, the rules of the football game were written, and it turned into an industrial game played in stadiums. "On October 26, 1863, representatives of 11 teams came together at the Freemans Tavern in London and prepared the first statute of football history containing 13 rules". Thus, the foundations of modern football were laid in the middle of the 19th century. On March 31, 1866, it was decided to play the match as 90 minutes. The decision stipulated that football teams would be on the field with 11 players, 1 of whom was a goalkeeper, was added to the rule booklet on 14 June 1897 at the end of the 19th century (Dilmen, 2015, p. 15).

At the end of the 19th century, the rules of the football game, which was organized in a way close to its current form, were finalized. This game, which can be learnt and followed easily by everyone, is an event that is open to the interest and viewing of many people despite the mathematical definition and limitations of the players. In this respect, football is a sport of contemplation" (Ankaralıgil & Kartal, 2013, p. 134). Efforts to organize football as a show started at the beginning of the 20th century, and many countries participated in these efforts. 207 countries are members of the International Association of Football Associations (FIFA), which was founded in Paris in 1904 and is now headquartered in Zurich, Switzerland. The aim of FIFA is to ensure that the game of football, the rules of which were arranged in England, to be sustained within the same discipline. For this reason, all matches are registered by FIFA and it is referred as the worldwide authorized institution of football. In order for football to reach the masses, organizations such as the 'World Cup' are organized with the participation of countries from various parts of the world. Another organization where the greatness of football as an industry is showcased, is the 'European Football Championship'. The 'European Football Championship', which has been held every four years since 1960, is organized by UEFA. Founded in 1954 and having 52 members, the "Union of European Football Associations" (Union of European Football Associations) UEFA is the organization that governs football in Europe. Established on 15 June 1954, the number of members of UEFA, which was 25 at the beginning, has increased to 55 today. In addition to all the states in Europe; Russia, Israel, Kazakhstan, Armenia, Georgia and Azerbaijan are also members of UEFA. (TFF İş Ortakları, 2022).

The rapid development of professional sports with spectators such as football in the 20th century predates broadcasting. Television was developed to spread and satiate this cultural habit, but it became very effective in a short time (Williams, 2003, p. 55). Television has an important role in the broadcasting of big football organizations to large audiences and their continuation by winning their love. Live broadcasting of football matches on television started for the first time in England, where the rules of football were written and recorded, and league-style matches were played according to these rules. The BBC (British Broadcasting Corporation), which started broadcasting television since the end of 1936, was in pursuit of broadcasting that attracted the attention of the masses. During this period, football was the organization that attracted the most attention. The first attempt at televising football matches was made in 1937, when the recorded broadcasting of the match between Arsenal and Everton. When this broadcast was appreciated by the audience, the cup match played between England and Scotland on April 9, 1938 was broadcasted live. Although England had secured the championship before this match, which Scotland won 1-0, it attracted a great deal of attention from the audience on the broadcast television (Karakuş, 2017).

It evaluated all kinds of options to attract viewers in connection with television's rating and advertising concerns (Bolat & Çakın, 2018, p.319). It has been understood that football is a suitable tool for the narrative structure of television since the first match broadcast, which won the admiration of the television audience, and from this date on, the match broadcasts on the television continued increasingly. Football played a leading role in this bilateral relationship that feeds on each other. The attractiveness of football was used to increase the number of viewers of television broadcasts. This interesting game has also led to an increase in the number of television buyers over time. In 1994, television viewers watched an average of six World Cup matches, and the number of television receivers in the world increased considerably thanks to football and television began to enter every home. In the same year, an American journalist asked "Which is more important: Brazil's victory or the US occupation?" to a citizen in Haiti, who was struggling with major problems in terms of food and shelter and he replied to the question as follows:" 'We are hungry every day. We have a lot of problems. The Americans say every day that they will invade our country. But the world cup is only held once in every four years' (Kuper, 2003, p. 391-392).

The contents of football matches in television broadcasting operating on the triple trivet have always been interesting, leading to the increase in the hardware of television technology and the development in terms of infrastructure. With the development of technology, television broadcasts that used to be transmitted from terrestrial broadcasts only, reached every corner of the world thanks to satellite broadcasts. Today, football match broadcasts can be watched on various platforms such as satellite broadcasting, terrestrial digital and internet. The roles between the television football duo have changed, and as a result of the ease of access to football broadcasts from all channels, television has begun to undertake the carrier of football.

NARRATOR OF FOOTBALL MATCHES BROADCASTED ON TELEVISION

People love stories and they get attached to them. In this context, it is possible to say that the post-truth phenomenon is fully compatible with human nature. This is because people always prefer power to truth and they aspire to rule the world rather than trying to understand it (Altun, 2022, p. 260). While mass media dominate the world on the one hand thanks to its technological structures and access power, it also directs the masses under the influence of the story. Using the power of the image, television has maintained its place for nearly a century and is accepted as the storyteller of the contemporary world as a mass media tool (Parsa, 1999, p. 23). In a structure where seeing is equated with believing, television produces the narrative visually.

Television creates the electronic image language by processing image and sound together. Electronic image language, which gains momentum with electronic imaging techniques, is formed by all kinds of colors, sizes and iconic expressions. The fact that the developments in the technical field helped to convey various images, just as in the cinema, also helped in the creation of the electronic image language. Although the language desired to be created is a kind of technological and technical thing, the product created creates an aesthetic expression (Uğurlu, 2008, p. 43). For this reason, a three-dimensional technical and aesthetic narrative is realized by using elements such as camera, light, sound, graphics and decor on the two-dimensional television screen.

The hidden power of television is the image. This is because the human brain processes visual information 60000 times faster than written information (3M Corporation Research, 2001). Television has the feature of creating what is called the real effect with the image, showing it and making people believe in what it shows (Bourdieu, 2000, p. 25). When the camera shows us something, it is there and it is real. This is the power of the image, but what we understand from the image may be completely wrong (Foss, 2012, p. 51). The attention of the viewers is tried to be kept on the television screen with the images flowing for 24 hours. Viewers watch the world through the camera, which is a technical tool.

When we look at the world through the lens of a television camera; it is seen that the world is classified on our behalf, put in order, enlarged or reduced by drawing a frame, colored, and arguments about the appearance of the world are produced (Postman, 1994, p. 19).

Audio is used to simultaneously support what the image tells. Ellis argues that sound is needed in addition to image in order to keep the attention of the audience awake (1992, p. 129). The fact that people believe what they see, remains incomplete if it is not supported by sound. When we consider the silent movies, the lack of expression is understood more clearly. It is reported that during the silent film screenings, the film is supported by the music played in the movie theater and a narrator is needed. The sound used in the broadcasting field consists of three elements: words, effects and music. Words that convey information directly to the audience, natural sounds belonging to the place where the event takes place, called the effect from the objects in that place, and the sound of music targeting the emotions and thoughts that interpret the event (Kars, 2003, p. 131) form the sound side of the television narrative in a technical sense.

One of the most interesting productions in television streaming is live broadcasts. It is in the nature of television to be there in that moment and to convey the events as they are. It is up to the camera to decide which story to tell, what 'reality' to present to the audience; because every design setting (representation) of reality requires a choice and an evaluation. The live TV broadcast falls very close to the cinema-truth poetics. In other words, although the reality is tried to be transmitted as close as it can be, it seems meaningful only when a form is given to the flow (İlerialkan, & Yılmaz, 2015, pp. 82-84). This leads us to the Aristotelian story line. It is a perfect entanglement poetics to describe live shooting with Aristotelian poetics as this is the very poetics that gives the drama or the novel its well-established traditional structure (Eco, 1992, p. 147, 149). In fact, live broadcast is also a television production. Just like in a novel, a story is told; event takes shape, develops, and ends. Instead of just a pen, camera, using the image, is the storyteller. The camera angle is the director's personal style. With the emergence of this style, the area that the audience will see is determined. The camera angle determines whether the viewer approaches the subject, moves away, looks from high or low (Kılıç, 2003, p. 54).

One of the most striking and important productions in the television narrative is football live broadcasts. Football live broadcasts overlap almost exactly with the narrative features of television. Football is an enthusiastic sport that appeals to everyone with its easy-to-understand and simple structure. Television also meets the expectations of the football audience as a mass media that appeals to everyone. The knowledge that football is a game is available to all viewers. Therefore, viewers watch a match with a different reality than it is in the stadium. The television audience is out of the field and the present time, and has to be content with what the camera shows (Adanır, 2007, p. 40).

Technically speaking, it is possible to easily follow the displacement of the ball and the players, which are the subject of the game, through the camera, in football broadcasts made from a certain area, namely stadiums. In cases where fixed cameras are not sufficient, innovative moving cameras are used to ensure that the viewer does not break away from the narrative. Replays of pre-recorded camera movements from different angles can fast forward or rewind time to fill free time during the match. In addition, the images of the audience selected for the broadcast in order to support the television narrative also support the football narrative. In that form, live football matches transform the football game into a television production. Football has ceased to be a game played on the field depending on certain rules and has turned into a carnival where many interesting non-football images from the stadium are conveyed during the match (Şeker & Gölcü, 2008, p. 125).

Carnival is a normal state of insanity that is exempt from all laws and restrictions (Bakhtin, 2005, p. 289). This situation, which Bakhtin describes, is liberated by the specific freedoms gained by the rituals and festivities of the carnival (Dentith, 2005, p. 84). The structure of football, which turns into a carnival in stadiums, reaches everyone on the television screen via live broadcast. The audience participates in the carnival from their seats at home. The complex structure of the carnival is football matches, which have been rearranged for the television audience, and a simple and entertaining narrative language has been created for easy reading.

Another element of football live broadcasts being suitable for the television narrative is the dynamic broadcast flow thanks to the displacement of the ball. Football has a content where other matches and discussions are experienced every week, but the narrative does not end. When the topics of one week are over, the topics related to the next weeks are started to be discussed. When the season is over, the topics related to the new season take the order. Therefore, football is an uninterrupted, unending subject and it fits with the most basic narrative feature of television (Şeker & Gölcü, 2008, p. 118-119).

MATCH BROADCASTS EXHIBITING THE USE OF TECHNOLOGY

Social interests determine the direction, function and speed of technical progress (Habermas, 1993, p. 50). This intense interest in the use of technology is also reflected in the preferences of individuals (Günay & Çakın, 2021, p. 30). Since the football is a game loved by the society, its broadcast on television is also watched with interest. In order to keep the attention of the television audience in front of the screen, the latest developments and innovations in television technology are used in the production of football broadcasts shown on television. Experienced production teams that broadcast football matches use technological innovations in accordance with the narrative of the match, as they know that millions of people follow the live broadcast.

The narrative created visually during the live broadcast of football matches is technically presented by combining it with sound elements. The enthusiastic voice of the speaker commenting on the match is sometimes accompanied by the commentator as an expert, and the excitement is tried to be kept alive without interruption. One of the indispensable elements of football matches broadcast on television is the effect, that is, the natural sound of the environment. The noise of the crowd coming to the match and the sound of hitting the ball are the factors affecting the television audience (Gökçe, 1997, p. 259). This sound is broadcasted as loud as possible without suppressing the voice of the speaker. Thus, the uninterrupted participation of the television audience in watching is clinched. Sound technicians place effect microphones at different points of the stadium so that the effect sounds are adjusted and broadcasted in accordance with the atmosphere of the environment. During the broadcast, the control of the microphones is carried out through a sound mixing table inside the broadcast vehicle. Sound technicians are very careful during the live broadcast. This is because undesirable sounds and hums are not welcomed by the audience as they will spoil the narrative.

There are many elements to be interested in for the spectators who go to watch the match when the match pauses at the stadium, but for the spectator watching the match on the television screen, attention should be kept constantly awake, and the act of watching should be ensured. Therefore, when the game stops or it is played at low tempo, it is necessary to keep the audience busy and keep their interest alive. For this reason, the match watched on television is a television production rather than a football match. Television productions require a production. Therefore, numerous and featured cameras with different lenses installed in stadiums, wide area lighting, narration of the match by a speaker, picture recording devices with high technical features for replaying the positions, the score of the match given graphically, statistics and player promotions serve for the effort of turning a football matches into a television production.

Objective time, which is shared as real in live football matches, evolves into subjective time thanks to the director's preferences and the display of these preferences with technology. It is possible through technology to draw attention to an important detail during the match or to show a detail that is even overlooked. Today, the coexistence of television technology and sports broadcasts is mostly observed in football matches. "The biggest factor in the rapid industrialization of football and its reach all over the world is digital broadcasting technology" (Akşar, 2005, p. 30). In addition to graphic-animation applications, which are an indicator of digital broadcasting technology, the latest technologies and advanced and innovative camera applications are used during football matches.

Dozens of cameras accompany the shooting, apart from the image of a pilot who follows the displacement of the ball. Cameras located in different places show color images during the match. For example, a close view of a foul committed by a football player gives the details of the event better. Thus, high-energy colors and sounds make the movement on the screen more energetic than continuous long shots. Close-up position replays given during the match broadcast can also be used to create a new rhythm by interrupting the flow of the event and to focus the audience's attention on the event (important moment) that requires repetition (Uğurlu, 2008, p. 40). Every moment during the match is recorded with cameras with high resolution and featured lenses to be shown again later.

All these arrangements made during the live broadcast of the match are turned into a visual feast by using innovative cameras. The aim here is for the viewer to focus completely on the broadcast they are watching without missing any details. Underneath this aesthetic concern lies the truth created because of the identification of objective time with subjective time.

Innovative Cameras

Compared to other live broadcasts, more cameras with more sophisticated features are used in match broadcasts. Umberto Eco says that during the live broadcast, he was selected by and through at least three cameras by the director's choice (1992, p.142). Football matches can also be shot with three cameras, but in this case, it is not possible to talk about a broadcast that the audience is used to. The spectators expect to watch the positions from different angles and see the details from inside the field, except for the displacements of the ball. For this reason, there are at least six cameras in even the smallest match production, and it is aimed to monitor the matches from different angles in a visual variety. The number and variety of cameras increase in proportion to the size of the production (Sirer, 2020, p. 77-78). Cameras with large lenses are preferred for close-ups.

Different and innovative cameras are used in major football organizations such as the Champions League and the World Cup. In the Champions League match broadcasts, at least fourteen cameras in HD standard and 16/9 scale, eight in slow motion, one in 75X and three in 55X are used until the quarter finals and sixteen cameras, four of which have super slow motion, eight of which have slow motion features, two of which are 75X and three of which are 55X are used for the broadcasting the matches after quarter finals (UEL, 2015/16, p. 19).

Since it is not possible to get close to the players and the technical committee during football matches, it is not possible to use the camera with the help of an apparatus or cameras placed in various mechanisms are used. One of the most seen cameras in stadiums is Jimmy jib. Jimmy jib is a crane type camera that is seen behind the goals and the camera moves up and down by being tied at the end of an arm. It is used to follow the position closely during the match.

During the football match broadcast, it is important that the camera follows the side of the field without shaking. These positions are shot by using a camera called 'Steadicam' and worn by the cameraman. Thus, "fluid and natural movement is provided by absorbing the shocks and without being shaken" (Bornwell, 2011, p. 75). With this camera, the players in the ceremony can be shot from close-up and eye level before the match starts. During the match broadcast, player substitutions can be followed. In addition, the Steadicam is the only camera that can be used for entering the pitch before or after the match for shooting purposes.

The spider camera, launched for the 2008 European Football Championship, is an innovative camera system that moves across the four corners of the pitch. The Spider Cam system has HD (high resolution) image quality and 360-degree mobility, connected to wires suspended on the stadium floor, moving with a sliding system (Fenerbahce.org, 2022). In this way, it can bring the positions on the field to the screen from an upper angle, and it creates a perspective where the audience can see the whole field.

Bird's-eye views taken with drones before and after match broadcasts are also used. With the development of technology, drone cameras have been used in many different areas recently. Football matches also pioneered these innovative cameras. The use of drones during the match broadcast is prohibited by UEFA, as it is considered a distraction.

The 'Hawk-Eye' used during football matches was used in football matches as the predecessor of VAR (Video Assistant Referee) technology. It has accompanied the match broadcasts with the thought that "images obtained from the goal line will be instantly delivered to the match officials and controversial positions will be resolved thanks to this technology without objecting to the referee" (ligtv.com, 2022) thanks to technology.

VAR (Video Assistant Referee) Application

The idea that "a technology is needed to resolve controversial positions in football matches was actually the result of the referee's decision to continue despite the ball crossed the goal line in the famous Germany-England match played in the second round of the 2010 World Cup, in the shot taken by Frank Lampard… In this direction, FIFA first used what is known as "Goal Line Technology" during the Club World Cup in 2012". During this period, the "Goal Line Technology" developed by Hawk-Eye Company and used in matches laid the foundation of the Video Referee System to be used in positions that could affect the course of the match. Shortly after this development, the VAR (Video Assistant Referee) System started to be used in matches (goal.com, 2018). Sony Sports has placed Hawk-Eye technology, which is an important part of their work, as a VAR (Video Assistant Referee) System, which is called digital refereeing in many countries of the world in a short time (Hawk-Eye Innovations, 2022).

The VAR (Video Assistant Referee) Application, which was tried for the first time in the friendly match played between Italy and France on September 1, 2016, was used for the first time in 2018 at the World Cup held in Russia in an official tournament. After being used in the World Cup, it was officially used in matches in seven countries in Europe in 2018 (goal.com, 2018). In Turkey, one of the countries where football has made its presence felt as an industry, VAR (Video Assistant Referee) application has started to be used in Super League matches with the 2018-2019 Season (TFF, 2018).

The executor of the predetermined rules in football matches is the referee. "The referee represents the system, and no one can change his decision on the pitch. Opposition to his decision is resolved through various degrees of punishment, starting with a warning, as in opposing the system (Erdoğan, 2008, p. 34). Just like the players, the referees can make mistakes from time to time. Considering that the referee is a human being, it is possible to miss some situations in the field of play. However, it is desirable that the final decision maker is always error-free. For this reason, a small detail that is overlooked by the referee is made the subject of long discussions after the match and finds wide coverage in the media. With the development of technology, referees, who wanted to make fewer mistakes, started to appear on the field with equipment that they could communicate with each other and comment on positions immediately. These systems, which provide verbal communication between them, have evolved into video communication over time, with the image taking place in all areas of life.

With the VAR (Video Assistant Referee) Application, which is thought to bring justice, quality and transparency, it was planned to correct obvious mistakes in the decisions that changed the course of the match and to be used in overlooked serious events such as goal, penalty/penalty, direct sending out and showing a card to the wrong player. The final decision was always with the referee and only the referee could request the VAR (Video Assistant Referee) Application during the match. In the face of this demand, the referees working in the video operation room (VOR) and controlling the images conveyed their decisions to the referee of the match (TFF, 2020).

The VAR (Video Assistant Referee) System in Turkey is located at the Riva Facilities of the Turkish Football Federation. Thanks to the "Media Transfer Network" (MTN) technology, the infrastructure of which was created by Telekom via fiber optic cables, the images of the cameras in the stadiums where the matches are played are sent to the VAR (Video Assistant Referee) Room at Riva Facilities with a delay rate of less than a second. There are 9 VAR (Video Assistant Referee) stations at Riva Facilities. The images are transported to Riva Facilities at the speed of light, with redundancy and error-free, with fiber cables that transfer video and audio from stadiums in different geographies where the match is played. It is also possible to communicate via fiber network with TV broadcasting vehicles (TFF, Hawk-eye, 2018).

The commentators have been separated into two groups regarding the implementation of the VAR (Video Assistant Referee) System in the matches. Some of them thought that using technology was necessary and that it improved football. Thirty-two years after his goal, which he described as the 'hand of God', Diego Maradona defended the VAR (Video Assistant Referee) Application, saying "technology brings transparency and quality, and provides positive results to teams that think about the attack and take risks" (TFF, 2022). On the other hand, some commentators who internalized football said that VAR extended the duration of the game. The statistics emphasized that the VAR (Video Assistant Referee) system extended the match time by only 60 seconds on average, which constituted only 1.34% of the total match time. However, during the match, 2 minutes 57 seconds were spent for substitutions, 8 minutes 51 seconds for free kicks, 7 minutes and 2 seconds for throw-ins, 5 minutes 45 seconds for goalkeeper kicks, and 3 minutes and 57 seconds for corners (TFF, 2020). However, all this time was considered due to the nature of the game. There were also those who described VAR (Video Assistant Referee) as "the funeral ceremony of football" (Dizdar, 2019, p. 522) with the thought that it adds artificiality to the game. Despite all these discussions, a technological eye was added to the game that pointed to the real truth. Although people witness the same event, they perceive it differently according to their own interests and perspectives. In this case, the numerous comments made about the contact of two players during the match make sense. As a result, perception is to make direct contact with sensible things through feelings (Roux, 2013, p. 32).

REINTERPRETED REALITY IN FOOTBALL PROGRAMS

Football is actually the only area in society where reality is not subject to negotiation: the ball is either inside or outside (The Guardian, 5.12.2016). The final decision is made at that moment by the referee, who is the decision maker during the match. However, after the match ends and the referee blows the final whistle, football-related programs start, in which ninety minutes are negotiated for long hours. In these programs, life is negotiated through football. While Albert Camus stated that 'he learned everything he knows about life and morality from football' (Ağaoğlu, 2017), he actually associated the hopeful side of life that will end in death with football.

Football, which is accepted as the mirror of life, is carried out not through experiences but through words conveyed in the postmodern age. Heidegger identified this situation as a situation where the border between truth and untruth is blurred and these two cannot be separated from each other completely, but cannot be substituted for each other (Benesh, 2021, p.51). In football programs, the audience has no desire to learn the truth. Even though the audience knows the truth, sometimes it is not in their interest to know it. For this reason, the field of negotiation in football-based programs leaves its place to the search for superiority over each other. The guests of the program are in an effort to establish dominance throughout the program by interrupting each other after the discourse of impartiality. This is an effort to come forward with discourse rather than truth. In other words, it is possible to comment for hours on an objective situation that is not subject to negotiation. According to Keyes truth is a relative situation and gains value according to the narrator in postmodern society (2021, p.148).

Making a match commentary on television means "a community alienated from the reality of football, reproduces and circulates a mechanical football discourse through television through television" (Şeker & Gölcü, 2008, p. 124). Comments made in this context consist of an effort to attract some supporters and increase their visibility. Although everyone watches the same image on the television screen, everyone perceives it differently in accordance with their point of view. Although the footage is repeatedly shown by the director from different angles, there is no perfect recording or point of view. There is definitely a dead spot. This situation constitutes the basis of the rightness of the audience. Although the camera best shows the velocity of the ball, the television screen eliminates perspective, making it difficult to understand the actual distance. For this reason, the idea of a perfect image that will enlighten the viewer by presenting the event as it really is in its pure form seems like a dream for now (Roux, 3013, p. 32). In fact, there is no need for facts in the post-truth age, more precisely, facts can be changed, distorted and reshaped (Crăciun, 2017), and as a free society, individuals have decided to live in a post-truth world with their free will (Tesich, 2021, p. 25).

CONCLUSION

Television, which was depicted by Postman as 'entertainment that kills'; expresses the truth, like time itself, about the communication techniques invented by man himself, and as a product of the conversation he has with himself through these techniques (1994, p.34). Today, the postmodern world is seen as a virtual reality environment that replaces symbols and images, real or concrete, rather than a real society (Bolat, 2019, p. 43). Therefore, individuals witness that the truth is reproduced over and over again through communication tools such as the programs we see on the television screen in the postmodern period. Television, which has an important place among communication tools, is still at the forefront with its visuality and easy accessibility. Television, which has been in the living space for nearly a century, has completed its transformation in technical terms.

Television is a good storyteller as a medium. The stories told to the society in a flow space are presented as a result of a visual knowledge. Individuals who have this knowledge through the act of watching can easily read the images through the television screen. Eco says that the presentation of reality on the television screen is made through the camera, and a flow is made by choosing among the cameras showing different things (1992, p. 147). The most striking productions in the television stream are the live broadcasts that claim to transfer the images that are there at that moment. The live broadcast also coincides with the narrative of truth. The most followed and popular live broadcasts on the television screen are football matches.

Television has been in close relationship with football since the beginning of the 20th century's, when football audience started to emerge. The compatibility of the presentation of football as a visual feast on the field with the narrative structure of television has highlighted the football live broadcasts among television productions. Broadcasting live from anywhere in the world via satellite broadcasts and transmitting these broadcasts live in the last quarter of the 20th century, have brought television to the fore in bilateral relations, and after this period, television paved the way for the spreading of football. However, the football matches broadcasted on the television screen are not exactly the same as the football played on the field. Due to the fluidity of the television narrative, a narrative is created by choosing from many cameras and different angles seen by these cameras during the match broadcast. Cameras are placed where the audience in the stadium can best follow the match. Depending on the importance of the match, the match is followed by up to thirty cameras. During the match broadcasts, a selection of innovative cameras with different features is made to enrich the match visually.

During the matches played in the stadium, the tempo is not reduced in the match watched on the television screen when the ball stops, and the same enthusiasm is tried to be maintained. Therefore, continuity of the attention of the audience is ensured with the speaker describing the match for the television broadcast, the atmosphere sound given by the microphones placed in the four corners of the stadium, and the heavy screenings that can be given instantly during the broadcast as a result of the development of television technology. Recently, it has been processed and shown on the screen with computer-aided images without missing any details. The latest innovation in this regard is the computer-aided applications that are implemented as line technology and leave no room for mistakes by calculating millimetrically whether the ball crosses the line or not. The most advanced of these applications is VAR (Video Referee Application), which has been used in football matches in many countries since the 2018 World Cup.

Increasing the number of cameras or applying camera applications equipped with innovative technologies is nothing but an effort to increase the visibility of football by mediating it with technology. The camera reproduces itself by reproducing its own reality through the television screen. However, it is not possible to place cameras in every corner of the pitch to please the audience. This is because the displayed images are presented by selecting. This situation always leaves a question mark in mind and leads to the production of productions on which possible scenarios are written in another time period, such as commentary programs made after the match.

Football mediated by technology on the television screen is actually a simple game. No matter how many cameras are used for shooting, the television narrative is not a mixed production. The underlying fact that it is loved and stands out so much is that it is simple enough for everyone to understand, no matter how embellished it is. VAR (Video Assistant Referee) technology, which has been used in football matches recently, supports the football narrative presented on television in an instrumental sense.

Football match broadcasts are the common denominator of people of all ages and levels. Although it is integrated with technology, television, which is a means of entertainment and relaxation, integrates with football, which serves the same purpose. Apart from the football matches broadcast on television, football programs in which position analyzes are made before, at the end of the match and even throughout the week also have a large number of viewers. Although the positions discussed in these programs are viewed from different camera angles and the images of these cameras are processed by computer, the only truth is that the viewers have a good time. For this reason, it becomes more important to reinterpret it with television narrative rather than whether the ball touches it or not. Because for the audience who supports the team in front of the television screen, there is definitely a view close to itself and another angle that the camera does not see.

Although a quarter of a century has passed since Maradona's controversial goal in 1986, technological developments have not changed the football-truth relationship. Although the football game and the positions in the game are analyzed technically as a result of technological progress, there is definitely a topic to talk about due to the nature of television. This is because it is necessary to fill the 24-hour flow on television. Football matches are demanding and expensive productions. It is aimed to fill the flow by spreading the football programs held in front of and at the end of the match over the hours. The context of technology is also used instrumentally in the programs made by considering all the elements of football. Increasing the attractiveness of the match, which is expected from football programs, is to polish this expensive production, and while doing all this, to support the television narrative and to create more audiences.

In the postmodern age, truth and non-truth are not questioned. People are not interested in whether the world shown through communication tools is real or not. This situation helps the truth to be bent and change shape. The camera, which acts as a visual mediator of communication, plays an important role in the displacement of truth from the point of view. Every new arrangement in television productions, such as innovative cameras mediated by technology, is used to support the television narrative. Football matches, which reach a large number of viewers with their simple narrative among television productions, are the productions in which the technological developments in this field are exhibited the most. In this context; it is thought that the football game, which is accepted as a commodity of consumption culture with its narrative integrating with technology, will continue its existence in the future and reach a key position in the new universes created.

REFERENCES

Adanır, O. (2007). *Audio and Visual Meaning Production* [İşitsel ve Görsel Anlam Üretimi]. Turkey: +1Book Publications.

Ağaoğlu, M. (2017). *A Keeper in a Nonsense World: Albert Camus [Saçma Dünyada Bir Kaleci: Albert Camus].* Üvercinka Journal. August.

Akşar, T. (2005). *Industrial Football [Endüstriyel Futbol].* Literatür Publications.

Altun, F. (2022, January). A Critical Approach to the Post-Truth Narrative in the Framework of Sociological Theory. *Research Article. Journal of Erciyes Communication.*, *9*(1), 249–267.

Ankaralıgil, N., & Kartal, H. (2013). Game, Ideology and Consumption: The Transformation of Football from Entertainment to Consumption in the Context of Mass Media [Oyun, İdeoloji ve Tüketim: Kitle İletişim Araçları Bağlamında Eğlenceden Tüketime Futbolun Dönüşümü]. *New Thoughts Journal, 7*(April), 125–144.

Aydın, C. & Aslıtürk G. E. (2017). Creation in the Framework of Mythology and the History of Religions: Reflections on the Sistine Chapel Ceiling Frescoes [Mitoloji ve Dinler Tarihi Çerçevesinde Yaratılış: Sistine Şapeli Tavan Freskolarına Yönelik Düşünceler]. *İdil Journal, 6*(30).

Bakhtin, M. (2005). Rabelais and His World: carnival and grotesque (Ç. Öztek, Trans.). Ayrıntı Publications.

Benesch, K. (2021). Is the Relationship between Truth and Post-Truth a Relationship between Modernism and Postmodernism? Heidegger, the Humanities and the Death of Common Sense [*Hakikat ile Hakikat Sonrası İlişkisi Modernizm ile Postmodernizm İlişkisi midir? Heidegger, Beşeri Bilimler ve Sağduyunun Ölümü]. Cogito Journal, 104,* 49–66.

Bolat, N., & Çakın, Ö. (2018). Violence as a Marketing Motif in Television Series: The Example of the Black Sea Series You Tell. In Virtual Media Violence and Social Traumas. HEGEM Publications.

Bolat, N. (2019). *Post-modernizm, inside: Communication in the Age of Posts [Post-modernizm içinde: Postlar Çağında İletişim]* (M. N. Erdem & N. K. Şener, Eds.). Literatürk Publication.

Bourdieu, P. (2000). On Television (T. Ilgaz, Trans.). Cogito Publications.

Corporation Research. (2001). *3M Corporation Research.* http://www.3m.com/meetingnrtwork/readingroom/meetingguide_press.html

Crăciun, A. (2017). *New challenges of communication in the age of post truth.* ttps://euprera.org/2017/07/01/new-challenges-of-communication-in-the-age-of-post-truth/.

Dentith, S. (2005). *Bakhtinian Thought: An Introductory Reader.* Routledge.

Dilmen, D. (2015). *Why 11 People, Why 90 Minutes [Neden 11 Kişi, Neden 90 Dakika]* (Vol. 4). Fitbol Journal.

Dizdar, C. (2019). VAR is the funeral of football! [VAR, futbolun cenaze merasimidir!]. *TRT Academic Journal, 4*(8).

Eco, U. (1992). The Open Work (Y. Şahan, Trans.). Kabalcı Publication.

Ellis, J. (1992). *Visible Fictions Cinema Television Video.* Routledge.

Erdoğan, İ. (2008). On Studying Football [Futbolu İnceleme Üzerine]. *Journal of Communication Theory and Research*, (26), 1–57.

Fenerbahce.org Archive. (2022). https://www.fenerbahce.org/haberler/arsiv/orumcek-kamera-stadimizda

Foss, B. (2012). Narration Techniques and Dramaturgy in Cinema and Television (M.K. Gerçeker, Trans.). Hayalperest Publication.

Goal.com. (2018). *What is video referee application (VAR)?* [Video hakem uygulaması (VAR) nedir]. https://www.goal.com/tr/haber/video-hakem-uygulamasi-var nedir/1n1vfg3dgig3o18pdz6c7ll42q

Gökçe, G. (1997). *Television Program Production and Directing [Televizyon Program Yapımcılığı ve Yönetmenliği]*. Derin Publication.

Günay, M. A., & Çakın, Ö. (2021). Changes in Consumer Behaviors in the Covid 19 Pandemic Process. In G. Çalışır & E. Diker (Eds.), *The Changing Face of Communication Covid-19 Process [Covid 19 Pandemi Sürecinde Tüketici Davranışlarında Yaşanan Değişimler, içinde: Covid-19 Sürecinde İletişimin Değişen Yüzü]* (pp. 10–334). Eğitim Publications.

Habermas, J. (1993). Technique and Science as Ideology (M. Tüzel, Trans.). Yapı Kredi Publications.

Habertürk. (n.d.). *The 'hand of God' story was a symbolic 'revenge'* [Tanrı'nın eli" hikayesi, sembolik bir 'intikam'dı]. https://www.haberturk.com/tanri-nin-eli-hikayesi-sembolik-bir-intikam-di-maradona-1986-dunya-kupasi-ndaki-golu-anlatti-2882076-spor

Hawk-eye innovations. (2022). https://www.hawkeyeinnovations.com/about

İlerialkan, D., & Yılmaz, R. (2015). Script: How to Write? How They Write [Senaryo: Nasıl Yazılır? Nasıl Yazıyorlar?]. *Alfa*.

İnal, R. (2008). *Globalization and Sports [Küreselleşme ve Spor]*. Evrensel Publication.

Karakuş, S. (2017). *Lived 79 years ago: The first football match to be televised live* [79 yıl önce naklen: Televizyondan canlı yayınlanan ilk futbol maçı]. https://www.gzt.com/zpor/79-yil-once-naklen-televizyondan-canliyayinlanan-ilk-futbol-maci-2798065

Kars, N. (2003). *Let's Make a TV Program, Let Everyone Watch [Televizyon Programı Yapalım, Herkes İzlesin]*. Derin Publication.

Keyes, R. (2021). The Post-Truth Era, Lying and Deception in Today's World (D. Özçetin, Trans.). Tudem Publication.

Kılıç, L. (2003). *Image Aesthetics [Görüntü Estetiği]*. İnkılâp Publication.

Kuper, S. (2014). Football is Never Just Football (S. Gürtunca, Trans.). İthaki Publication.

Ligtv.com Archive. (2022). *The hawk's eye is being tried for football* [Şahin gözü futbol için deneniyor]. http://www.ligtv.com.tr/haber/sahin-gozufutbol-icin-deneniyor

Macmillan Contemporary Dictionary. (1988). ABC Publication.

Parsa, S. (1999). Television Semiotics [Televizyon Göstergebilimi]. *Editing Journal.*, *16*, 15–28.

Postman, N. (1994). Amusing Ourselves to Death (O. Akınhay, Trans.). Ayrıntı Publication.

Roux, M. (2013). Socrate en Crampons (B. Yanık, Trans.). Tekin Publication.

Şeker, M., & Gölcü, A. (2008). Reproduction of Football on Television [Futbolun Televizyonda Yeniden Üretimi]. *Communication Theory and Research Journal.*, *26*, 111–129.

Serim, Ö. (2014). *Football Art [Futbol Sanatı]*. Bence Book.

Sirer, E. (2020). *The Language of the Image in Football Broadcasts [Futbol Yayınlarında Görüntü Dili]*. Kriter Publication.

Talimciler, A. (2009). Within the (un)changing) States of Male Identity: The Overlooked Area in: Formation of Male Identity in Turkey: Sports/Football [Erkek Kimliği'nin Değiş(meye)n Halleri içinde: Türkiye'de Erkek Kimliğinin Oluşumunda Göz Ardı Edilen Alan: Spor/Futbol]. Beta Publications.

Tesich, S. (2021). The Regime of Lies. *Cogito Journal, 104,* 23–28.

TFF. (2018). *Hawk-Eye CEO Carter: TFF VAR Center is one of the best in the world* [Hawk-Eye CEO'su Carter: TFF VAR Merkezi dünyanın en iyilerinden biri]. https://www.tff.org/default.aspx?pageID=248&ftxtID=29704

TFF. (2020). *VAR (Video Assistant Referee) Handbook.* https://www.tff.org/Resources/TFF/Images/MHK/VAR.pdf

TFF. (2022). *İş Ortakları. FIFA Fédération Internationale de Football Association.* Work Partners. https://www.tff.org/default.aspx?pageID=356

The Guardian. (2016). *The scoreboard never lies: why sport in a post-truth world matters more than ever.* https://www.theguardian.com/sport/2016/dec/05/sports-distraction-post-truth-world

Uğurlu, H. (2008). *Constructing the Concept of Time in Live Broadcasts on Television [Televizyondaki Canlı Yayınlarda Zaman Kavramının Yapılandırılması].* Galatasaray Üniversitesi İleti-ş-im Journal.

Williams, R. (2003). Television, Technology and Cultural Form (A. Ulvi Türkbağ, Trans.). Dost Publication.

ADDITIONAL READING

Hardt, H. (2004). *Myths for the masses. An essay on mass communication.* Blackwell Publishing. doi:10.1002/9780470774335

Kuper, S. (2016). *Football Against The Enemy.* Orion Books.

Walters, R. L. (1994). *Broadcast Writing Principles and Practice.* California State University.

KEY TERMS AND DEFINITIONS

Football Match: A football match is a team sport played with a distinctive spherical ball between two teams of eleven players. In a match consisting of 90 minutes divided into two forty-five-minute halves, the team that manages to score more goals than the opposing team wins, but if the number of goals scored is equal, the match is ended in a draw.

Football Program: Football is a game played between two teams, officially of eleven players each, on a field one hundred yards long with goals at each end, in which points are made by getting a ball across the opponent's goal line. Football refers to a number of team sports that involve, to varying degrees, kicking a ball to score a goal. The football program is also a program in which football-related comments are made, controversial positions and analyzes about football are made.

Image Language: Image is a representation or likeness of a person, animal, or thing. The television image creates the electronic image language by presenting both motion and sound together. Electronic image language, which gains momentum with electronic imaging techniques, is realized by means of all kinds of colors, sizes and iconic expressions. The fact that the developments in the technical field helped to convey various images, just as in the cinema, also helped in the creation of the electronic image language. Although the language to be created is a technological and technical thing, the product created creates an aesthetic expression.

Live Broadcast: A live broadcast, also called a live transmission, generally refers to various types of media that are broadcast without a significant delay. The most common seen media example of the live transmission is a news program or a news broadcasting. Other types of live broadcasts include live television.

Sports: Any game that requires physical activity and involves a degree of competition, as baseball, football, bowling, or basketball. Sports (US) are all forms of usually competitive physical activity or games which, through casual or organised participation, aim to use, maintain, or improve physical ability and skills while providing entertainment to participants, and in some cases, spectators. Usually the contest or game is between two sides, each attempting to exceed the other. Some sports allow a tie game; others provide tie-breaking methods, to ensure one winner and one loser. A number of such two-sided contests may be arranged in a tournament producing a champion. Many sports leagues make an annual champion by arranging games in a regular sports season, followed in some cases by playoffs. Hundreds of sports exist, from those between single contestants, through to those with hundreds of simultaneous participants, either in teams or competing as individuals. In certain sports such as racing, many contestants may compete, each against all with one winner.

Technology: Application of scientific knowledge and advances to practical purposes. Any use of materials or objects, as tools, to serve human needs.

Video Camera: A video camera is a device that captures moving image information from live environments and encodes it into data that can be converted or converted to electronic visual media. A typical digital camera consists of a lens, image sensor, storage media, and many other features that can be found in other cameras (such as scalable aperture, filters, and flash). Video technology dates back to the mid-twentieth century, with the first videotape recordings used in television broadcasts in the early 1950s. At the same time, digital technology was developing in the field of computer programming. However, video remained an analog format for the next few decades. The main difference between analog and digital media is that the former is a continuous stream whereas the latter consists of discrete values (digits) representing picture information. Analog video cameras were initially huge and difficult to use, but evolved into portable "camcorders" in the 1980s. Eventually, camera devices adopted the ability to record digital information, and digital video replaced most other motion picture formats as its quality surpassed that of previous analog formats. Most camcorders now available on the consumer market are digital camcorders. The digital format allows for easy editing and sharing of video.

Chapter 8
"Not Ignoring the FoMO (Fear of Missing Out) Effect" as a New Way to Persuade Consumers to Buy

Aybike Tuba Özden
https://orcid.org/0000-0002-3133-3620
Ondokuz Mayıs University, Turkey

ABSTRACT

FoMO (The fear of missing out) was noticed by marketers and started to be used on consumers. FoMO is an anxiety disorder that is defined as not being aware of exciting things when not being looked at, or missing out on the experiences of others. Although the FoMO effect has a negative meaning, businesses manage to use this concern to their advantage. Limited production, shortage of products in stock, short-term discounts, showing the number of people interested in the same product, promotions offered as opportunities not to be missed are among the efforts of businesses to persuade consumers through FoMO. It is seen that the literature on FoMO in the field of marketing is limited. This study aimed to examine the relationship between FoMO and consumption and to evaluate the relevant literature. For this purpose, the findings, results, and evaluations obtained by examining the experimental and conceptual studies in the relevant literature were synthesized.

INTRODUCTION

Today's communication technologies are developing at a great pace. Thanks to these technologies, information can easily spread all over the world. This rapidly developing technology significantly changes the lives of consumers. Undoubtedly, this change also affects consumption habits. Platforms such as the internet, social media and virtual reality are turning into platforms that take precedence over stores or shopping malls. Businesses try to retain their existing customers and gain new customers through the communication they establish with consumers and the experiences they give them. However, technological

DOI: 10.4018/978-1-7998-9251-9.ch008

developments make this process increasingly complex. Therefore, businesses have to look for new ways to persuade consumers. Marketers began to develop methods to attract consumers' attention without ignoring the FoMO effect. FoMO is an anxiety disorder that is defined as missing the news (Przybylski et al., 2013, p. 1842). It can be said that the power of accessing all kinds of information quickly, together with the Internet, creates this anxiety. As a matter of fact, FoMO is a psychological problem of the people of the new world. Consumers are so accustomed to obtaining information from the outside world that they cannot stay away from the internet for fear of missing something. For example, charging of smartphones, computers or tablets has become a primary need for many consumers. Buses, parks, restaurants and even streets can be used as environments where these smart devices can be charged. It can be said that one of the reasons for this primary need is related to FoMO. Because every consumer whose device's battery is low or whose battery is running out is afraid of missing out on developments. Today, the product variety is very large. Businesses trying to be different and visible among such diversity have to add attraction to their products. Consumers exposed to such diversity and appeal may wish to have them all. As such, FoMO is the desire to have everything and not miss anything. The development of technology and the desire to be constantly up-to-date caused by social media platforms have started to cause a kind of anxiety in consumers. Especially the fear of missing the developments shared on the internet has led to the emergence of a concept called FoMO (The fear of missing out) in the world. Businesses can also transform this anxiety into purchasing behavior.

Herman conducted the first study on the use of the FoMO effect in marketing. Herman identified this concept while working on marketing and branding methodology in 1996, then conveyed how it could be used in terms of marketing through a scientific article, and then FoMO entered the Oxford English Dictionary in 2013 (Kaçik & Acar, 2020, p. 76). Afterwards, the FoMO effect was used in the field of marketing to persuade consumers to buy. Many strategies, such as keeping the number of stocks limited, making a limited number of sales, and satisfaction comments from those who bought the product, were produced using the FoMO effect. It can be thought that with the technological developments, the effect of FoMO may differ or it may affect more people. One of the ways to catch up with the future is to understand the present. For this reason, it is necessary to understand the reflections of FoMO effect in the field of marketing today. It has been observed that there are not enough studies on FoMO, which is a new phenomenon (Hayran et al., 2020, p. 1; Elhai et al., 2021, p. 206). Therefore, this study aims to synthesize research on the FoMO effect and its use in marketing. At the same time, various suggestions have been developed for future research and businesses on the subject. It is thought that this study will present a different perspective to researchers and practitioners related to FoMO, which is thought to have different uses in the field of marketing in the future.

In the first part of this study, it is explained what the FoMO effect is and what kind of reflections it has on consumers. Then, how the FoMO effect is used in the marketing world is emphasized and the results of the research done in the relevant literature are mentioned. Finally, various suggestions for future studies were developed and a general evaluation and discussion was made in the conclusion part of the research.

BACKGROUND

With the Internet and web technologies, information has become easily and quickly accessible. With Web 2.0 technologies, consumers have begun to interact over the internet. In this process, which is called the social web, individuals and institutions can produce content on the internet that others can see or contribute to. Technological developments have taken web technologies to a much higher level and enabled consumers to communicate with machines with Web 4.0. In fact, with Web 5.0, communication with machines that can think and feel in the future seems possible. As a matter of fact, the point reached in artificial intelligence technologies shows that this process is not far away. These technologies have inevitably affected consumers and their consumption habits.

For example, consumers can clean their homes remotely with smart vacuums. Consumers, who can learn about the products finished in the refrigerator through smart cabinets, can also adjust the temperature of their homes remotely. Smart toothbrushes can personalize the brushing process by communicating with consumers' smart phones, and they can share the information acquired by these devices with the dentist. Smartphones, which have become a basic need for many consumers, have turned into assistants that offer many services such as banking, shopping, socializing or education. Virtual reality environments called metaverse are similarly platforms where you can play games, shop, organize museum tours, and organize weddings or concerts.

Therefore, it is possible to talk about a new world order where everything is digitized. Thanks to smart machines, consumers can have all kinds of information about both their private and social areas. The fact that they are so aware of all the developments can lead them to the fear of missing out on the developments. There is a fast-paced life outside and it is of great importance for some consumers not to be deprived of it. In particular, social media is an effective platform that consumers use to learn about what is going on in the outside world. Social media is defined as a group of internet-based applications that are built on the ideological and technical foundations of Web 2.0 and allow the emergence and modification of user-generated content (Whiting & Williams, 2013, p. 363). It can be said that social media environments are among the prominent socialization environments of today. A strong social media account can be measured by the number of followers. As a matter of fact, consumers do not want to miss the likes and comments of their followers regarding the shares they have made. As a result, it can become a need for consumers to be aware of the developments, both for the follower and the follower.

Prepared by We Are Social and Hootsuite; According to statistics made within the framework of platforms such as the internet, social media or e-commerce, the number of internet users worldwide is 4.6 billion (Kemp, 2021). According to this report, consumers in the world spend about 7 hours a day on the Internet and 2.5 hours on social media. 92.6% of internet access is done with smart phones. According to the report, the age group that uses social media the most is between the ages of 25-34 and the time spent on social media has increased 1.5 times in the last 5 years. The most used social networks; It is in the form of Facebook, Youtube, Whatsapp, FB Messenger and Instagram. Looking at these statistics, it can be seen how much the internet and social media influence consumers. Such intense use of the Internet and social media has led to the emergence of various psychological problems. For example, fear of being deprived of a smartphone/device (nomophobia) or being without internet (netlessphobia) are new generation psychological disorders (Yıldırım & Kisioglu, 2018, p. 473). Among these is the type of psychological disorder called "fear of missing out", abbreviated as FoMO.

FOMO EFFECT

Worries such as missing out developments or not hearing about the experiences of others can be called FoMO. Especially through the internet and social media, a life flowing in the outside world is shared.

Other lives in this outer world are usually exciting and joyful. Consumers can share the places they visit, the food they eat, the activities they experience, their friends, their trips, what they wear, what they read or their shopping moments, in short, all their lives on social media. For consumers who are exposed to these shares, there is an intriguing life flowing on their screens. Following these lives, doing like them if possible, being different if it is not possible to be like them, but being aware of what "they" do can be among the primary expectations of today's consumers. FoMO is being in pursuit continually not to miss out any information about the life flowing.

FoMO was first conceptualized by using self-determination theory developed by Ryan and Deci (cited by Ehai et al., 2021, p. 205). According to this theory, consumers have an inherently consistent self, they tend to improve psychologically and they thrive to overcome the existing barriers (Ryan & Deci, 2000, p. 68). However, this autonomy needs to be supported in the environment they belong to. Consumers need intrinsic motivation to achieve self-actualization and they can direct their intrinsic motivation by being encouraged when they feel socially connected to others (Elhai et al., 2021, p. 205). Przybylsk et al. (2013) applied this theory to FoMO and stated that FoMO is a negative emotion arising from unmet social relationship needs. Przybylski et al. (2013, p. 1842) defined FoMO as individuals' fears, concerns and worries about losing contact with events. FoMO is a fear that other people are having fun without us and therefore it is the state of staying constantly connected not to miss things. In psychology, FoMO is discussed as an obsession and a kind of severe symptom (Riordan et al., 2015, p. 5).

Herman (2019) defined FoMO as a fearful attitude that occurs in consumers for missing out existing opportunities and joy created by opportunities. According to the author, FoMO is individuals' concentrating their attention on the empty half of the glass. According to Riordan et al. (2015, p. 2), FoMO is the restless and often all-consuming feeling of the thought that others are having rewarding experiences. The idea that other consumers are having fun without you creates FoMO (Przybylski et al., 2013, p. 1841). This idea can make individuals feel obligated to follow other people continually in the digital world and not to miss out anything. Especially social media use can cause consumers to experience FoMO (Beyens et al., 2016, p. 1).

FoMO is associated with both general psychological needs (such as consumers' needs to identify with their status, to be recognized by others and the need for interpersonal connection) and also social belonging (not to be separated or isolated from the group) (Kang et al., 2019, p. 4). It is thought that in today's conditions, digital environments have created social spaces and the desire to belong to a group has begun to shift to taking part in internet environments, apart from taking part in real social spaces. The fear of not belonging to a group can bring along the fear of exclusion. An indispensable part of FoMO experience is social pressure (Hodkinson, 2016, p. 4). Therefore, not being separated from the group is important for consumers. Indeed, it has been found that young people who need popularity experience more FoMO (Beyens et al., 2016, p. 1). In fact, it is found that consumers experience FoMO even in fun activities (Hayran et al., 2016, p. 468) and it can be said that consumers who experience FoMO enjoy instant experiences less.

Consumers may experience FoMO due to their feelings such as being liked and approved by others to feel good and not to be excluded by others (Riordan et al., 2015, p. 5). As a matter of fact, it can be seen that consumers with a high sense of belonging have increased FoMO levels (Beyens et al., 2016; Browne et al., 2018). When these consumers distance themselves from what others do, they may worry about not being like them and not being accepted for not being like them. The fear of missing out developments may cause these consumers to feel incomplete and tired. Trying to follow the instant notifications coming to these smart phones and having knowledge of these developments is a tiring activity both mentally and physically. FoMO causes complaints in consumers such as headache, shortness of breath or chest pain (Baker et al., 2016, p. 279). FoMO is also a process that decreases life satisfaction of consumers (Przybylski et al., 2013, p. 1844).

When studies conducted on FoMO are examined, it can be seen that it is associated with various emotional states. For example, FoMO has been found to be associated with stress (Elhai et al., 2016, p. 509) and depression severity (Oberst et al., 2017, p. 51). In this case, it can be said that consumers experience stress or depression due to the feeling of missing out shares they are not included in. Oberst et al. (2017, p. 58) stated that digital addiction can be decreased by increasing self-esteem and developing social skills. Problems such as anxiety, sleep disruption, lack of concentration or social media addiction are psychological problems that may occur as a result of FoMO (Milyavskaya et al., 2018, p. 725; Alutaybi et al., 2020, p. 1). According to the results of another study, it was found that FoMO is positively associated with having repetitive thoughts in the mind (rumination), boredom and anxiety (Elhai et al., 2018, p. 289). As a result, the fear of missing out what happens drives consumers to more widespread internet use (Beyens et al., 2016). In summary, Hoşgör et al. (2017, p. 215) stated that the most common situations in literature related with FoMO are the following:

- FoMO increases social media use.
- Facebook, Instagram, Twitter and Snapchat have an effect on FoMO.
- FoMO is more common especially in young men.
- Individuals with FoMO level have lower satisfaction with life.
- Consumers with low competence and autonomy levels tend to have FoMO.
- Continually checking on notifications to smart phones affect FoMO.
- Consumers who use social media in the classroom during lessons have higher FoMO level.

FOMO EFFECT AND CONSUMPTION

According to Herman (2020), abundance of product alternatives that consumers are faced with leads them to the desire to have everything. Herman (2000) stated that among the many product options offered to the market, when consumers cannot consume these options, they will experience the feeling of missing out on the opportunity they desire and they will tend to consume all the offers in the market, especially the ones which are scarce (Zhang et al., 2020, p. 1620). This theory of Herman was supported with subsequent studies. Hodkinson (2016, p. 2) stated that when it first emerged, FoMO was a concept specific to popular culture and young people and it expressed a personal weakness. According to the author, consumers show commercial, cognitive and emotional reactions to FoMO (Hodkinson, 2016, p. 6).

With the developing technology, businesses can produce a large number and a large variety of products. Therefore, it is not possible for businesses to stay away from these channels. Consumers who try to make decisions in such a wide range of products may show a great effort to obtain information about the product or brands. This effort can also create an anxiety to be deprived of information. For example, buying a technological device can lead to a confusing problem today. The fact that technological products are diversified according to their features in addition to being constantly updated can turn into a process that makes it difficult for consumers to make decisions. A consumer who wants to buy a computer thinks that he can buy a much newer model by waiting for a few months. Therefore, following the market of this product and being aware of the developments can become a priority for this consumer or such consumers may try to follow the product others buy and the comments about these products. Information missed out may create concern and anxiety for them. As a result, these consumers may experience the fear of missing opportunities and falling behind, that is, FoMO. Consumers who experience FoMO can make decisions by looking at their peers and environment in their purchase decisions (Jood, 2017, p. 29). Businesses who have this information try to turn this anxiety experienced by consumers into selling products. For example, businesses share the number of consumers who buy products. Consumers can make decisions to buy not to fall behind people who buy that product. Similarly, the comments of people who buy the product are also very important. For this reason, businesses first of all try to please the people who buy the product. Undoubtedly, the main reason for this effort is creating loyal customers. However, it has been found that consumers buy a brand not due to feelings of loyalty, but for not missing out on the service other loyal customers have received (Argan et al., 2018, p. 48). Comments of customers who are satisfied with the product made in digital environment are also important. Positive comments of customers who are satisfied can persuade other consumers. In their study, Park and Lee (2009, p. 334) defined the extent to which online reviews facilitate consumers' decision making process about a product as perceived benefit. Consumers can decide easier with these comments. For this reason, businesses can create a sense of losing and missing out in consumers who think about buying a product by specifying the number of comments and the points given to a product. It can be seen that experiences recommended by others create FoMO (Good & Hyman, 2021, p. 564). Continually following the comments of a product other consumers are satisfied with and even not missing out on the price or renewed comments about the product is important for some consumers. As a matter of fact, this follow can be a confirmation of what a right decision they have made.

As can be seen, there is a constantly flowing and self-renewing flow of information in digital environment. Being deprived of this flow of information is a source of anxiety and stress for consumers experiencing FoMO. Businesses create a situation that will cause anxiety and stress to consumers and then provide solutions to get rid of this anxiety and stress. It can be seen that FoMO affects consumers' intentions to purchase holiday (Çetinkaya & Şahbaz, 2019, p. 383). Hodkinson (2016:7) stated that travel packages are important among purchases on which FoMO is effective. For example, a consumer who wants to have a holiday with early booking researches hotels. However, hotel businesses limit the number of hotels consumers can go with early booking and they keep the date range of early booking short. In addition, giving the number of consumers who are searching the same hotel and limiting the number of people who can stay in that hotel with early booking are also causes of concern for consumers planning this holiday. Consumers who think that they do not have enough time to decide and that other consumers will buy the service until they make their decision try to act and decide quickly. For these consumers, there may be opportunities missed each moment they do not follow. As a matter of fact, Erciş et al. (2020) stated that FoMO has an effect on unplanned purchase. A positive correlation was also found between internet addiction and smart phone addiction and impulsivity (Mazhari, 2012; Kim et al., 2014).

Businesses who offer "unmissable opportunities" try to persuade consumers to make quick decisions and therefore to buy. It cannot be said that such promotions are new. However, the promise of "unmissable opportunities" can be much more effective in the digital world. It is possible to reach much higher number of consumers in digital environment. These consumers continually see advertisements for "unmissable opportunities" in front of the screen. In this case, the fact that consumers do want to miss the opportunities other consumers do not miss creates FoMO effect in consumers.

It cannot be said that the urge to learn what others are doing is a new phenomenon. However, learning so quickly about what others are doing is probably a new situation. The internet and social media continually give us information about what others are doing. In fact, individuals even share this information from their social media accounts without the need for third parties to provide it. For example, while the home lives and families of famous people, what they ate or where they went were a mystery to us in the past, they are no longer a secret. These famous people share this information with everyone on their own initiative. Lives of famous people have become accessible. Consumers who are following these accessible lives have begun to buy what they buy and do what they do to feel famous, rich, popular or known like them. However, these shares are so frequently made that it is important for consumers who are experiencing FoMO to follow not to miss out these shares. As a matter of fact, smart phones can transmit the shares of all lives that are followed with instant notifications. It is not surprising for businesses to use this situation to persuade consumers to buy. These famous people recommend products to their followers with influencer marketing. It is easy to come across "unmissable opportunities" among these recommendations.

Another practice of businesses marketing products with FoMO effect is specifying the number of stocks. Limited number of stocks can trigger consumers' sense of purchase before the stocks run out. Businesses create FoMO on consumers by creating a perception that they have insufficient number of products, that is, there may be a shortage in that area (Hodkinson, 2016, p. 12). Consumers who think that there will be a shortage in the product market they will buy are worried that others will buy the products they need to buy and therefore they are afraid of missing the shares of other consumers about the issue. Businesses create the perception in consumers that they have to hurry to buy their products and that the product will run out if they do not hurry up. Sometimes they limit the product to "only one person one product" to create this perception. However, there is a situation that needs attention regarding the perception of scarcity. When consumers perceive scarcity as a manipulative situation, the positive effect of scarcity on product evaluation diminishes (Lee et al., 2020; 2018, p. 281).

Businesses try to use FoMO effect by showing the products that are out of stock in product promotions made in the digital environment. For example, when consumers make a filtering about the size, colour or model of a product they want to buy, they encounter the products that are out of stock. Consumers who see the products others buy or consume may have increased urge to own those products. There is a filtering as "show the products in stock" in shopping websites. Even this filtering reminds consumers that there are products which are not in stock.

The relationship between hedonic consumption, which is the consumption habit of postmodern times, and FoMO also seems to be remarkable. Hedonic consumption can be summarized as consumers' making consumption because they enjoy consumption. Consumers can make hedonic consumption due to reasons such as fun, individual satisfaction, socializing, the feeling of belonging to another world, status or adapting to new trends (Arnold & Reynolsd, 2003, s.80-81). Results of studies conducted show that consumers consume social media in a hedonic way due to FoMO (Gürdin, 2019, p. 1273). In another study, it was concluded that the participants who gave the answer "it is a must for me" for social media have higher FoMO and hedonic consumption levels when compared with the participants who gave the answer "it is OK if I don't have it" (Çopuroğlu, 2021, p. 4317).

The feeling of belonging to a group may cause consumers to show similar behaviors with the group. Consumers may experience FoMO when they do not follow group behavior (Kang et al., 2019). For this reason, consumers can follow the developments related with the group they belong to and they may try to show the consumption behaviors they show. Not being excluded by the group may require showing behaviors that are compatible with the group. FoMO has a mediating effect in the relationship between problematic smart phone use and the fear of being evaluated positively or negatively (Wolniewicz et al., 2018, p. 618). Therefore, consumers may experience FoMO to be received positively by group members.

FoMO effect can show itself in different sectors when it comes to consumer behavior. Hodkinson (2016, p. 2) stated that FoMO effect is used to influence teenagers and young adults in sectors such as real estate, beer, clothing and female hygiene. Kim et al. (2020) found that FoMO is an important extrinsic motivation in sports activity consumption. The authors stated that the businesses providing sport services which position this service as a popular activity and the consequences of missing out this activity (being excluded, having no information about the subject) may have an effect on consumers by creating FoMO. Researchers working in another sector found that consumers with high FoMO levels visited the account profiles of SMEs more often and bought the products recommended by SMEs and that this situation had a positive effect on consumers' states of being happy (Lee et al., 2021). FoMO effect is also used in games of chance. Those who win high prizes in games of chance are promoted and a perception that they will not miss out on these prizes is created (Özen & Ortaç, 2020, p. 95).

Application such as Facebook, Instagram or Whatsapp offer opportunities for consumers to share time-limited content. For example, features such as content sharing that can be deleted automatically 24 hours later, the ability to delete a message sent to someone else within a specified time and content that does not allow copy may cause consumers to be constantly on the alert. In fact, any moment they are not looking, something can be shared and deleted before they can even they look at it. Therefore, it is important to be online all the time.

FUTURE RESEARCH DIRECTIONS

FoMO is a recent phenomenon. For this reason, although there are studies on FoMO, it can be seen that they are not sufficient in number (Hayran et al., 2020; Elhai et al., 2021). It is thought that this limited number of studies should be replicated and different factors related with the consumer behavior of FoMO should be addressed. Studies conducted show that FoMO effect can be used while persuading consumers to buy. However, it is thought that it will be useful to investigate how FoMO can be used in developing consumer habits that will serve sustainable societies such as sustainable consumption, organic food or energy saving. For example, research that will enable consumers to be more sensitive to carbon foot prints can be included through FoMO.

Research on how FoMO effect shapes consumer behavior on different occupational groups, social status or different cultures will enable a better analysis of consumer behavior. Consumers with similar cultural values show similar consumption habits (Assael, 1992, p. 356). Similarly, consumers with similar economic power show similar purchase behaviors (Hawkins et al., 2004, p. 114). In digital age, consumers have the power to dominate what is happening in the world; however, they tend to adapt to the group they belong to despite this. For example, Kang et al. (2019) found that there is an association between FoMO and herd consumption. For this reason, businesses in global market need to identify the cultural effects and differences of FoMO. For example, Elhai et al. (2021) compared the FoMO levels of German and Spanish participants. It is thought that these studies should be tested in different countries, ethnic origins and cultures so that they can be compared.

It is thought that the extent of FoMO effect in different sectors or different product groups is among the issues that need to be researched. For example, FoMO effect in luxury consumption products may be different when compared with other consumption products.

FoMO effect is measured with different scales (Przybylski et al., 2013; Cheever et al., 2014; Alt et al., 2015; Zhang et al., 2020). It is thought that FoMO levels or reactions of consumers can be measured with neuromarketing. Thanks to developing technology, it is possible to measure the hours consumers are under FoMO effect, how much time they spend on which web pages on the internet during these time periods or what reactions they give to which content (likes, comments, etc.). For example, the purchasing decision of a consumer under the influence of FoMO effect and the purchasing decision of a consumer who is not under this effect can be found by monitoring mobile data.

It is also thought that researching the association of FoMO effect with various factors will provide enlightening information to businesses and researchers. For example, the relationship between FoMO and factors such as price perception, ethnocentric tendencies and ethical values can be emphasized. In addition, there is a need to diversify research on the relationship between personality traits or life styles and FoMO. For example, Aydın et al. (2021, p. 1514) discovered that evening-type consumers are more prone to FoMO. Evening types are consumers who have trouble waking up in the morning, who feel more energetic in the afternoon and who are active in late hours of the day (Suh et al., 2017, p. 2).

The rush of not missing group experience may create FoMO. For example, consumers may boycott various products such as moral reasons, socio-cultural reasons or political reasons. One of the reasons for this boycott may be showing behaviors in accordance with the norms of the group one belongs to. Consumers who are sensitive in this regard feel obliged to follow the developments in digital environment or social media and they can show their consumption behaviors according to these developments. In this context, it can be thought that being prone to a purchase behavior such as boycott increases FoMO. For this reason, it is thought that studies should be conducted on the relationship of FoMO with factors such as nationalism, ethnocentrism or self-construal.

CONCLUSION

It is getting harder for businesses to be different in the eyes of consumers in such a wide variety of products. Businesses trying to be positioned in the minds of consumers in order to be different and to attract attention try to use communication with all its dimensions. Internet and social media have become the most prominent communication tools of our day.

Marketers can use FoMO as a motivation tool to guide the intention to purchase since consumers create an idea and emotion about the product with the information they have in the social media (Abel et al., 2016, p. 41). As a matter of fact, it can be seen that FoMO affects consumer behavior (Marie & Grybs, 2013, p. 263). There is a strong positive correlation between FoMO and the probability of purchase (Good & Hyman, 2020:336).

Rifkin et al. (2015) found that the pleasure expected from the experiences consumers thought they missed increased and 54% of these consumers experienced FoMO during consumption, 22% experienced FoMO before consumption and 30% experienced FoMO after consumption. These statistics about FoMO are an indicator that it is an important problem for consumers of our day. It can be said that Covid-19 pandemic or different extraordinary processes can increase digital addiction and this addiction can have an effect on FoMO. Koban et al. (2022:2) information developed FoMO and this situation was directed with the desire to know about the most recent pandemic information. Another situation is the perception of scarcity that occurs when consumers start to stock various products due to quarantines. Consumers who were exposed to news that some basic needs such as pasta and toilet paper were sold out in supermarkets formed queues to buy these products even if they did not need them. For this reason, it is thought that FoMO is a phenomenon that will keep its actuality.

Although FoMO has an impact on consumption for businesses, extreme fear can affect the well-being of consumers and therefore care should be taken while using FoMO in the field of marketing (Kim et al., 2020). As a matter of fact, like all disciplines, marketing discipline should also adhere to ethical values and should have values in which the welfare of consumers and the society should be a priority.

The future holds digital transformations that are no longer hard to imagine. It seems possible that with Metaverse world, with the virtual reality gradually settling in our lives and with this technology, cities and even all living spaces will turn into marketing areas. The systems of smart glasses that allow for environmental stimuli can soon become a popular application (Appel et al., 2019, p. 133). Perhaps the future in which consumers walking in streets will walk without even having to look around when they are in virtual reality environment. It is even possible to imagine a future in which criminals will be found with one look by combining smart lenses with face recognition systems. In the near future, with these smart lenses or glasses, just by looking around, maybe consumers will be able to see the managers of restaurants, the food in menus, price tags of shops, product options, the distance of their friends in terms of location, what they will experience before buying the products, in short, all their needs. With these reasons, FoMO created by the existing digital age may evolve in different ways or it may be observed in more consumers. As a result, digital transformation and how this transformation affects consumers should be understood well.

REFERENCES

Abel, J. P., Buff, C. L., & Burr, S. A. (2016). Social media and the fear of missing out: Scale development and assessment. *Journal of Business & Economics Research, 14*(1), 33–44. doi:10.19030/jber.v14i1.9554

Alt, D. (2015). College students' academic motivation, media engagement and fear of missing out. *Computers in Human Behavior, 49*, 111–119. doi:10.1016/j.chb.2015.02.057

Alutaybi, A., Al-Thani, D., McAlaney, J., & Ali, R. (2020). Combating fear of missing out (FoMO) on social media: The FoMO-R method. *International Journal of Environmental Research and Public Health, 17*(17), 1–28. doi:10.3390/ijerph17176128 PMID:32842553

Appel, M., Krisch, N., Stein, J. P., & Weber, S. (2019). Smartphone zombies! Pedestrians' distracted walking as a function of their fear of missing out. *Journal of Environmental Psychology, 63*, 130–133. doi:10.1016/j.jenvp.2019.04.003

Argan, M., Argan, M. T., & İpek, G. (2018). I wish i were! Anatomy of a foncumer. *Journal of Internet Applications and Management, 9*(1), 43–57. doi:10.34231/iuyd.407055

Arnold, M. J., & Reynolds, K. E. (2003). Hedonic shopping motivations. *Journal of Retailing, 79*(2), 77–95. doi:10.1016/S0022-4359(03)00007-1

Assael, H. (1992). *Consumer behavior and marketing action*. PWS-KENT Publishing Company.

Aydin, D., Selvi, Y., Kandeger, A., & Boysan, M. (2021). The relationship of consumers' compulsive buying behavior with biological rhythm, impulsivity, and fear of missing out. *Biological Rhythm Research, 52*(10), 1514–1522. doi:10.1080/09291016.2019.1654203

Baker, Z. G., Krieger, H., & LeRoy, A. S. (2016). Fear of missing out:Relationships with depression, mindfulness, and physical symptoms. *Translational Issues in Psychological Science, 2*(3), 275–282. doi:10.1037/tps0000075

Beyens, I., Frison, E., & Eggermont, S. (2016). "I don't want to miss a thing": Adolescents' fear of missing out and its relationship to adolescents' social needs, Facebook use, and Facebook related stress. *Computers in Human Behavior, 64*, 1–8. doi:10.1016/j.chb.2016.05.083

Browne, B. L., Aruguete, M. S., McCutcheon, L. E., & Medina, A. M. (2018). Social and emotional correlates of the fear of missing out. *North American Journal of Psychology, 20*(2), 341–353.

Çetinkaya, F. Ö., & Şahbaz, R. P. (2019). Sosyal medyada gelişmeleri kaçırma korkusunun kişinin tatil satın alma niyetine etkisi [The effect of FoMO on the intention of buying a holiday on social media]. *Türk Turizm Araştırmaları Dergisi, 3*(3), 383–402. doi:10.26677/TR1010.2019.168

Cheever, N. A., Rosen, L. D., Carrier, L. M., & Chavez, A. (2014). Out of sight is not out of mind: The impact of restricting wireless mobile device use on anxiety levels among low, moderate and high users. *Computers in Human Behavior, 3*, 290–197. doi:10.1016/j.chb.2014.05.002

Çopuroğlu, F. (2021). Tüketicilerin sosyal medya kullanımı, fomo ve hedonik tüketim arasındaki ilişki [The relationship between consumers' use of social media, FoMO and hedonic consumption]. *OPUS International Journal of Society Researches, 17*(37), 4298–4326.

Elhai, J. D., Levine, J. C., Alghraibeh, A. M., Alafnan, A. A., Aldraiweesh, A. A., & Hall, B. J. (2018). Fear of missing out: Testing relationships with negative affectivity, online social engagement, and problematic smartphone use. *Computers in Human Behavior, 89*, 289–298. doi:10.1016/j.chb.2018.08.020

Elhai, J. D., Levine, J. C., Dvorak, R. D., & Hall, B. J. (2016). Fear of missing out, need for touch, anxiety and depression are related to problematic smartphone use. *Computers in Human Behavior, 63*, 509–516. doi:10.1016/j.chb.2016.05.079

Elhai, J. D., Yang, H., & Montag, C. (2021). Fear of missing out (FOMO): Overview, theoretical underpinnings, and literature review on relations with severity of negative affectivity and problematic technology use. *The British Journal of Psychiatry, 43*(2), 203–209. doi:10.1590/1516-4446-2020-0870 PMID:32401865

Erciş, A., Deligoz, K., & Mutlu, M. (2021). Öğrencilerin FoMO ve plansiz satin alma davranişlari üzerine bir uygulama [A Study on FoMO and impulsıve purchasing behaviors of students]. *Atatürk Üniversitesi İktisadi ve İdari Bilimler Dergisi, 35*(1), 219–243.

Good, M. C., & Hyman, M. R. (2020). 'Fear of missing out': Antecedents and influence on purchase likelihood. *Journal of Marketing Theory and Practice, 28*(3), 330–341. doi:10.1080/10696679.2020.1766359

Good, M. C., & Hyman, M. R. (2021). Direct and indirect effects of fear-of-missing-out appeals on purchase likelihood. *Journal of Consumer Behaviour, 20*(3), 564–576. doi:10.1002/cb.1885

Gürdin, B. (2019). Sosyal medyanın hedonik tüketimi ve FoMO'nun gücü [Hedonic Consumption Of Social Media And FoMO's Power]. *Üçüncü Sektör Sosyal Ekonomi Dergisi, 54*(3), 1259-1278.

Hawkins, D. I., Best, R. J., & Coney, K. A. (2004). *Consumer behavior*. McGraw-Hill.

Hayran, C., Anik, L., & Gurhan-Canli, Z. (2016). Exploring the antecedents and consumer behavioral consequences of. ACR North American advances. In P. Moreau & S. Puntoni (Eds.), *NA - Advances in Consumer Research* (Vol. 44, pp. 468–468). Association for Consumer Research.

Hayran, C., Anik, L., & Gürhan-Canli, Z. (2020). A threat to loyalty: Fear of missing out (FOMO) leads to reluctance to repeat current experiences. *PLoS One, 15*(4), 1–17. doi:10.1371/journal.pone.0232318 PMID:32353059

Herman, D. (2019). *The Fear of Missing Out*. http://fomofearofmissingout.com/fomo

Hodkinson, C. (2016). 'Fear of Missing Out' (FOMO) marketing appeals: A conceptual model. *Journal of Marketing Communications, 25*(1), 1–24.

Hoşgör, H., Koç Tütüncü, S., Gündüz Hoşgör, D., & Tandoğan, Ö. (2017). Üniversite öğrencileri arasında sosyal medyadaki gelişmeleri kaçırma korkusu yaygınlığının farklı değişkenler açısından incelenmesi [Examination in terms of different variables of prevalence of fear of missing out among college students]. *International Journal of Academic Value Studies., 3*(17), 213–223.

Jood, T. E. (2017). *Missing the present for the unknown: the relationship between fear of missing out (fomo) and life satisfaction* [Unpublished doctoral dissertation]. University of South Africa, Pretoria.

Kaçik, S., & Acar, F. (2020). Üniversite öğrencilerinin gelişmeleri kaçirma korkusu (GKK) ve yaşam doyumu düzeylerinin demografik değişkenler açisindan incelenmesi [The evaluation of fear of missing out (FoMO) and the level of life satisfaction of university students in terms of demographic variables]. *Kayseri Üniversitesi Sosyal Bilimler Dergisi, 2*(1), 74–90.

Kang, I., Cui, H., & Son, J. (2019). Conformity consumption behavior and FoMO. *Sustainability, 11*(17), 1–18. doi:10.3390u11174734

Kemp, S. (2021, Jan). *Digital 2021: The latest insights into the 'state of digital'*. https://wearesocial.com/uk/blog/2021/01/digital-2021-the-latest-insights-into-the-state-of-digital/

Kim, D., Lee, Y., Lee, J., Nam, J. K., & Chung, Y. (2014). Development of Korean smartphone addiction proneness scale for youth. *PLoS One, 9*(5), e97920. doi:10.1371/journal.pone.0097920 PMID:24848006

Kim, J., Lee, Y., & Kim, M. L. (2020). Investigating 'fear of missing out' (FOMO) as an extrinsic motive affecting sport event consumer's behavioral intention and FOMO-driven consumption's influence on intrinsic rewards, extrinsic rewards, and consumer satisfaction. *PLoS One, 15*(12), e0243744. doi:10.1371/journal.pone.0243744

Koban, K., Neureiter, A., Stevic, A., & Matthes, J. (2022). The COVID-19 infodemic at your fingertips. Reciprocal relationships between COVID-19 information FOMO, bedtime smartphone news engagement, and daytime tiredness over time. *Computers in Human Behavior, 130*, 1–8. doi:10.1016/j.chb.2021.107175 PMID:35035063

Lee, J. A., Bright, L. F., & Eastin, M. S. (2021). Fear of missing out and consumer happiness on instagram: A serial mediation of social media influencer-related activities. *Cyberpsychology, Behavior, and Social Networking, 24*(11), 762–766. doi:10.1089/cyber.2020.0431 PMID:33877908

Lee, S. Y., Oh, S., & Jung, S. (2018). Influence of scarcity claims on product evaluation: The role of reversibility of decision. *Social Behavior and Personality, 46*(2), 281–292. doi:10.2224bp.6576

Marie, A., & Grybś, M. (2013). Modern trends in consumer behaviour in era of ecommunication. *Studia Ekonomiczne, 151*, 263–273.

Mazhari, S. (2012). Association between problematic ınternet use and ımpulse control disorders among Iranian university students. *Cyberpsychology, Behavior, and Social Networking, 15*(5), 270–273. doi:10.1089/cyber.2011.0548 PMID:22489545

Milyavskaya, M., Saffran, M., Hope, N., & Koestner, R. (2018). Fear of missing out: Prevalence, dynamics, and consequences of experiencing FOMO. *Motivation and Emotion, 42*(5), 725–737. doi:10.100711031-018-9683-5

Oberst, U., Wegmann, E., Stodt, B., Brand, M., & Chamarro, A. (2017). Negative consequences from heavy social networking in adolescents: The mediating role of fear of missing out. *Journal of Adolescence, 55*(1), 51–60. doi:10.1016/j.adolescence.2016.12.008 PMID:28033503

Özen, A. & Ortaç, S. (2020). Gelişmeleri takip edememe kaygısı (fear of missing out) ve piyasa örneklemleri [Fear of missing out and market samples]. *İzmir Sosyal Bilimler Dergisi, 2*(2), 92-97.

Park, C., & Lee, T. M. (2009). Antecedents of online reviews' usage and purchase influence: An empirical comparison of U.S. and Korean consumers. *Journal of Interactive Marketing, 23*(4), 332–340. doi:10.1016/j.intmar.2009.07.001

Przybylski, A. K., Murayama, K., DeHaan, C. R., & Gladwell, V. (2013). Motivational, emotional, and behavioral correlates of fear of missing out. *Computers in Human Behavior, 29*(4), 1814–1848. doi:10.1016/j.chb.2013.02.014

Rifkin, J., Cindy, C., & Kahn, B. (2015). FoMO: how the fear of missing out leads to missing out. In K. Diehl & C. Yoon (Eds.), *ACR North American Advances* (Vol. 43, pp. 244–248). Duluth, MN: Association for Consumer Research.

Riordan, B. C., Flett, J. A. M., Hunter, J. A., Scarf, D., & Conner, T. S. (2015). Fear of missing out (FoMO): The relationship between FoMO, alcohol use, and alcohol-related consequences in college students. *Journal of Psychiatry and Brain Functions, 2*(9), 1–7.

Ryan, R., & Deci, E. (2000). Self – Determination theory and the facilitation of intrinsic motivation, social development and well- being. *The American Psychologist, 55*(1), 68–78. doi:10.1037/0003-066X.55.1.68 PMID:11392867

Suh, S., Yang, H. C., Kim, N., Yu, J. H., Choi, S., Yun, C. H., & Shin, C. (2017). Chronotype differences in health behaviors and health-related quality of life: A population-based study among aged and older adults. *Behavioral Sleep Medicine*, *15*(5), 361–376. doi:10.1080/15402002.2016.1141768 PMID:27148632

Whiting, A., & Williams, D. (2013). Why people use social media: Uses and gratifications approach. *Qualitavite Market Research: An International Journal, 16*(4), 362-369.

Wolniewicz, C. A., Tiamiyu, M. F., Weeks, J. W., & Elhai, J. D. (2018). Problematic smartphone use and relations with negative affect, fear of missing out, and fear of negative and positive evaluation. *Psychiatry Research*, *262*, 618–623. doi:10.1016/j.psychres.2017.09.058 PMID:28982630

Yıldırım, S., & Kişioğlu, A. N. (2018). Teknolojinin getirdiği yeni hastaliklar: Nomofobi, Netlessfobi, Fomo [New diseases due to technology: Nomophobia, netlessphobia, FoMO]. *Sdü Tıp Fakültesi Dergisi*, *25*(4), 473–480.

Zhang, Z., Jiménez, F. R., & Cicala, J. E. (2020). Fear of missing out scale: A self-concept perspective. *Psychology and Marketing*, *37*(11), 1619–1634. doi:10.1002/mar.21406

ADDITIONAL READING

Alt, D. (2015). College students' academic motivation, media engagement and fear of missing out. *Computers in Human Behavior*, *49*, 111–119. doi:10.1016/j.chb.2015.02.057

Beyens, I., Frison, E., & Eggermont, S. (2016). "I don't want to miss a thing": Adolescents' fear of missing out and its relationship to adolescents' social needs, Facebook use, and Facebook related stress. *Computers in Human Behavior*, *64*, 1–8. doi:10.1016/j.chb.2016.05.083

Blackwell, D., Leaman, C., Tramposch, R., Osborne, C., & Liss, M. (2017). Extraversion, neuroticism, attachment style and fear of missing out as predictors of social media use and addiction. *Personality and Individual Differences*, *116*, 69–72. doi:10.1016/j.paid.2017.04.039

Elhai, J. D., Levine, J. C., Dvorak, R. D., & Hall, B. J. (2016). Fear of missing out, need for touch, anxiety and depression are related to problematic smartphone use. *Computers in Human Behavior*, *63*, 509–516. doi:10.1016/j.chb.2016.05.079

Elhai, J. D., Yang, H., & Montag, C. (2021). Fear of missing out (FOMO): Overview, theoretical underpinnings, and literature review on relations with severity of negative affectivity and problematic technology use. *The British Journal of Psychiatry*, *43*(2), 203–209. doi:10.1590/1516-4446-2020-0870 PMID:32401865

Herman, D. (2019). The Fear of Missing Out. http://fomofearofmissingout.com/fomo

Hodkinson, C. (2016). 'Fear of Missing Out'(FOMO) marketing appeals: A conceptual model. *Journal of Marketing Communications*, *25*(1), 1–24.

Przybylski, A. K., Murayama, K., DeHaan, C. R., & Gladwell, V. (2013). Motivational, emotional, and behavioral correlates of fear of missing out. *Computers in Human Behavior*, *29*(4), 1814–1848. doi:10.1016/j.chb.2013.02.014

KEY TERMS AND DEFINITIONS

Consumer: They are individuals, groups, or institutions that buy or have the capacity to purchase products to meet their wants and needs.

Consumer Behavior: It is the emotional, mental and behavioral reactions of consumers in the purchasing decision process.

FoMO (The Fear of Missing Out): It is the fear of not being aware of the events in the digital world.

Metaverse: It is a three-dimensional virtual space where social life, commerce and all interactions can be experienced in the virtual reality world.

Perceived Scarcity: It is the perception of consumers that the accessibility of the product they demand is decreasing.

Problematic Internet Use: It is the situation where consumers use the internet at a level they cannot fulfill their responsibilities and have problems in their social relations and cannot control it.

Social Media: They are online resources where the individual or corporate digital content can be shared.

Chapter 9
Truth Trying to Survive:
Reality Perception in Survivor Programs

Ufuk İnal
Ondokuz Mayıs University, Turkey

Elif Şevik İnal
https://orcid.org/0000-0002-7590-2258
Marmara University, Turkey

ABSTRACT

The place where most of us face the perception of reality in the pre-internet social life consists of a miraculous glowing box in the focal point of our rooms. Television is perhaps one of the most basic media tools that create our perception of reality by using the power of sound and image. The urge to believe what you see continues to make us addicted to this device. Television audience surveys in Turkey show that Turkish people watch television for an average of 4.5 hours a day. Considering that the average person works 8 hours a day and sleeps 8 hours, it is understood that people spend more than half of their free time in front of the television. With the use of the internet in all areas of social life, an average of 3 hours of leisure time consumption of people is devoted to social media. This situation reveals that television has a very serious competitor in directing our perception of reality. This study is about the construction of reality in the Survivor program, which is the most consumed competition program on Turkish television.

INTRODUCTION

What should come to mind when we say reality? Is today's society a society of reality? Should we start the discussion here? Is truth a subjective concept? Is there a concept of relative truth? In what context should we consider the concept we are discussing? All these questions are just a few of the dozens of questions we come across in order to make judgments about today's society. The reason behind the intense discussion of the concept lately is the artificial environment that we have to face today, namely the internet. So, is it right to blame the reality debate only on the internet?

DOI: 10.4018/978-1-7998-9251-9.ch009

Television is one of the essential devices that make up our perception of reality in daily life. Many studies conducted in academia reveal how, to what extent, and how this tool affects people. This study focuses on the intersection of television, reality, and social media, based on the studies. One of the central problems of this research is that a new form of influencing the audience replaced some of the audience that was only affected by television until recently. This audience, which can also be defined as a new generation audience or influencing audience, uses various web tools to influence television broadcasts. One of the most popular social media platforms, Twitter, is one of these tools. Therefore, this study focuses on the Survivor competition, a program with a high potential to influence the broadcast content of the audience. The importance of the reality created in the online environment emerges at this stage. Because in this medium, people can not only look at events from their windows by building their reality but also shape the perceptions of other users' reality. This possibility requires evaluating the concepts of television, social media, audience, and reality on a standard level.

NARRATIVE FORMS AND TELEVISION

Communication systems cover the process of creating specific coding systems and making sense of the designed coding systems. One of the essential communication tools of daily life, which we create to communicate, on which we reach consensus, is letters and graphic systems, that is, language. According to Özbay (2005, p. 68), language; Requires listening, speaking, reading, and writing skills. These four skills constitute the most crucial distinction distinguishing human beings from other beings. At the same time, language is an organism in which a person can express herself and what is going on around her.

Man is a social being, and the instinct to tell requires the construction of such structures. The construction process is a gradual process that takes time. Koç states that children can understand the primary graphic and sequencing structure of the language created when they are 3-4 years old. In the following periods, children gain the ability to differentiate and organize these graphics and sequences as more complex structures. After a while, they learn how to benefit from the rich possibilities of the language by establishing relationships of place, time and reason about the developments in their environment. They acquire this skill from the narratives they have known from the stories since their early ages (51: 1993).

Narrative is a form of construction. According to Atabek, the cornerstone of the construction process is communication. In this respect, narrative is accepted as one of the essential elements that make up culture like language (1992, p. 339). All kinds of experiences obtained from experiences are multiplied and shared with narratives. Çetin states that when people could not store their information with permanent texts such as writing, they used narratives to store, organize and transmit information (1999, p. 8). Yücel bases the narrative on words. According to him, it is possible to evaluate the statements containing the word as a kind of narrative (1988, p. 14). On the other hand, according to Yılmaz, a literary text is not a narrative; therefore, not every narrative may have a literary content (2017, p. 693). These two approaches constitute the primary distinction of narratology studies that focus on the theory of narrative structures.

The first approach to what a narrative is only accepted oral text transfers as narratives. The second approach considers any text that contains a story as a narrative. According to Yılmaz, scenarios such as novels, short stories, narrative poems, plays, films, and operas can be evaluated under the second category as a kind of narrative text. The narratives performed are plays, films, and operas. Screenplay, narrative poems, novels, and short stories are also written narratives (2017, p. 693). Considering that there are too many narratives in the world to count, as Roland Barthes mentioned, it can be observed that each new day welcomes the masses with a new type of narrative. Barthes' interpretation on this subject is based on language, which is the basis of the narrative. Language can be used through a variety of tools to create message content. In other words, in addition to verbal, written, and visual messages, even hand, arm, and head movements can be used to create messages, that is, as narrative tools (2005, p. 11).

Based on the discourse that narrative components can be transmitted through different channels, it seems reasonable to consider today's most common communication tools as visual and auditory narrative tools. It can be said that a sound is a form of construction in radio broadcasting. Likewise, visual and auditory elements constitute the entire narrative language of television productions. The images to be created will sprout over the texts. These texts are translated into the language specific to television. In other words, descriptive elements based on writing, like in a novel or story narrative, are not used in this narrative form. In television productions, a kind of influence on the mental level is used with certain usage forms of audio-visual elements (Yılmaz & Erdem, 2016:244; İlerialkan & Yılmaz, 2015, pp. 21-25).

The Narrative Structure of Television and Reality

Television can be defined as a device that creates a narrative using visual and auditory elements. However, this definition will not suffice to explain the primary function of television. Because television is a structure that influences the mind with the light clusters, it contains the visuals and sounds it reflects on the screen. In this structure, the visuals are repeated, reflected in sync with the sounds, and aimed to influence the audience. Thanks to its visual narrative power, television is ahead of other mass media in its power to influence the masses (Taskiran & Yilmaz, 2015, p. 7; Gürer, 2016, p. 69).

Television is a tool that puts people in the center. The images projected on the screen provide the best visual perception with various camera uses (Gürer, 2016, p. 72). Camera technologies can reflect a limited area. For this reason, a part of the visual field captured by the camera should be chosen so that it can be quickly completed in the human mind. The pieces selected from the existing universe are built in line with the thought desired to be created in the human mind.
Aziz describes the narrative characteristic of television as follows:

- The existing universe is miniaturized.
- Icons appearing on the screen indicate parts of the general.
- Sound is a helpful element in designing this universe.
- There is no complete silence.
- It has an aspect that makes the person passive (2006- 65).

This language that Aziz describes is created by blending it with reality. Television feeds on reality. With visual and auditory expression techniques, the audience builds a reality on the audience or reflects the reality as it is (Gürer, 2016, p. 69). These visuals, built within the boundaries of reality, flow away before the audience has a chance to think that they are deception or fiction. At this point, Millerson states that the audience is not willing to think about this issue either. At this point, the audience's expectation is more about whether the content is interesting, entertaining, gripping, intriguing, or enjoyable than its relationship with reality (2009, p. 7). Gürer and Gürer point out that today individuals tend to have emotional needs rather than vital needs. This situation has caused individuals to seek pleasure. Television is experienced as a result of seeking pleasure (2017, p. 1172).

The process of feeding on reality is shaped by imitating or identifying. In the tiredness of daily life, individuals adopt and prefer television content that they reach effortlessly. The experiences presented to individuals through different stories eliminate their loneliness and distract them from the sense of responsibility and stress (Özel ve Durmaz, 2021, p. 367). In this process, the audience may tend to imitate the characters they see on the screen daily. In this way, the audience is affected by the content they are exposed to at the maximum level. In connection with the exposure process, he can perceive the reality he sees on the screen as his reality after a while. This situation can be explained by the effect of fast getting used to the television and other mass media. Television offers high-speed information without allowing the viewer to question. The rapid presentation of separate parts of life out of context accelerates this process (Emir, 2003, pp. 144- 145).

The audio-visual world of television leads the audience to emulate and emulate what they see on the screen. The interaction rate increases gradually, primarily when it works with a dramatic narrative structure combined with the screen's lives, characters, atmospheres, and emotions. The atmosphere designed on the screen reflects the relationship between reality and the life that the audience dreams of. Careful life patterns keep the goals and expectations of the audience alive, renew them and satisfy their pleasure (Gürer & Gürer, 2017, p. 1172).

The natural flow of daily life within the narrative structure of television causes the audience to create shared expectations by playing with the perception of reality. A new world is presented to the audience with fiction and non-fiction content. This world, where the boundaries of reality and fiction are thoroughly eroded, is the entertainment expectation of the audience. Entertainment is the main theme of today's commercial television broadcasting. In order to reach large audiences, commercial televisions feature content based on reality shows, commercial films, soap operas, competitions and comedy programs. On the other hand, in increasing competition, innovative, dynamic, and hybrid formats have begun to emerge. Within the framework of the requirements of the modern world, television programs tend toward breakthroughs in terms of content and technique. This situation brings with it breakthroughs. The use of the internet and new media instruments have enabled television programs to come into existence in different forms (Gürer, 2016, pp. 69- 91).

In the new order, along with the narrative structure of television, there are also changes in the audience. The use of Web 2.0 and 3.0 is becoming more and more common day by day. This ensures that the audience can easily be included in the television content. In this system, mediated by social media platforms, television viewers have now reached the position of being both affected and influenced. The new audience, which Bolat describes as an active audience, can produce and design its content (2020, p. 123).

THE POST-TRUTH CONCEPT

The general orientation in research on the concept is shaped by the axis of politics, media, and social sciences. The effect of the concept on society and how this power is used can be accepted as a common point of academic studies. The general opinion in the literature is that the concept of Post-truth emerged with Keyes. However, current research reveals that this concept is based on a different basis. In 1992, Serbian-American writer Steve Tesich used the concept of post-truth in an article. The meaning it attributes to the concept is giving up on reality and ignoring reality. However, Keyes attributed a political meaning to this concept as it is known (D'Ancona, 2017). For this reason, it is essential not to ignore the fact that the concept is shaped in the hands of different disciplines.

Economists have defined this concept as having no basis of truth but is believed to be accurate. This is the general opinion about the definition of the concept. In this context, it can be said that the idea of the post-truth world, which is frequently spoken today, points to a worldview where "every individual's opinion is considered to be at least as important as the other's, and therefore everything is subjective. Of course, the effect of social media in the creation of such an environment is enormous. The use of social media by millions of people, the enormous width of the information network due to the structure of the system, and the incalculable speed of information flow are the most significant factors in the formation of this system. However, it would be a wrong approach to say that only social media allows subjective information flow. Because in today's media age, it is evident that the media tools that we describe as traditional use social media connections, which are individual production tools, as a news source (Prado, 2018, pp. 7- 9). As Oxford Dictionary editor Casper Grathwohl stated, the concept was born and continues to evolve in social media environments where the level of credibility is gradually decreasing (Petters, 2018, p. 145).

Hannah Arendt emphasized that the point on which today's society can be called a post-truth society is not just a break with traditions but that this is an inevitable acceleration. On the other hand, Tracy B. Strong, who works in political thoughts at Southampton University, discussed the use of right and wrong in politics and Trump's discourse in the preface he wrote to Baron's book. At the center of the discussion, he emphasizes the importance of the context of truth. According to Strong, it is not a matter of discussion unless proper validation is required. The meaning loaded on it determines the context of the truth. To take the example of Trump, Trump is saying the wrong thing. Although he knows that what he is saying is wrong, he disapproves of it. However, he does not hesitate to say what he knows to be wrong as if it were true. At this point, the context gains value. Because the truth and falsity of what is said according to its contexts are related to the situation encountered. Therefore, in this discussion, an attitude emerges that if a lie is used for a purpose, its accuracy does not matter. In this regard, Trump's spokesperson said that "anything is true if enough people believe it." discourse clarifies the meaning created on the concept (Baron, 2018, pp. 10- 12).

After the Trump incident, a video taken at the Adventist Church during a woman's coronation ceremony attracted attention. The speeches in the video contain slander and hate speech against women's priesthood. It is claimed that those who support women to become priests serve the devil. Although this video does not resonate as much as the Trump case within the scope of post-truth, it is shown as a practical advertisement example (Manners, 2017, p. 15). These and similar examples show that social media messages have begun to guide perception management. This power that social media has in its content has also attracted the attention of media tools that can direct the perception of society. As Şen stated, traditional media tools incorporate new forms every day. This situation changes the distribution and consumption of media outputs (2021, p. 57). New media environments, where the source and target of the message that we are familiar with from traditional media tools change direction from time to time, offer a space that they have not experienced before. In this space, where the message flow is instantaneous and bidirectional, individuals eliminate geographical boundaries. This situation provides the formation of a global cultural network in which new common values sprout. Thus, this space triggers the creation of new possibilities in the media. With the change in individuals' media consumption habits, the media produces new forms of production (Kılınç, 2017, p. 122).

SURVIVOR PROGRAM AND NARRATIVE STRUCTURE USED

Television programs refer to the combination of images prepared using the television's technical features within the appropriate broadcast zone, in line with the determined target audience, for specific purposes (Bolat, 2016, p. 75). Therefore, it contains many types and format features. The program that will be focused on in this study is Survivor Allstar 2022. Survivor is a program format that has been translated into a competition format for the process of experiencing wildlife by a group of people. It has been projected on television screens in different parts of the world since the 90s. The format of the program is shaped in line with the cultural values and the concern of being watched in the regions where it is broadcast. Survivor, as Gürer emphasizes, is a hybrid genre that includes both reality show and game show features. In one of the first examples of the species published in Australia, two groups of humans were released into the wild. Competitors were given only materials such as matches and knives and were expected to survive. Competitors had to build their own shelters, find food and feed themselves, and ensure their safety by being protected from the wild. Competitors found water sources, built wooden shelters, and had to eat everything they could find, from various fish to monkeys, not to starve. This method has been preferred to carry the program to the heights of reality. In fact, in the British version of the program, the contestants unwittingly caught and ate an endangered crocodile species. In the American version of the program, the contestants had to eat things like maggots and giblets to be successful and not be hungry. Such uses preferred in the competition are the items that fill the content of the reality show theme. On the other hand, competition elements are also used in the program. What is expected from the teams is to win the determined competition games. Winning these games based on physical strength and struggle is not enough for them to win the competition. Contestants, however, must win the appreciation of the audience. Because the audience can determine the future of the contestants in the program. For this reason, attention is paid to ensuring that the contestants prefer to participate in the program and have their counterparts in the target audience.

In the competition, where physical appearance and popularity are as important as fighting power, names such as models, singers, social media phenomena, cinema, and theater actors are included in the teams. The potential of each preferred competitor to create a fan base is emphasized. This part of the work is the program's link with social media. Competitors with popularity are supported through social media. This situation leads to the inclusion of the audience in the program content. While the viewers determine the contestants' future from the SMS numbers determined for the contestants, they try to influence the voting behavior of other program viewers with the tags (Hashtag) they create on social media.

The possibility of creating a sensation with the relations and discourses of the contestants selected by considering the demographic data is not overlooked. The conflict elements necessary for the average television viewer to stay on the screen can also be established through the relationships of these characters. The audience on social media discusses conflicts in the program through the program label.

Regional values are used in determining the teams that will compete in Survivor programs. In order to create a competitive environment, the competitors were determined according to their races in the United States. In a different program broadcast in the region, the teams were divided according to their mental and physical strength. Since the competition requires physical struggle, the competitors are mostly chosen from people with a sports background. In Survivor, published in Turkey, competitors are selected from national and international professional athletes such as swimmers, athletes, football players, rowers, boxers, and wrestlers. It can be said that the selected athletes are positioned as a representative from each branch. This shows that the influence of the competitors on the audience in their branch is considered essential. It has been seen that the athletes of the clubs with the most supporters in football, traditional or social media in other branches, or those who have the potential to be, are preferred. Thus, to meet the expectations of the target audience, a wide-ranging competition group is formed.

In Turkey, Survivor has been organized by Acun Medya, headed by Acun Ilıcalı, since 2006. The program was broadcast on Show TV for five years and was successful in ratings. The program, whose broadcasting rights were transferred to Star TV in 2013, was broadcast on this channel for two years and increased its screen success. In 2015, Acun Ilıcalı crowned his success in television programs by establishing his channel. Acun Ilıcalı, who bought the TV8 channel, also established the TV8.5 television channel and broadcasted the Survivor program on these two channels. The program is broadcast in primetime on TV8, six days a week. The Survivor Panorama program, in which the topics in the program are discussed, appears on the screen every day of the week during the daytime. In addition to these, the Survivor Extra program, which includes former contestants, is broadcast immediately after the program. On the other hand, the Survivor Panaraoma program is broadcast on TV8.5 screens just before the Survivor program starts. Repetitions of the program can be watched on the TV8 website. Another communication organ belonging to Acun Media is the website called acunn.com. On this website, essential details that are not broadcast on television are presented to the audience. This website presents essential details that are not broadcast on television to the audience. Thus, the program is presented to the audience on different platforms in the form of transmedia storytelling (İnal & Şevik, 2017, p. 200).

In Survivor, published in Turkey, two teams are formed every year among famous names and selected volunteers from the public. In this year's version of the program, famous and volunteer contestants who received the best grades in Survivor programs, previously broadcast in Turkey, took place. For this reason, the name of the program has been determined as Survivor All Star. 36 contestants compete in the program this year. Since the competition games are based on strength and struggle, reserve players are also included in the program, where many injuries are experienced. In addition, there are players instead of the disqualified contestants for not following the rules. So far, 26 as ten substitutes appear to have been involved in the competition.

The competition rules require players to be successful both as a team and individually. Winning the team game is vital in two ways. The first is about which team the eliminated competitor will be selected from. Another importance is related to supply support. Competitors obtain support supplies that can fill their bellies by winning team games. In addition, there are also individual competitions. The competitors try to win the immunity prize in these competitions by competing individually. Candidates who win the immunity award are formed from the qualifying pot. In the elimination system, the audience also plays a decisive role. Who will be eliminated from the team that lost the team game first determines the friends' votes for that team? The names of the candidates to be eliminated from the team are determined. The determined names must be chosen from those who do not have an immunity award. The competitor who receives the least of SMS among the competitors entering the qualifying pot leaves the competition. At this point, the social media messages of the audience come into play. Social media tags play an essential role in the narrative structure of the program. The label of the program changes every broadcast period. This year, the social media tag of the program has been determined as #survivor2022allstar. This label is kept on the screen from time to time during the program. It is expected that the audience who produces discourse about the program will meet with a single stakeholder. This will enable the content produced in traditional media to be strengthened in various ways by social media environments.

In this study, the descriptive analysis method, a frequently used research method in the field of social sciences, was used. The universe and sample of the study were determined through the #survivorallstar2022 tag. The number of tweets sent from the day the SMS sending event started (5.03.2022) to the day it ended (09.03.2022) in the competition was obtained from www.brand24.com data. According to the data obtained from the site, this tag was used 513,285 times during the SMS sending activity. In quantitative research, the sample of the universe of this size is stated as 370. The most interacting 370 messages were categorized according to various themes in this context. In the research, some of the tweets posted on the #survivorallstar2022 hashtag, which was determined institutionally by the Survivor AllStar Turkey competition, were examined. Tweets were randomly selected under the popular tweets tab on Twitter.

Table 1. Types of profiles interacting through the tag

#survivorallstar2022	370	
On behalf of Contestant Fans	44	Seems to be a supporter in profile. Not understood to be biased in profile.
On behalf of Survivor Fans	12	
People who changed their name	4	
Changing both	3	
People Who Changed Profile Photo	45	
Independent Individual	262	Not understood to be a supporter as a profile.

The table above calculated the tweets shared with the hashtag #survivorallstar2022 by what kind of profiles were produced. These profile types consist of primarily independent individuals. The category of independent individuals refers to the absence of any guiding or partisan content about the competition in the profile photo or profile name. In the category of those who changed their profile photo, there are individuals whose profile photo is one of the contestants. The category of those who changed their name refers to the profiles in which the profile name has been changed to match the terms of the contestants. Those who changed both their profile photo and their name were named as those who changed both. On behalf of Survivor fans, the category is a classification with a profile photo and messages about the survivor contest. It includes profiles based on supporting a determined competitor in the category on behalf of the contestant fans.

The second important element in the categorization is related to the bias or neutrality of the messages of the determined categories. Individuals whose profile photo and profile name do not influence the contest or the competitor are described as "not understood to be a supporter as a profile." In the category "Apparently as a supporter as a profile," it is expressed that the user's profile photo or name consists of text or images about the contest or the contestant.

Table 2. Engagement rates of tweets

Number of Tweets	**370**	**Total**
Retweeted	364	7398
Liked	367	79.027
Answered	145	1238

In the table above, 370 messages, which are thought to represent the total number of tweets between the dates when the voting started and ended, were examined. The data shows that 364 of 370 tweets were recirculated, 367 were liked, and 145 were answered. On the other hand, it is seen that 364 messages were retweeted 7398 times, 367 liked messages were liked 79,027 times in total, and 145 replied messages were replied to 1238 times.

THE EFFECT OF REALITY CREATED ON TWITTER ON THE *SURVIVOR* CONTEST

Survivor All-Star 2022 started this season on January 15, 2022. According to the data obtained from the www.getdaytrends.com website, the #SurvivorAllStar2022 tag has succeeded in entering the country's plan on the days and hours of the broadcast. Almost every day the program was broadcast, this label became the plan, and thousands of people became partners in this interaction network.

In the examination, it was observed that many non-corporate accounts were used in the name of the competition. Except for the anonymous accounts, it was seen that all of the candidates participating in the contest had one or more fan pages. In addition, it has been observed that some individuals following the competition have attached the candidates they support to their profile photos or next to their names. Individuals, supporters of the contestants, fan pages, or simple individuals produced various discourses through the program's social media hashtags. These discourses are the realities of individuals themselves. Therefore, these realities can have a manipulative effect on other individuals.

When we look at the tables, it is understood that the interaction day of the messages created by the audience during the voting period is high. According to Table 2, even only 370 messages seem to have been recirculated 7398 times. It is seen in Table 1 that 108 of the 370 messages produced are from the fan base following the program. Twelve of this number are accounts that only produce content for the Survivor program. It is not thought that these accounts will affect voting and changing the program content.

On the other hand, 44 of the 108 people drew attention to the fan pages of the contestants. It can be predicted that these accounts will be followed by the audience that already supports a specific competitor. In terms of the power to influence the program content, it is a fact that the fan pages can control the voting potential with the content they produce. However, it is thought that it will not change the existing voting opinion. It is estimated that those who follow these pages already have the potential to vote for a competitor. Therefore, it can be said that the activities of fan pages to increase voting status will have a negligible effect on television content.

According to the research findings, it was determined that 52 people used their names, images or both in a way to remind them of the competitor. It can be said that this audience, which produces content on the determined label, is the most objective segment in the category of 108 people, who seem to be biased in terms of profile. The objective concept mentioned here arises from the fact that these profiles use accounts that state that they support the competitor, albeit partially instead of an individual account. It can be said that these content producers did not create their accounts to support this competitor. This shows that the contestants selected for the program impact the audience. This effect brought the audience to the size of a competitor fan and a fan. Therefore, the power of this audience to influence and change the voting potential of different individuals will be higher than others.

According to the data obtained, it is seen that 262 of the 370 messages examined were produced by individuals independent of the competition as profiles. In other words, the purpose of using these accounts is not just to generate messages for this program. Therefore, the content created by these people will not reach only Survivor-loving audiences. It turns out that people who have no ties to the program will be exposed to these messages. In this context, it can be said that 262 independent profiles create a more robust interaction environment than the accounts that make up the remaining 108 messages. It is thought that this situation directly affects the reach of the program messages to a vast audience. It can be said that the fact that the program tags are among the tags with the most potent interaction on the day they are broadcast is directly related to this situation. The findings obtained from the research indicate that almost all of the posts made on the created tag have the potential to receive interaction. This can be explained by the fact that the program is interesting. It is seen that the content shared through the program tag has a powerful potential to change the reality perception of the audience. This research conducted during the qualifying period shows that the future of the contestants can be determined by sharing this tag. It is thought that survivor, which contains the features of Reality Show and documentary genres, gradually thins the boundaries of reality and fiction on the audience. It has been observed that the audience reproduces the reality part of this story, which also exists, through the contents created on social media, with their perception. Therefore, the fiction produced in the traditional medium has become a reality in the minds of the audience. After passing this fact through his filter, the audience supports the reality construction of the people related to the subject by putting it into production on social media channels. At this point, it is seen that this transformation has become an indispensable part of the monitoring process.

CONCLUSION

Survivor is one of the most-watched reality shows on Turkish television. To examine the program on a daily post-truth level, its extensions on the Twitter platform were reviewed for a certain period. During the research, it was revealed that the hashtags created on behalf of the program, especially on the broadcast days, were one of the most popular topics. Messages sent to the label opened on behalf of the program were evaluated under common themes. The obtained data reveal that some of the messages sent under the label are manipulated, and some are for entertainment purposes. On the other hand, all of the messages sent serve to reconstruct reality in the social media environment. Individuals combined their subjective realities with objective data and shared them through the labels created on behalf of the program. Moreover, this reality narrative structure was created based on visual and auditory elements in a fictional tool. In other words, the reality created on television, which is fiction based on it, has been disconnected from the context of reality intertwined with virtual reality. The Survivor competition program examined is content open to the guidance of the audience. When evaluated in this context, it can be seen that the messages sent under the program label aim to highlight the candidate supported in the program. In the sample examined, it can be said that the audience feeding the label serves this purpose not only with their discourse but also with their profile photos and profile names. Some individuals use the names and images of the candidates they support on their profile pages and discourses. On the contrary, it has been seen that some of them produce discourse without giving any clue about the candidate they support. This situation is associated with the objectivity of the created reality. However, it is clear that individuals who prefer both approaches have the power to create a manipulative effect. From the point of view of the structure forming the narrative, the use of social media tags in the program's content has created a profit in every respect. The discourse created in a traditional media tool has had a strong impact in online environments. This seems to have increased the impact and the level of appreciation of the program. Both cases have proven the success of the program. In all this content bombardment, only reality has been lost.

REFERENCES

Atabek, Y. (1992). Narrative by Theorists [Kuramcılara Göre Anlatı.]. *Kurgu Dergisi, 11*, 339.

Aziz, A. (2006). *Television and Radio Broadcasting* [Televizyon ve Radyo Yayıncılığı]. Turhan Yayıncılığı.

Baron, I. Z. (2018). *How to save politics in a post-truth era*. Manchester University Press. doi:10.7765/9781526126832

Barthes, R. (2005). *Semiotic Adventure* [Göstergebilimsel Serüven] (R. Mehmet & R. Sema, Trans.). Yapı Kredi Yayınları.

Bolat, N. (2016). Effect of Image Tekniks in The Fact that Feudal Content Series Do Not Reach High Audience in Modern Turkey: Karagül Series [Modern Türkiye'de Feodal İçerikli Dizilerin Yüksek İzleyiciye Ulaşmadında Görüntü Tekniklerinin Etkisi: Karagül Dizisi]. *Middle Black Sea Journal of Communication Studies, 1*(2), 69–86.

Bolat, N. (2020). The Impact of The Technical Transformation of Television on Content. Televizyonun Teknik Dönüşümünün İçeriğe Etkisi. In E. Sirer (Ed.), *Yeni İzlence Yeni İzlerkitle* (pp. 107–126). Literatürk.

Çetin, Z. (1999). *The Introduction of a Narrative Form, The Novel, to Cinema* [Bir Anlatı Formu Olan Romanın Sinemaya Uyarlanması]. Marmara Üniversitesi Sosyal Bilimler Enstitüsü Radyo Televizyon ve Sinema Anabilim Dalı Doktora Tezi.

D'ancona, M. (2017). *Post Truth The New War on Truth and How to Fight Back*. Ebury Press.

Emir, İ. Y. (2003). *Image in Mass Communication* [Kitle İletişiminde İmaj]. İletiş-im Kitapları.

Gürer, M. (2016) Narrative Structure of Television and Hybridization In Television Programs [Televizyonun anlatı Yapısı ve Televizyon Programlarında Hibritleşme Süreci]. *International Peer-Reviewed Journal of Communication and Humanities Research*, 69-94.

Gürer, S. Z., & Gürer, M. (2017). The Sunumu of "Pretentious Consumption" on the Axis of Lives Designed on Television: An Example of a Bold and Beautiful Series [Televizyonda Tasarlanan Hayatlar Ekseninde "Gösterişçi Tüketimin" Sunumu: Cesur ve Güzel Dizisi Örneği]. *Uluslararası Sosyal Araştırmalar Dergisi, 10*(51), 1160–1173.

İlerialkan, D., & Yılmaz, R. (2015). *How to Write a Script, How Do They Write?* [Senaryo Nasıl Yazılır? Nasıl Yazıyorlar?]. Alfa Yayınları.

İnal, U. & Şevik E. (2017). Facebook Usage of Turkey's 10 Most Listened Radios. [Türkiye'nin En Çok Dinlenen 10 Radyosunun Facebook Kullanımı]. *Ulakbilge Sosyal Bilimler, 5*(9), 199-230.

Kılınç, U. (2017). Create It! Extend It!: Evolution of Comics Through Narrative Advertising. In R. Yılmaz (Ed.), *Narrative Advertising Models and Conceptualization in the Digital Age* (pp. 117–132). IGI Global. doi:10.4018/978-1-5225-2373-4.ch007

Koç, A. A. (1993). Conceptual and Linguistic Development of Narrative Structure [Anlatı Yapısının Kavramsal ve Dilsel Gelişimi]. *Dilbilim Araştırmaları Dergisi, 4*, 51–60.

Manners, B. (2017). Being Adventist in A Post-Truth World. *Advntist Record,* 14-15.

Millerson, G. (2009). *Production and Management on Television* [Televizyonda Yapım ve Yönetim]. Tur-Gen Yayınları.

Özbay, M. (2005). Writing as a Science and Culture Transceasor [Bilim ve Kültür Aktarıcısı Olarak Yazı]. *Hacettepe Üniversitesi Türkiyat Araştırmaları Dergisi, 2*, 67–74.

Özel, S., & Durmaz, T. (2021). Next Generation Monitoring Practices: Watching [Yeni Nesil İzleme Pratikleri: Tıkınırcasına İzlemek]. *Marmara Üniversitesi Öneri Dergisi, 16*(55), 363–388.

Petters, M. A. (2018). *Education in a Post-truth World. In Truth, Fake News*. Springer.

Prado, C. G. (2018). *America's Post-Truth Phenomenon*. ABC-Clio, LLC.

Şen, O. (2021) Robot Journalism [Robot Gazetecilik]. In Gazetecilikte Uzmanlaşma alanları (pp. 57-75). Pelikan Yayınevi.

Yılmaz, R. (2017) Typology of Metaleptic Uses in Television Advertisements [Televizyon Reklamlarında Metaleptik Kullanımların Tipolojisi]. E-gifder, 5(2), 691[704.

Yılmaz, R., & Erdem, M. N. (2016). *Traditional and Digital Advertising in 150 Questions* [150 Soruda Geleneksel ve Dijital Reklamcılık]. Umuttepe Yayınları.

Yılmaz, R., & Taskiran, N. Ö. (2015). A Modal For Mind- Device Dialectic and the Future of Advertising in the Social Age. In N. Ö. Taskıran & R. Yılmaz (Eds.), *Handbook of Research on Effective Advertising Strategies in Social Media Age* (pp. 1–16). IGI Global Publications.

Yücel, T. (1988). *Summer and Life* [Yazın ve Yaşam]. Yol Yayınları.

KEY TERMS AND DEFINITIONS

New Generation Audiences: With the increase in internet and social media usage, passive tracks express the change of the audience. New tracks consist of individuals influenced by mass broadcast content and influence those contents.

Post-Truth: The new reality of the online world appeals to the senses. A new space where emotions replace reality.

Survivor: It is a television show that combines reality show and competition format.

Television and Narrative: Expresses the story structure created by using the unique features of television.

Twitter: A communication platform that destroys geographical boundaries where the masses can make their voices heard.

Chapter 10
The Construction of the Social Roles Attached to Women in TV Commercials Through the Narrative

Nilay Tan Çakır
Ondokuz Mayis University, Turkey

Recep Yılmaz
https://orcid.org/0000-0003-3406-2755
Ondokuz Mayis University, Turkey

ABSTRACT

This study is aimed to show how the gender characteristics attributed to women reflect in the advertisement narratives and how these construct through narratives. The first part of the study is presented the concept set related to the subject. In the second part, an analysis by adhering to the conceptual framework is drawn by the literature review. In this section, television commercials, which are first in Turkey, are analyzed despite the upward trend in digital media and advertising investments. In the 2019 Crystal Apple advertising competition, 16 commercial films that received the Crystal Award in the TV and Cinema category were determined as a sample. In the study, the paradigms that form the basis of the qualitative research approach are accepted. In addition to the narrative analysis method, it also supported content analysis. The research results reveal the essential components of the advertising narrative, the roles attributed to women in television advertisements, and how they are constructed through narrative.

INTRODUCTION

When the components of narrative are examined, it can be seen that "story" and "discourse" are the most crucial concepts which are used define narrative. H. Porter Abbott uses the term "narrative" to refer to the combination of story and discourse and defines these two components of narrative as "Story is an event or

DOI: 10.4018/978-1-7998-9251-9.ch010

sequence of events, and narrative discourse is those events as represented" (2002, p. 16, cited in Herman et al., 2005, p. 469). In order to study the structure of a text or make a structural description, narratologists decompose the components of narrative and attempt to identify their function and relationship. Narratology has a significant place in the literature worldwide. The fundamental approaches to the narrative analysis used in the present work is primarily based on Manfred Jahn's studies. He is an eminent scholar in the fields of narrative theory, narratology, and narratological film analysis (Jahn, 2015). In addition, the works of David Herman (Herman et al., 2005) and Marie-Laure Ryan (Ryan, 2004), both of whom address the approaches in classical and modern narrative theories together, made big contribution to the present study. As for the works in Turkish literature, we benefited from Bahar Dervişcemaloğlu's study in which the components of narratology were addressed in detail (Dervişcemaloğlu, 2014), and Nedret Tanyolaç Öztokat's study (Tanyolaç Öztokat, 2005) was chosen as the reference for narrative analysis.

Several theoreticians including Barthes (1975), Chatman (1990), and Bal (1985) argue that anything that tells a "story" is a narrative, regardless of its genre. Manfred Jahn also held the same opinion with those scholars in his study. He claimed that narrative involves anything that tells or presents a story (Jahn, 2015, pp. 43-48). From this perspective, it can be said that advertisements which present a story may also be considered as a type of narrative. According to Herman et al., it's the medium which determines whether an advertisement has a narrative structure or not. In this respect, radio and television, which present a story world mimetically, are appropriate media for narration (Herman et al., 2005, pp. 52-53). In Escalas's study conducted in 1998, content analysis of tv advertisements was performed, and it was found that approximately one fourth of all tv ads at that time were in the form of narrative. To her, advertisements tell stories because stories involve, captive, and entertain consumers. Apart from all these, stories communicate with consumers and persuade them (Escalas, 1998, pp. 267-268). In this consumer age, advertising narratives have a significant role for both advertisers and agencies in terms of persuading consumers. In addition, the scholars conducting interdisciplinary studies in communication sciences argue that advertising narrative is a field of study with a high growth potential. The works of Jennifer Edson Escalas (Escalas,1998), Chingching Chang (Chang, 2012), Rashmi Adaval (Adaval, 1998) and Recep Yılmaz (Yılmaz, 2014) also contributed to the design of this study since they acknowledge advertisements as a form of narrative.

When you simply read/watch a text with a story, it would be difficult for you to ascertain that the text structurally involves a number of elements. However, when considered as a narrative and broken up to its components, a text would provide you with several findings. As an example, let's have a look at the introductory text for the advertisement of Profilo XXL Refrigerator (Profilo, 2020):

I came up through the ranks. I got the sunlight, the water. Well, naturally, I grew a bit large. And I succeeded in the end; I became the champion. I thought everyone would chase after me once I went to the city, but they say I will not fit in their refrigerator.

The qualities that makes this text a narrative is not limited to the fact that it involves a story and a character. For instance, there is a narrator in this text who narrates the story to us. In addition, there are several elements which reflect the narrator's voice: The narrator uses the first person singular "I", and he/she is a character in this story, which makes it a homodiegetic narrative. In the following parts of the text, several other elements such as the lead character's being a watermelon will also be evaluated. We can mention a variety of concepts and relationships that are intertwined in the narrative. The point is that there are a number of assumptions, expectations, questions, and interpretations along with those concepts.

A more holistic approach could be adopted for all these concepts through a better understanding of the fundamental approaches in narrative theory, the media of the story, and the structures produced by the society. The present study benefits from narratology for the basic approaches used for analysis, while it is based on the fields of advertising and gender for the evaluation of the sample advertisements. In this respect, it has an interdisciplinary characteristic.

THE SOCIAL ROLES IMPOSED ON WOMEN IN TV ADVERTISEMENTS

Television is one of the most widely-used mass media. It has a crucial role in terms of gender issues and the determination of gender-based roles since it disseminates these roles to the society and has an undeniable socio-cultural power. It represents women with a traditionalist point of view in a variety of productions including tv series, movies, advertisements, and magazine and entertainment programs (Bolat, 2018, pp. 1685-1686).

The transformation of the family structure and women's role in the society is a revolt against the dominant state of myths and their established status. For this reason, advertising agencies and media employees need to use new gender myths to give the impression that they in harmony with working women, single moms, and "new" sensitive and respectful men. Those new myths do not fully disregard the old myths, of course. However, they omit some pieces from a series of concepts and replace them with new ones (Fiske, 2011, p. 188). As Fiske asserted, the transformation of the family structure and women's role in the society is bound to be manifested in the advertisements. While investigating how the social roles imposed on women in television advertisements are constructed through narratives, we found in this study that myths – which are one of the *signifying* elements – were also effective in this respect.

Due to the customs and the sexist attitude adopted in the course of time, the society assigns women domestic roles as wives and housewives. Television advertisements generally depict women as wives, mothers, daughters, or sisters and assign them different roles based on a sexist division of labor. As for women's employment in the advertising sector, a study conducted in 2002 with the employees of forty advertising agencies revealed that the creative crew of thirty-five of those agencies consist completely of male employees, while the rate of male and female creative staff was equal only at five of them. Besides, of sixty-three producers working at those agencies, only fourteen of them were female. Art directors consisted mostly of male employees: only two agencies had an equal number of male and female art directors. In the light of these findings, Mengü emphasizes that the language and discourse men use for women reflects patriarchy. To her, the power and status items that compose women's gender identity are produced by the patriarchy (Çakar Mengü, 2007, pp. 126-129). Considering all these findings and arguments, we can say that the patriarchal structure starts with the production process of the advertisements, and the roles assigned to women in advertisements are determined predominantly by men.

Advertisements construct our consumerism, needs, and desires by using the dominant codes in the societal sphere. The dominant codes in the advertisements restrain women's roles to domestic life, baby care, and family issues taking place in the everyday life. Advertising texts developed using such codes establishes and manipulates women with respect to socioeconomic and ideological aspects (Ercan, cited in Çakar Mengü, 2007, p. 145).

In a previous study where 489 television advertisements winning an award in nine Effie competitions held in Turkey between 2007-2018 were analyzed, the manner in which gender-based roles were portrayed in advertisements were examined. The study was carried out with the collaboration of Bahçeşehir

University (BAU) Department of Advertising and the Association of Advertisers (RVD): The Platform for Gender Equality in Advertisements. The lead character's gender, dominant role, the type of the argument he/she uses, marital status, age, minimum degree of clothing, bodily figure, basic environment, interaction with children, role as a working person, role as a home-maker, and the stereotype he/she reflects, the gender and number of supporting characters, and voiceover's gender and the type of the argument he/she uses. The obtained results revealed that only 35% of the lead characters in the sample ads were women, and the majority of those ads comprised cleaning, household, and cosmetic products. In addition, 89% of the voiceovers were men, while this rate was only 10% for women. As for the leading characters' marital status, 44% of women were portrayed as married, while only 23% of men were married. Nearly half of the women lead characters (43%) were depicted in a domestic environment, and only 10% of them were represented in a workplace. The stereotypes presented in those advertisements were in harmony with the traditional gender roles: women are mainly busy with household chores or their bodies. Another significant finding is that the stereotypes such as "carrier man" and "womanizer/macho man", both of which are traditionally associated with masculinity, displayed a downward trend while "family man" stereotype was on the rise. The most interesting finding of the study is that 21% of the male lead characters didn't have any stereotypical characteristics. In fact, women were portrayed only in certain roles, whereas men were represented in various ways (RVD, 2018).

Thanks to the social values and cultural attributes, television advertisements maintains the social structure and reconstruct it. Gender roles are presented in tv ads within the framework of this social structure. Women have two different qualities for advertising agencies: first, they are the target audience; second, they are objects used to persuade and impress the target audience. In a study conducted in Turkey by Eda Sezerer Albayrak in 2014, the use of woman image in television advertisements was addressed and analyzed in terms of motherhood and wifehood, beauty and attractiveness, and being a working woman. The results of the study revealed that women are presented in two different worlds: the first being the place where men are present, and the second one being a world of their own where they are busy with their duties as mothers, wives, and housewives. Women are generally depicted as a tool belonging to the private sphere and having roles that involve private sphere. In other words, they act in accordance with their gender roles (Sezerer Albayrak, 2015, pp. 117-122).

METHOD AND IMPLEMENTATION

Research Question

The roles that the society impose upon women also influence the way women are represented in advertisement films. The present study questions how these roles are constructed through narratives. Within this context, the manner in which feminine roles are established in advertising narratives was investigated. The issue of gender in advertisements has been addressed in a number of studies in Turkey. However, there are very few studies which dwells on gender in advertising narrative and narrative analysis. Although the number of studies on advertising narrative is vast in the international literature, there's still a huge lack in Turkish literature in this sense. The master's thesis named "*Gender Frames and Glocalization: A Comparative Study of Nigerian and Turkish Advertisements*" and written in 2019 studies the transformation of global brands' advertising narratives that center on gender equality in the process of localization. In another one named "*The Effects of Animation on the Television's Publicity to The Narration Advertisement*" and issued in 2008, signs were analyzed in terms of narration, implementation, and language. Nevertheless, the literature lacks a study that performs narrative analysis and offers a comprehensive perspective on advertising narrative.

The studies in Turkish literature that deal with advertising and narrative together are as follows: The article written by Rengin Küçükerdoğan in 2013 named "*Narrative Structural Analysis and Narrative Spaces in Advertising Media*" addresses person, time, and space – the three elements which are present in all narratives – in advertising narratives (Küçükerdoğan, 2013, pp. 8-16). The paper presented by Recep Yılmaz in 2017 named "*The Use of Women's Image as a Narrative Element in Ads*" performs a semiotic analysis of women's image in advertising narrative and reveals that women are given various roles in advertisements (Yılmaz, 2017, p. 23). In Nur Erdem's article issued in 2017 named "*Culture, New Consumer Capitalism, and Advertising Narrative in the Digital Age*" (Erdem, 2017, p. 254) and in two works of Recep Yılmaz namely "*Structural Transformation of Advertising Narration in Turkey at Digital Era*" (Yılmaz, 2017, p. 261) and "*Typology of Metaleptic Uses in TV Commercials*" (Yılmaz, 2017, p. 694), advertising texts were addressed as a type of narrative. These studies could be considered as prominent works in the fields of advertising and narrative in Turkey. Nevertheless, there's still a huge lack of research in these fields. In this respect, the present work, which benefits from the narrative elements of TV advertisements will contribute to the literature.

The Aim and Significance of the Study

This study aims to demonstrate how gender-based attributes imposed upon women in TV advertisements are reflected in advertising narratives and how these advertisements are constructed through the narrative by means of analyzing recent TV commercials. To this end, a structural analysis of the sample TV advertisements was performed, and the manner in which gender-based roles of women are presented in TV advertisements was determined. This study raises some questions including "Can each and every TV advertisement be regarded as a form of narrative?", "What are the basic components of advertising narrative?", and "How are the roles, stereotypes, and emotional characteristics of women established through narrative?" and seeks answers to them.

The original value and significance of the present study lies in the fact that although the literature worldwide is focusing more and more on advertising narrative, Turkey still lacks researches that carry out narrative analysis of the structure of advertising films. In this respect, since this study makes use of narrational elements of television advertisements, we presume that it will make a significant contribution to the literature.

The Scope of the Study

The sample of the present study comprises the tv advertisements awarded with a Crystal Apple for TV and cinema categories in the 2019 Crystal Apple Awards, an annually held competition that gives awards on advertising. The reason behind choosing these advertisements was to include a variety of advertising films in different categories and to set forth the current state of the social roles imposed on women in those films. Such roles were addressed in various aspects, rather than limiting the scope of the study to a small number of categories or brands. In this respect, recent advertising films were chosen in order to demonstrate the current state of this issue in Turkey.

The underlying reason why TV advertising films were preferred in this study is that the rate of investment in TV advertising is considerably higher than the investments in digital media in Turkey (46% for TV investments and 33.3% for digital media investments, according to The Estimation Report for 2019 Year-end Investments in Media and Advertising in Turkey). The investment shares of outdoor, press, radio and cinema advertising for the year 2019 were 9.4%, 6.5%, 3.7%, and 1.1%, respectively (Turkish Association of Advertising Agencies, 2019). Despite the upward trend in digital media and advertising investments, TV still remains the leading advertising media in Turkey. Because it appeals to both visual and auditory senses, television has always been effective on the target audience and thus got the biggest share in media and advertising investments, even before the digital age. In addition, tv advertisements are a symbol of power and reputation for advertisers and brands due to their high cost and persuasive nature.

The Method of the Study

The paradigms that form the basis of qualitative research approach were adopted in the present study. In this process, "point of view" is significant, and it is acknowledged that there is no single "truth" or "right" for events and facts. Instead, multiple realities and different and various perceptions exist (Yıldırım and Şimşek, 2016). In this study, descriptive method was used, and data collection was performed using document analysis. The sample TV advertisements comprise the research data for analysis. The sample of the study consists of the sixteen advertising films analyzed through document analysis. These sample films were selected using the criterion sampling method, which is a purposive sampling method.

The analysis method used in this study is based on the method suggested by Nedret Tanyolaç Öztokat in her book "*Yazınsal Metin Çözümlemesinde Kuramsal Yaklaşımlar*" (Theoretical Approaches in the Analysis of Literary Texts). Similar to the literary analysis methods, structuralism was used in this study. The analyses were basically centered on "structure" and "meaning" which is present in that structure (Tanyolaç Öztokat, 2005). Advertising films were examined in terms of several aspects including narration, the role of the narrator, narrative characters, temporality, spatiality, description, polyphony, narrative levels, and thematic spheres.

In addition to the narrative analysis method, content analysis was also used in this study. In this respect, a content analysis was performed by determining the lead character's gender, his basic environment, and the voiceover's gender.

FINDINGS AND INTERPRETATION

The findings obtained in the present study, the objective of which is to demonstrate how the gender roles imposed upon women in TV advertisements are presented in the narrative and how these advertisements are constructed through narrative, are summarized in this section.

The TV Advertisement for the 155th Year of Ziraat Bank – Yeşilçam[1]

In this advertisement, which was prepared specially for the 155th year of Ziraat bank, the massages constituting the meaning and emphasized in the organization of the text were as follows: There may be good and bad days in the routine flow of life. We need hope and courage to stand and deal with the challenges we face. Such hard times and challenges can be overcome through social solidarity.

When we examine this advertisement in terms of gender, we see there is discrepancy and inequality in the selection of the characters' gender with regard to labor division and power relations. For instance, a mother prepares the kids for school, while men work in the factory. A woman opens the curtains of the house, while a man pulls up the shutters of a shop. In addition, the working women are confined to only a few workplaces like office, fashion shop, and restaurant. Men, on the other hand, are represented with professions requiring physical labor. On the basis of such a discrimination lies the general social conception that there is power imbalance between men and women and the identity imposed on men.

The lead male character of this advertisement is depicted as a person who is a guiding spirit and authority figure and his basic environment is his workplace. The voiceover is also a male character.

Peros Advertisement – Peros: Maids' Choice, Not Celebrities

In this TV advertisement, a laundry detergent is advertised and Saba Tümer, a Turkish female TV programmer, is the lead character. However, the story changes when her maid tells Saba that "she" has the say in deciding the detergent to be used. The maid's profound knowledge on Peros is emphasized in the advertisement.

Celebrities are generally used in laundry detergent advertisements only for attracting attention to the product because they generally have maids in their house who help them with the household chores. In this respect, the message of the advertisement is that since maids have more knowledge on chores than their employers, they are the real bosses when it comes to household chores.

As was shown in the previous studies, just like most other household and care product advertisements, the lead character here is also a female character. Once again, the basic environment of the lead female character is "home" and her basic role is to carry out household chores. Although the lead character is female, the voiceover is male. It was reported in previous studies that male voiceovers are more frequently used in advertisements than female voiceovers, which is one of the biggest inequality issues in terms of gender representation.

Atasay Advertisement – Wear What Suits You

In this advertisement, a number of women endeavor to do something in different places and for different purposes. At the same time, in a melodic tone, the voiceover tells the aims of the characters in the advertisement film. In Turkish language, the verb "wear" means to wear jewelry and to be bent on something. In this advertisement, the word "wear" is used as a pun: the characters' wearing jewelry and being bent on achieving their aims. By using pun, a rhetoric figure of speech, the message of the advertisement is conveyed through a catchy manner. The fundamental message of this advertisement is that there are women out there who have high ideals and make great effort to achieve them.

In addition, another important message is that women can have great goals in spite of the stereotypes attributed to them and will struggle to achieve these goals by putting their heart in them. Women's struggle to realize their goals do not necessarily mean that they have to neglect their self-care.

When we look at the narrative characters, we can see that they are all women. As was reported in the study where Eiffe awarded tv advertisements between the years 2017 and 2018 were examined, the second biggest category in which women characters are preferred in the advertisements is fashion/clothing/accessories with a rate of 80%. In this advertisement, which was also awarded with a Crystal Apple for fashion and accessories category, only female characters and a female voiceover was used.

Showing women in a variety of social environments, this advertisement does not restrict women's place to home or workplace. As can be seen in the findings on spatiality, the spheres used in this advertisement are also different from the typical conventional state. An example to the depiction of women in a nonconventional gender role is that a woman character is shown looking at the sky while dancing in a night club rather than working in a laboratory with a serious image.

The lead character of Atasay advertisement is female. She is predominantly ambitious, target-oriented, strong, and hardworking. Her basic environment is social life spheres. The voiceover of the advertisement is also a woman.

Turkcell Advertisement – Metin Oktay: "Just Look at the Road When on Road"

Awarded with a Crystal Apple for social responsibility category, this advertisement presents a story between Emre Akbaba (a Turkish footballer) and Metin Oktay (a legendary Turkish footballer who died in 1991 in a car accident). In the film, the main idea is not to deal with your mobile phone while driving. In this context, it shows a car trip and a nearly missed car accident.

The basic messages of this advertisement are as follows: We shouldn't use our mobile phones while driving. Negative experiences can be avoided if we follow the advice of people who have had such experiences.

The lead character of this advertisement is male. The predominant roles attributed to him are giving advice and sharing experience. His basic environment is the car and the road. There is no voiceover in the advertisement.

Axe Advertisement – Put in Your Pocket; You'll Need It

Awarded with a Crystal Apple for cosmetics, self-care and beauty category, this advertisement portrays a young man who is stranded on a deserted island and creates a comfortable environment for himself with some struggle. When a woman comes to the island, he uses the Axe deodorant in his pocket and suddenly becomes very attractive. The advertisement emphasizes the importance of being always well-prepared and in terms of your self-care.

When we look from the gender perspective, we can see that both male and female characters are presented with their sexual attractiveness, male attractiveness being more obvious. The lead character is male, and he performs duties that require physical strength and shows his skills, which reflects the social roles imposed on men. The female character, on the other hand, is delicate and represented only with her beauty. The underlying reason behind preferring those contrasting roles is the social acceptance that there is a power imbalance between men and women. The lead character is predominantly portrayed as a survivor and a skillful and well-prepared person. His basic environment is the nature. The voiceover is also male.

Nescafe 3 in 1 Advertisement – More Famous Than the Celebrity

In this advertisement, which was awarded with a Crystal Apple for beverages category, Kerem Bursin (a famous Turkish actor) plays as himself. The story of the advertisement is that the new content and packaging of Nescafe even surpasses Kerem Bursin's fame as a celebrity figure.

The lead character of this advertisement is also male, which backs up the argument that the majority of lead characters in advertisements are male. Women characters, on the other hand, were presented as fans of Kerem with an admiring smile on their faces. The basic environment of the lead character is a café. The voiceover is male.

Turkcell Advertisement – The Cat Dripping From Upstairs

Awarded with a Crystal Apple for technology services, this advertisement of Turkcell promotes its limitless fiber Internet campaign. A variety of visuals accessed through the Internet such as cat videos, nostalgic movie characters, home workout videos, search engines, social media websites, and video streaming websites were used in the advertising film. They were narrated by using wordplays like "leak out online" or "drip". In addition, a man who has become famous in Turkey with a video that went viral also appears at the end of the advertising film. In this advertisement, the main message is that our homes get more entertaining with the use of limitless Internet.

The lead character is male, his basic environment is home, and he is portrayed as a wonderer family member. The voiceover is male.

Eti Canga Advertisement – "The Messy" Publicity Campaign

In this advertisement, which was awarded with a Crystal Apple for food category, the characters speak using completely scrambled words. The advertisement introduces 10 new packaging of the product and uses the neurological finding that even though we encounter scrambled words, our brain will comprehend them correctly as long as the first and the last letter of a word are in correct places.

The lead character speaks in totally scrambled words. The message is that just like it is possible to get yourself understood even when you speak this way, it's possible for messy people to find what they look for. In other words, even though a person is messy, he/she can still have the insight to remember the place where they've left something.

When looked from the gender perspective, we see that the lead character is male, just as the case in the majority of advertisements. The messy people in the advertisement are male, and their messiness is depicted as normal, and they have no problem showing their messiness to other people, which is another issue needed to be questioned in terms of social identity context. The lead character is male, he is portrayed as a young and messy person, and his basic environment is home. The voiceover is male.

Boyner Advertisement – Mother's Day Campaign

Awarded with a Crystal Apple for the fashion and accessories category, this advertisement basically implies that mothers perceive things in a manner far from reality. In the film, a child plays a musical instrument, and his mom listens to him with admiring eyes although it's obvious from his brother's face that he is playing the instrument not so well.

With regard to gender, this advertisement presents women at home since its target audience is women and the theme is Mother's Day. However, the representation of women mostly at home in the advertisements demonstrates the social status imposed upon women. As can be seen in most advertisements, women are mostly presented in a domestic environment while men are pictured in a variety of environments.

The voiceover of this advertisement is female, which makes it exceptional according to the finding that 89% of the voiceovers in advertisements are men, while this rate is only 10% for women. This data was obtained in a study performed with the collaboration of Bahçeşehir University (BAU) Department of Advertising and the Association of Advertisers (RVD): The Platform for Gender Equality in Advertisements. The lead character, however, is the boy playing the instrument, which means once again a male lead character is used in an advertisement. His basic environment is home.

Koç Holding Advertisement – How Great It Is to Love You

This advertisement, which was awarded a Crystal Apple for the corporate image category, pays tribute to Ataturk on his death anniversary on November 10th by using his photos. People's photos taken with Ataturk's pictures stream in the advertisement. A touching version of the song "Eyes Smizing with Love" is played while photos are streamed throughout the film. The basic theme of this advertisement is to commemorate Atatürk with respect and yearning. When looking from the gender perspective, we didn't encounter any gender inequality. The lead character is male, and his basic role is leadership. He is portrayed in various social spheres. There's no voiceover in the advertisement. The song used in the advertisement is performed by a female singer.

Ford Advertisement – The Biggest Ford Trucks F-Max

In the commercial, which won the Crystal Award in the category of automotive and automotive products in 2019, in the type of cinema and tv, it is explained that there is a big world inside F-Max. Here, the breadth of the product is highlighted by a colorful story. Thanks to a platform, tours are organized for tourists from all over the world. Cycling, marching band, athletics team, wedding procession, dance team, drone, motorcycle, horse, and astronaut seem to pass through the vehicle. The basic meaning of this advertisement film is examined, provided with a story that shows that many things can pass through the car.

In terms of gender, although there is a truck advertisement, there are also women in most character groups. However, the fact that the protagonists are male shows that this advertisement cannot stand out from the other majority. The voice-over is also male.

Koç Holding Advertisement – Biennial 2019

This commercial film received the Crystal Award in culture, art, media, broadcasting, and entertainment in tv and cinema in 2019. In the commercial, which draws attention to the proliferation of plastic waste with an allusive method, the representative of the 7th Continent makes a press statement. The biennial, which deals with the relationship between art and ecology, aims to draw attention to the wastes caused by humanity.

When we look at it in terms of gender: The gender of the 7th Continent representative is uncertain. In this film, where the representatives of the state are generally men, it is seen that the representative of Istanbul is male. Equality is observed in the distribution of men and women in the meeting and press team.

The gender of the protagonist in the commercial is uncertain. The character is wrapped in plastic bags and does not engage in dialogue. The actions of the protagonist are narrated by a narrator. The narrator in the story is a woman. At the end of the story, the voice-over calling the brand is male. In this context, it can be said that the distribution of men and women in the film is balanced.

Filmekimi Advertisement – Despite This Advertisement

This commercial, which received the Crystal Award in culture, art, sports, media, broadcasting, and entertainment at the 2019 Kristal Elma, addresses art and cinema lovers in a sincere and humorous way. Expressions such as "We are at your service with our export surplus and award-winning films, comfortable halls and friendly staff" are included in the advertisement film. Instead of an artistic promotion, it is aimed to attract attention by applying the opposite.

The first part of this commercial that we examined; is poor image quality, clichéd stereotypes, voices that speak the marketer's language, irrelevant music (game mood), and poor typography. The message that creates the primary meaning in the commercial is that the advertisement is terrible. In the second part, the poor quality of the ad was once again emphasized with the phrase "despite this advertisement." When we examine it in terms of gender, no finding can be commented on. There is no protagonist in the filmekimi commercial. There are both male and female voices.

Finish Advertisement – Let Bahar Smile

This commercial film received the Crystal Award in the tv use category. The commercial was initially designed as a product placement in the "Kadın/Woman" series. It was broadcast in the commercial of the series and was watched as a continuation of the series. In the commercial, the character Bahar eats with her children. Then she says she will wash the dishes, forgetting that she has a dishwasher. She smiles at the reminder of his children.

When we examine it in terms of gender, the female protagonists showing in the home environment and taking care of their children show parallelism with the findings obtained in previous studies. The primary setting of the mother character is shown as the house. Again, in the advertisement with the female main character, a male voice-over accompanied her.

A101 Advertisement – E Cheap Campaign

This commercial film won the Crystal Award in tv and cinema, retail, sales, and e-commerce categories in 2019. In the commercial, a mother and her two children are shown shopping in an A101. It is emphasized that this market with cheap products is everywhere.

When we examine it in terms of gender, we see the mother taking care of her children and buying children's products. We know the existence of the maternal role imposed on women. In the A101 commercial, the protagonist's gender is female, and her primary role is motherhood. Its immediate environment is the market. In previous studies, it has been observed that since the 1980s, women have started to be primarily responsible for shopping instead of men. In this respect, we see that grocery shopping is among some changing social roles. The voice-over is male.

Even when the woman can find a place for herself in the advertisement as the protagonist, the male voice accompanies her. The clearest inequality seen in the ad regarding gender is in the choice of voice-over. As in many studies, it is seen that male voice-over is used more frequently than female voices. In the study in which tv commercials that received awards in the last ten years at Effie were examined, the rate of male voice-overs was 89% in Turkey. In 75% of the commercials in which the main character is female, it has been determined that the voice-over is male (RVD, 2018). This commercial film we examined is also in line with this research.

Allianz Advertisement – Allianz Life Cycle

This commercial film received the Crystal Award in the bank, insurance, and financial services in tv and cinema in 2019. In the commercial, it is emphasized that similar situations are experienced in various periods of life, such as infancy, childhood, youth, and old age. On the one hand, the growth of a baby; on the other hand, showing the old age of a person and their being parallel to each other constitute the primary meaning.

When we look at it in terms of gender, we see that there are male protagonists. The fact that the care and care work is also done by men shows that this role, which is mainly attributed to women, can change. Sensitive and respectful men are also featured in advertisements, thanks to the changing new gender myths. The primary roles of the protagonists are to be father and son. Its main environments are various indoor and outdoor spaces. The voice-over is male.

CONCLUSION

It's undeniable that the transformation of the family structure and women's role in the society would be reflected in advertisements. The present study investigates how the social roles imposed on women, behavior patterns, and emotional traits are constructed through narrative in tv advertisements.

One possible answer to the research question "Can each and every tv advertisement be regarded as a form of narrative?" might be as follows: Advertising films that tells a story could be considered as narrative, as it is signified in the definition of narrative. On the other hand, the informative or sale-oriented advertisements that do not have a story and thus cannot be deemed as a form of narrative. For this reason, we can say that not every tv advertisement is narrative. Narrative involves anything that tells or presents a story. All of the sample advertising films analyzed in this study can be considered as narrative since they are fictional, have stories, and presents events in a real-like manner. Because these award-winning advertising films involves stories, they influence consumers and appeal more to their emotions.

Another research question was "What are the basic components of advertising narrative?". In his study conducted in 2019, Yılmaz formed an analytic base in order to identify how the components of narrative are reflected in advertisements and to analyze how they could be used in researches on advertising. He addressed the components of narrative including narration, concentration, narrative states, narrative time, verb tenses and moods, chronotypes, characters, and discourses and how all these components are reflected in advertisements. Likewise, based on those components, the present study also analyzes the sample advertising films in terms of mimesis and diegesis, narrative and narration, narrator, narrative characters, temporality, spatiality, polyphony, and narrative levels. It was seen that all these components are present in most of the sample advertising films. However, there aren't any narrators in some of them. In some other sample films, the story doesn't involve any polyphony. And, one advertising film does not have a lead character.

Myths have a significant place in the analysis of the roles imposed on women in tv advertisements. Advertising agents need to make use of those gender myths in order to depict working women, single moms, and sensitive and respectful men. Since advertisements are somehow considered as the naturalization of culture, this naturalization process takes place along with myths. Women's role as mothers and wives is deemed as their natural role, and this conviction is reproduced in advertisements.

When we look at the gender roles attributed to women and men in advertising films, we can see that labor division and power relations are the main factors determining the selection of the characters' gender. In Ziraat Bank advertisement, for instance, it was a woman who prepares her children for school whereas the factory workers consisted mostly of men. A woman opens the curtains of her house, while a man pulls up the shutters of his workplace. The working women are represented in only a small variety of workplaces including office, fashion workshop, and restaurant. Men, on the other hand, generally work at jobs requiring physical labor. The general social conviction that there is power imbalance between men and women and the identities attributed to men and women by the society form the basis of this discrepancy. Atasay advertisement, however, is exceptional in this respect. A female mountain climber is depicted in a hairdresser as a well-groomed lady. Similarly, a science woman who is working on finding a new galaxy is portrayed dancing in a night club. Besides, the spaces used in this advertisement are different from the traditional and typical spheres where women are generally represented.

As for the gender of the lead characters in the sample advertising films, 10 of them were male, while 4 of them were female. In one of the sample films, the lead characters' gender is indefinite. In Filmekimi advertisement, there is no lead character. Different from the other sample advertising films, this advertisement does not have any lead character.

When we evaluate the dominant roles of the lead characters, we see that the basic roles of the female lead characters in Peros, Finish, and A101 advertisements are to perform household chores and buy groceries. The domestic duties such as housework and grocery shopping are women's responsibility in these advertisements. In Alianz advertisement, on the other hand, we see the male lead character taking part in childcare and looking after his sick father, both of which are the duties generally attributed to women.

Of all the sample advertising films, 10 of them had male voiceovers (narrator), 3 of them had female voiceovers, one of them had both male and female voiceovers, and 2 of them didn't have any voiceovers. Female voiceovers were used in Boyner, Atasay, and Biennale advertisements. According to the data obtained in a study performed with the collaboration of Bahçeşehir University (BAU) Department of Advertising and the Association of Advertisers (RVD): The Platform for Gender Equality in Advertisements, 89% of the voiceovers in advertisements are men, while this rate is only 10% for women. The abovementioned three sample advertisements are exceptional in this respect.

As was reported in previous studies, female lead characters are preferred in the advertisements of domestic, cleaning, and self-care products. Besides, male voiceovers are used in the advertisements where lead characters are female. Among the 16 sample films analyzed in this study, only 4 of them had female lead characters. The voiceovers used in 3 of those ads were male, and only one was female, which is one of the biggest inequality issues in terms of gender representation. Even if women have a leading part in an advertisement, male voiceovers accompany them. The results obtained in this study revealed that the most obvious problem in the advertisements in terms of gender equality is the selection of the voiceovers. As was reported many other researches, the number of male voiceovers outweigh that of female ones.

In Turkcell advertisement, only one gender is represented. Although the theme is Bairam, all characters in the film are male since the story is about football. In contrast, only female characters are used in Atasay advertisement. Therefore, we may presume that the brand and product are the determining factors in the selection of characters' gender.

In Axe advertisement, masculine attractiveness is highlighted, which is contradictory to the case in the majority of advertisements where feminine attractiveness is emphasized. In this advertisement, the lead character is male and performs tasks that require physical strength and shows his skills. This also reflects the social roles attributed to men. The female character, on the other hand, is depicted as a delicate woman and represented only with her beauty. The basis of such discrimination is the social conviction that there is power imbalance between women and men.

Sexist division of labor, role distribution, behavior patterns, and emotional traits are created by the social structure (families, schools, media etc.). Therefore, in order to redistribute and transform these roles, the discourse of ideological structures and advertisements, in particular, should be analyzed in the first place. Revealing how the social roles imposed upon women through narrative in tv advertisements, the present study will contribute significantly to achieving this transformation.

REFERENCES

Adaval, R., & Wyer, R. Jr. (1998). The Role of Narratives in Consumer Information Processing. *Journal of Consumer Psychology*, *7*(3), 207–246. doi:10.120715327663jcp0703_01

Allianz Turkiye. (2019, Oct 8). *Allianz Life Cycle* [Video]. YouTube. https://www.youtube.com/watch?v=D9L6WkhZz3w

Atasay Jewelry. (2018, Dec 17). *Wear What Suits You* [Video]. YouTube. https://www.youtube.com/watch?v=gwrssbRWJfo

Axe Türkiye. (2019). *Put in Your Pocket; You'll Need It* [Video]. YouTube. https://www.youtube.com/watch?v=vygySn0T-8w

Bolat, N. (2018). Erkek Egemen Bir Dünyada Kadının Medyada Temsiliyeti Üzerine Bir İnceleme: Eşkıya Dünyaya Hükümdar Olmaz Dizisi Örneği [An Analysis on the Representation of Women in the Media in a Male-Dominated World]. *Gümüşhane Üniversitesi İletişim Fakütesi Elektronik Dergisi*, *6*(2), 1676–1703.

Boyner. (2019, May 2). *Mother's Day Campaign* [Video]. YouTube. https://www.youtube.com/watch?v=gOMYQcPP_cw

Çakar Mengü, S. (2004). *Televizyon Reklamlarında Kadına Yönelik Oluşturulan Toplumsal Kimlik* [Social Identity Created for Women in Television Advertisements]. İstanbul Üniversitesi İletişim Faültesi Yayınları.

Chang, C. (2012). Advertisements and Narrative Processing. In Advertising Theory (pp. 241–254). Routledge.

Dervişcemaloğlu, B. (2014). *Anlatıbilime Giriş* [Introduction to Narratology]. Dergah Publications.

Erdem, M. N. (2017). *Dijital Çağda Kültür, Yeni Tüketici Kapitalizmi ve Reklam Anlatısı* [Culture, New Consumer Capitalism and Advertising Narrative in the Digital Age] [Conference presentation]. 1st International Conference on New Trends in Communication, Istanbul, Turkey.

Escalas, J. E. (1998). Advertising Narratives: What are they and how do they work? In Representing Consumer: Voices, Views and Visions (pp. 241–254). Routledge. doi:10.4324/9780203380260_chapter_9

Eti. (2018, Oct 5). *"The Messy" Publicity Campaign* [Video]. YouTube. https://www.youtube.com/watch?v=m7WpFeZrLp8

Finish Türkiye. (2018, Nov 21). *Let Bahar Smile* [Video]. YouTube. https://www.youtube.com/watch?v=BXyP-3s4Ubc

Fiske, J. (2011). *İletişim çalışmalarına giriş* [Introduction to communication studies]. (S. İrvan, Trans.). Pharmakon Publications.

Ford Trucks, T. R. (2018, Nov 16). *The Biggest Ford Trucks F-Max* [Video]. YouTube. https://www.youtube.com/watch?v=HmfS_ZlMh9Q

Herman, D., Jahn, M., & Ryan, M. L. (Eds.). (2005). *Routledge Encylopedia of Narrative Theory*. Routledge.

İstanbul Kültür Sanat Vakfı. (2018 Sep 26). *Despite This Advertisement* [Video]. YouTube. https://www.youtube.com/watch?v=C_Kzw768hfw

Jahn, M. (2015). *Anlatıbilim* [The Narratology] (B. Dervişcemaloğlu, Trans.). Dergah Publications.

Koç Holding. (2019, Sep 12). *Biennial 2019* [Video]. YouTube. https://www.youtube.com/watch?v=oJ6-ZNtrBk8

Küçükerdoğan, R. (2016). Anlatısal Yapı Çözümlemesi ve Reklam İletişimde "Anlatı Yerlemleri" ['Narrative Locations' in Narrative Structure Analysis and Advertising Communication]. *Dilbilim Dergisi*, *2*(30), 5–18.

Nescafe 3ü1 Arada. (2018, Oct 22). *More Famous Than the Celebrity* [Video]. YouTube. https://www.youtube.com/watch?v=iAR-zcIFhOQ

Peros Temizlik. (2018, Oct 28). *Maids' Choice, Not Celebrities* [Video]. YouTube. https://www.youtube.com/watch?v=nZTXWX1li8E

Profilo. (2020, May 20). *Profilo XXL Refrigerator Advertising* [Video]. YouTube. https://www.youtube.com/watch?v=3xB8IEIPQvo

RVD. (2019). *Türkiye'deki Effie Ödüllü TV Reklamlarının 10 Yıllık Toplumsal Cinsiyet Eşitliği Karnesi Özet Bulgular*. https://www.rvd.org.tr/uploads/2019/02/effie-kisa-arastirma-raporu.pdf

Ryan, M. L. (2004). Metaleptic Machine. *Semiotica*, *1*(4), 439–469. doi:10.1515emi.2004.055

Sezerer Albayrak, E. (2015). Televizyon Reklamlarında Kadın İmgesi Kullanımı [Using the Image of Women in Television Ads]. In G. Ağrıdağ (Ed.), Türkiye'de ve Dünya'da Kadın Araştırmaları. Çukurova Üniversitesi Basımevi.

Tanyolaç Öztokat, N. (2005). *Yazınsal Metin Çözümlemesinde Kuramsal Yaklaşımlar* [Theoretical Approaches to Literary Text Analysis]. Multilingual.

Turkcell. (2018, Nov 6). *The Cat Dripping from Upstairs* [Video]. YouTube. https://www.youtube.com/watch?v=5o-SANBtkAg

Turkcell. (2019, May 30). *Just Look at the Road When on Road* [Video]. YouTube. https://www.youtube.com/watch?v=n_p9pfu9LWc

Turkish Association of Advertising Agencies. (2019). *Türkiye'de Tahmini Medya ve Reklam Yatırımları Raporu.* https://www2.deloitte.com/content/dam/Deloitte/tr/Documents/technology-media-telecommunications/turkiyede-tahmini-medya-ve-reklam-yatirimlari-2019-ilk-6-ay-raporu.pdf

Türkiye'nin Reklamları. (2018, Oct 15). *A101 E Cheap Campaign* [Video]. YouTube. https://www.youtube.com/watch?v=W_-MbqiFELo

Yapı Kredi. (2018, Nov 9). *How Great It Is to Love You* [Video]. YouTube. https://www.youtube.com/watch?v=cR_HbU52Svk

Yıldırım, A., & Şimşek, H. (2016). *Sosyal bilimlerde nitel araştırma yöntemleri* [Qualitative research methods in the social sciences]. Seçkin Publications.

Yılmaz, R. (2014). *Anlatı Yoluyla Dünyanın Zihinsel Yeniden Kurulumu: ''Palto'', ''Dönüşüm'' ve ''Hayvan Çiftliği'' Romanlarının Alımlama Pratikleri Üzerine Bir İnceleme* [Mental Reconstruction of the World through Narrative: A Study on Reception Practices of "The Overcoat", "The Metamorphosis" and "The Animal Farm"] [Unpublished doctoral dissertation]. Kocaeli Üniversitesi Sosyal Bilimler Enstitüsü İletişim Bilimleri Anabilim Dalı.

Yılmaz, R. (2017). Reklamlarda Bir Anlatı Öğesi Olarak Kadın İmgesinin Kullanımı [The Use of the Image of Woman as a Narrative Element in Advertisements]. In M. Talas & E. Yalçınkaya (Eds.), *4th International Congress on Social Sciences, China to Adriatic*. Academic Press.

Yılmaz, R. (2017). Televizyon Reklamlarında Metaleptik Kullanımlarının Tipolojisi [Typology of Metaleptic Uses in TV Commercials]. *Gümüşhane Üniversitesi İletişim Fakültesi Elektronik Dergisi*, *5*(2), 691–704.

Yılmaz, R. (2017). *Türkiye'de Reklam Anlatısının Dijital Çağdaki Yapısal Dönüşümü* [Structural Transformation of Advertising Narrative in Turkey in the Digital Age] [Conference presentation]. 1st International Conference on New Trends in Communication, İstanbul, Turkey.

Ziraat Bankası. (2018, Dec 25). *''Yeşilçam'' Advertising* [Video]. YouTube. https://www.youtube.com/watch?v=bm63JYzlGfA

KEY TERMS AND DEFINITIONS

Character: S/he is a narrative person and an element of narrative theory.

Narrative: Anything that tells or presents a story.

Narrative Analysis: The analyzes mainly focused on the "structure" and the "meaning" that exists in that structure.

Narrator: A person who narrates something, mostly a character who tells the events of narrative.

Qualitative Research: In this process, "perspective" is important, and it is accepted that there is no single "correct" or "correct" for events and phenomena.

Social Roles: The role people play as members of a social group.

Structuralism: It is a method for the interpretation and analysis of human cognition, behavior, culture, and experience that focuses on the oppositional relationships between elements.

Television: One of the most widely used mass media. It has a crucial role in terms of gender issues and the determination of gender-based roles since it disseminates these roles to the society and has an undeniable socio-cultural power.

ENDNOTE

1 This work is derived from the master's thesis named "The Construction of Social Roles Attributed to Women through Narrative in TV Commercials" and supervised by Assoc. Prof. Dr. Recep Yılmaz.

Chapter 11
Spin Doctor in the Post-Truth Era:
"Our Brand Is Crisis" Movie Example

Betül Başer
Ondokuz Mayıs University, Turkey

ABSTRACT

Today, the reaction of the masses towards the lies of the politicians brings together a new process rather than the politicians lying to the masses. In the post-trust era, the insignificance of the truth, politicians reflecting the lies as if they were the truth, and the masses believing in such reflections represent such a process. In this era, politicians render excuses to cover up the truth without having any feeling of guilt. There are spin doctors that work to enable the politicians to realize these purposes. The purpose of spin doctors is to manipulate the media and the public opinion and to reveal the aspects of events to benefit their own political targets rather than as these events are. In this study, the Our Brand Is Crisis movie will be considered in the context of spin doctor tactics usage in the post-truth era. The purpose of this study is to reveal the cinema representation of the spin doctor tactics in the post-truth era and to discuss the spin doctor concept and tactics with sample scenes.

INTRODUCTION

Today, the reaction of the masses towards the lies of the politicians brings together a new process rather than the politicians lying to the masses. In the post-trust era, the insignificance of the truth, politicians reflecting the lies as if they were the trust, masses believing in such reflections represent such a process. In this era, politicians render excuses to cover up the truth without having any feeling of guilt. There are spin doctors that work to enable the politicians to realize these purposes. The purpose of spin doctors is to manipulate the media and the public opinion and to reveal the aspects of events to benefit their own political targets rather than as these events are. Spin doctors attempt to block the criticism against the individuals or institutions they represent to reach the target audience or to turn the event in favour of the represented individuals or institutions if they fail to prevent the criticism (Kundakçı, 2014, p.

DOI: 10.4018/978-1-7998-9251-9.ch011

313). Spin doctors know what type of news the journalists choose, how to feed the journalist with a new story every day and benefit from stories well by using surprising tactics. Various spin doctor tactics are employed to bring the masses into a psychologically convenient state. In this study, the "Our Brand Is Crisis" movie will be considered in the context of spin doctor strategy usage in the post-truth era. The purpose of this study is to reveal the cinema representation of the spin doctor strategies in the post-truth era and to discuss the spin doctor concept and strategies with sample scenes. For the analysis, the "Our Brand is Crisis" movie is selected with a purposeful sampling method. The content analysis method is implemented and the spin doctor tactics in the movies are evaluated by considering sample scenes. This study focuses on the ways of presenting the spin doctor tactics in the post-truth era with content analysis and attempts for systematic inference according to identified criteria.

GENERAL OVERVIEW OF POST-TRUTH CONCEPT

The term "post-truth" is the combination of the words "post" which means after and "truth" which means reality. The "post-truth" word was selected as the word of the year by the Oxford dictionary in 2016 and this term is related to the reactions of individuals according to emotions and beliefs rather than the truth itself (Oxford Learner's Dictionaries, 2016). The Arabic word "hakikat" (truth) comes from the word "hakk". The truth word which is the opposite of the superstitious word signifies reality, trueness, fixity and absolute. The truth which does not merely signify reality explains a measure and judgement related to the reality (Zabcı, 2021, p. 15). When we talk about the post-truth era, the "post" preposition is not used to refer to an era beyond the truth in temporal terms. In the post-truth era, the "post" preposition is used to express the decreased importance of truth rather than going beyond the truth. This concept that explains the start of a post-truth era states that what individuals are expected to believe is not the scientific data but the emotions, ideologies and political prejudices (Bezembinder, 2018, p. 45). The post-truth concept was commonly used during the Brexit process which represents the United Kingdom leaving the European Union and the US presidential elections which Donald Trump won and the increased usage of this concept played a significant role in this term being accepted as the term of the year (Kocabay Şener, 2019, p. 394). September 2016 issue of The Economist magazine declared that the world entered to "post-truth politics" era. One of the important events that laid the ground for this explanation was the disputed election period of Donald Trump. Donald Trump commonly adopted a propaganda strategy with unfounded news during the election campaign period. The development that made the post-truth concept and Donald Trump's election campaign important was the fact that Trump won the election (The Economist, 2016).

Harsin (2015, p. 331) defines post-truth as the "regime after trueness". The post-truth concept is more than simply bending the truth and it is about how important truth can be to impact the visibility and participation of the politician. The consecutive recent developments formed the conditions for the post-truth and the important factors that led to the post-truth are as follows:

- Decomposition of the media structure and media's failure to act as a "gatekeeper".
- Inability to trace the source of the online information and stop the dissemination.
- Internet algorithms.
- Clickbait.
- Economic, technological, political and socio-cultural developments.

According to Keyes, humanity that leaves in a post-truth era today reveals excuses to cover up the truth to save themselves without feeling any guilt (Keyes, 2017, p. 22). The lie concept which can be evaluated as the opposite of the truth concept has always been a factor since the existence of humanity. Today, the reactions of humanity toward lies started to decrease and untrue information or fake news is normalized. The post-truth concept that first emerged in the political field was positioned everywhere where there are people, accelerated and expanded by increasing its impact with the internet following the developments in the communication technologies and sustaining this state by showing its destructive power (Delal & Abanoz, 2021, p. 274).

The reaction is important in the post-truth process that includes lies and deception. In this process, the lies become ordinary and the easiness for individuals to adopt the lies increases. The truth started to lose its value due to discourses of politicians that do not reflect the truth and that are easily accepted by the masses (Uluk, 2018, p. 93). The reaction of the masses towards the lies of the politicians brings together a new process rather than the politicians lying to the masses. The insignificance of the truth and the acceptance of the masses lies as long as the lies match their prejudice, views and thoughts represent this process. The masses take a position against the lies as if they are true and advocate for these lies (Alpay, 2020, p. 29). The fake content in the post-truth era is identified with the political figures using populist discourse. However, the post-truth concept does not signify distorting the truth to manage the masses with populist discourse and fake news alone (Güven, 2020, p. 23).

GENERAL OVERVIEW OF SPIN CONCEPTS

The term spin is the abbreviation of "Significant Progress in the News" words. The verb means "to turn, twist, spin, revolve and rotate". This term has a wide usage area including various sports fields (Özgen & Bayraktar, 2014, p. 2). The spin concept is commonly used in sports games in American cultures such as baseball and cricket. Here, throwing the ball to the opposite side of the opponent is defined as "spin". Due to this move in the game, the teammates of the player in the game can catch the ball for superiority. This unexpected move might surprise the opponent team (Lilleker, 2013, p. 266).

William Lewis Safire, an American public relations practitioner who approached the topic from a political point of view and is considered the author of the American presidents, highlights that this term is used as "deceiving" in a negative sense in the United States of America since the 1950s. Today, this represents "polishing the reality" (Safire, 1996). Spin is the art to disrupt and go around the events when the reality is revealed (Foa, 2006, p. 206).

The term spin was first used unwittingly as a public relations phenomenon which the public relations experts of the military institution Strategic Defense Initiative (SDI) in the mid-1980s for the first time against the accusation of this institution in the US were impractical (Görgün, 2006, p. 307). The press release prepared by the public relations experts of the Strategic Defense Initiative spun the truth by using techniques such as choosing, filtering or framing the truth to reflect the information suitable for the interest of the institution, writing the information that will benefit the institution among the existing information or expressing this information in the press releases, talking about unproven truth, using softer words rather than stronger words and creating an agenda with the press release. A spin doctor is especially used by the individuals who apply spin in a planned way (transferred from Bricknell. by Görgün, 2006, p. 307). The spin doctor that gives the best curve or twist to a statement or phenomenon prefers to twist the information, distort its shape, change and skew the information rather than a decent communication and therefore, deceive the target audience (Nel, 2005, p. 280).

GENERAL OVERVIEW OF SPIN DOCTOR CONCEPT

The term Spin Doctor was first used in 1984. This term was used in the Political Dictionary book by William Safire in the editorial department of The New York Times for activities related to election campaigns that led Reagan to be re-elected (Wilcox et al. 2000, pp. 11- 12). This represents an informed and intelligent middle class other than the leaders and journalists who are aware of the media's power. The concept aims to manipulate the media and public opinion. In addition to political spin undertaken to influence the media, this practice expands to the activities of P.T. Barnum who is one of the pioneers of public relations, the preferences of media experts to set the agenda and policies undertaken by the institutions to eliminate all the negative events in case of crisis (Özgen & Bayraktar, 2014, p. 2). The messages are twisted to achieve better results and moreover, organized in a completely different way most of the time (Seitel, 1998, p. 2). Spin doctors do not always lie. Sometimes they rebuilt the truth. Some are fabrication and others are not. But the most effective approach is when individuals do not realize something is a lie (Erdoğan, 2006, p. 300). Although not all the words of a spin doctor are lies, the spin doctor only uses a portion of the truth and fades the rest of the truth.

The most famous spin doctor in the UK was Alaster Campbell who was the campaign consultant of Tony Blair between 1994 and 2003. Campbell played with words to legitimize the Iraq war in the eyes of the public (Kundakçı, 2014, p. 312). Betül Mardin, the connoisseur of public relations in Turkey, states to refer to some of the public relations experts as spin doctor practitioners as these individuals play a key role in politics (Görgün, 2006, pp. 307- 308).

The purpose of spin doctors is to reveal the aspects of events to benefit their own political targets rather than as these events are. Words, flyers, images and banners are prepared for the political targets. Today, these are shared with the public after certain editing processes including the newsletters and internet portals. Spin Doctor distorts the truth, explain the events differently than they are, prevent the public to access the true information with fake and false documents, deceives journalists and shift the minds of their political opponents to other subjects to neutralize them (Lilleker, 2013, p. 266). In other words, spin doctors attempt to block the criticism against the individuals or institutions they represent to reach the target audience or to turn the event in favor of the represented individuals or institutions if they fail to prevent the criticism. For example, the spin doctor can be one step ahead of the news and turn scandalous news of a sports team that might be in the headlines due to a betting game and turn this into a routine sports news (Kundakçı, 2014, p. 313).

The success of the spin doctor comes from the talent to use the mass communication tools. It is possible to consider this as a sort of public relations activity as these activities change and guide the perception of the masses, take them under their influence and include activity field for direction. Spin doctors have the skills to reflect true events differently. The steps taken by the power and other power elites make the power oner more advantageous and moreover, push the masses to accept these steps. While doing that, these groups sometimes adjust the voice tone of the presidents on the radio for more influential speech and re-organize the truth in others (Mavioğlu, 2012). Thus, they do not reveal the reality to the masses and skillfully hide the real sides of the events. With that, they broadcast different messages to the public to change their perspective and misguide the public. Thus, they attract the attention of the masses and strive them away from the truth (Güler Yılmaz, 2014, p. 203).

Today, especially during and after the election campaigns, politicians need experts to consolidate their images. They desire to highlight their strengths and the weakness of their opponents. While the Spin Doctor works like an invisible president in politics, they face the camera as the spokesperson of the president in the media (Kundakçı, 2011, p. 319). The main purpose of mass communication tools is to inform society. These tools have certain effects on the masses. While these tools inform the masses, it is a fact that they function as guiding a common belief and value judgements (İnal, 2016, p. 89). Today, the developments in information and communication technologies also brought the digitalization process (Şen, 2021, p. 72). In other words, the rapid access to information in today's world enables spin doctors to use different media to reach the public.

Spin doctors apply various tactics by using different media. Some of these tactics are the media impact technique, opponent definition technique, someone from public technique, events for public opinion technique, staging fake events technique, justification of lies technique and confession with denial technique (Güler Yılmaz, 2014, p. 215; Ker Dinçer & Başok, 2014). In this study, these techniques will be analyzed based on scenes from "Our Brand is Crisis" movie.

OUR BRAND IS CRISIS MOVIE ANALYSIS WITHIN SPIN DOCTOR IN THE ERA OF POST-TRUTH CONTEXT

Purpose

The purpose of this study is to discuss the spin doctor tactics in the era of post-truth based on samples. In line with this purpose, the study attempts to analyze how the theoretical knowledge is reflected to practice by investigating how spin doctors analyze the target audience in the most detailed way to change the opinions of individuals with the spin process.

Limitations

This study that focuses on the spin doctor tactics in the era of post-truth is limited to spin doctor tactics considering an election campaign in Our Brand Is Crisis movie. The content analysis method selected by the researcher is another limitation of this study.

Method and Sample

This study is a descriptive study investigating the spin doctor tactics in the era of post-truth based on discourses in Our Brand Is Crisis movie. The content analysis method is implemented and the spin doctor tactics in the movies are evaluated by considering sample scenes. Content analysis is a flexible method that enables a set of the analytic approach to impressionist, intuitive, interpretive analysis as well as systematic, solid textual analysis (Hsieh & Shannon, 2005, p. 1277). This study focuses on the ways of presenting the spin doctor tactics with content analysis and attempts for systematic inference according to identified criteria. "Our Brand Is Crisis movie is selected with a purposeful sampling method to analyze within this framework. In the purposeful sample selection, each selected unit is knowingly and consciously selected by the researcher. If each unit in the universe does not have the equal right of selection at the sample selection stage, this is called purposeful sampling. The reason for the purposeful sampling method is to choose the units that are believed to represent a universe with another discourse that has average properties (Gurtan, 1982, pp. 41- 42). Accordingly, the convenience of Our Brand Is Crisis movie for spin doctor tactics will be evaluated.

Findings

This section of this study reveals the findings obtained from the content analysis method on the Our Brand Is Crisis movie. The findings of this study include the evaluation of spin doctor tactics in the movie. The movie tag is given in Table 1.

Table 1. Our Brand Is Crisis movie tag

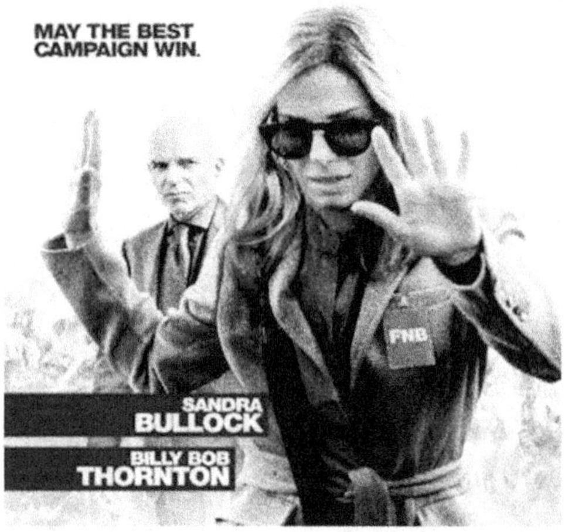	**Director:** David Gordon Green **Scenario:** Peter Straughan **Producer:** Grant Heslov, George Clooney **Cast:** Sandra Bullock Billy Bob Thornton Anthony Mackie Joaquim de Almeida Ann Dowd Scoot McNairy Zoe Kazan **Director of Photography:** Tim Orr **Montage:** Colin Patton **Music:** David Wingo **Distributor:** Warner Bros. Pictures **Release Date:** 11/09/2015 **Duration:** 107 minutes **Language:** English **Budget:** 28 million dollars

The Plot of The Movie

The movie adapted from Our Brand is Crisis documentary is about the American election campaign tactics in South America. The president of Bolivia is about the be elected. The former president must choose a campaign manager who is an "expert" for the possibility to win but "expendable" for the possibility to lose. Therefore, the former president hired Jane Bodine who won a lot of elections but was obsessively defeated by her opponent Pat Candy. Candy is the campaign manager of the other presidential candidate. Bodine will fight against her opponent and get the chance to regain her successful career. The movie provides examples of how the ideas and thoughts of individuals can be directed and how the agenda can be manipulated by using mass communication tools within the framework of the fight between campaign managers. The election campaign which started twenty-eight points behind resulted in success with the effective strategies of Bodine.

Movie Analysis

Our Brand Is Crisis movie uses media impact, opponent definition, someone from the public, show towards the public opinion, staging fake events, justification of lies and confession with denial techniques. The explanations of the techniques will be evaluated and analyzed by using sample scenes from the movie.

Media Impact Technique

Media has had an increasingly important and vital position in almost every individual's life from the past until today. When the relationship between media and political communication is considered, it is possible to talk about a relationship highlighted by mutual interaction. Each technique used in spin doctors' efforts undertaken toward the media relationships is closely related to Media Impact Technique. Actors in politics always need the news to be published, thus, they can transfer the ideas and thoughts adopted by large masses and most of the time, adopt media as a unidirectional communication process tool to me memorable (Oktay, 2022, p. 101). Spin doctors who keep this truth in mind play an important role to forward news about the political actors they represent to media institutions to publish this news with their positive relationships with media workers. (Günay, 2015, p. 74). The movie starts with an interview with Bodine who is a spin doctor. When Bodine is asked how important honesty is, the answer was, "*Reality is politics is relative. Everything I told the voters to be real is real.*" In this scene, the fact that politicians can transfer a distorted version of reality to the public is revealed. The scene in which Castillo's vote was projected as 8% in the movie has the following dialogue: "*Castillo's past is a bit too much; he did some bad collaboration... I mean our job is to take a presidential candidate that the voters do not like, rebrand him and sell him...*" This dialogue is given as an example to show what individuals who will serve the news to the media can do, and how can this individual change public opinion.

Opponent Definition Technique

The opponent definition technique can be applied differently depending on the conditions. Theoretically, this technique almost always consists of messages containing general verbal expressions. Opponent Definition Technique: which is commonly used for propaganda purposes aims to attack the opposition at a personal level by addressing the prejudices of the target audience instead of legitimate comments and this simply consists of attracts towards an individual or idea (Shabo, 2008, p. 47). When the opponent definition technique is considered from a spin doctor's perspective, putting the opponent with different ideas in a difficult situation, humiliating or expressing new statements to leave the opponent in the background are common practices, especially during the election period (Ker Dinçer & Başok, 2014, pp. 312- 313).

Bodine says the following words to win the election:

Bolivia might be living the worth period of its turbulent history. We are at a turning point. And the people of Bolivia must make a choice. There is Rivera on one side. Without principles, without experience. An opportunist sitting and waiting in the corner as his country is dissolved but there is also senator Castillo who can be elected. You might not like him. You might think he is an arrogant scum but he is a fighter. He is incredibly brave. He is really experienced. He is solid and he is your only chance. We are trying to save the lives of people. But this has gone beyond an election and turned into a crisis. And our brand or what we sell is a crisis.

This scene used the opponent definition technique. After Bodine's speech, Castillo makes a public announcement. And the votes go up from 8% to 10%.
The following dialogue of Bodine is an example of the Opponent Definition Technique.

We will do Rivera what none of the politicians will want to experience. We will define him with a certain identity. We will attack him like this: We will say he is a fraud; corrupt and inexperienced person and he is lying and we will call all of the major newspapers every day and we will feed them Rivera's story with a spoon. We will search every word he says, everyone, he talks and every vote he casts. And we will look for ways to use what we have found against him.

This dialogue shows that an opponent can be easily tainted and the votes can be influenced by changing the public opinion.

Someone From Public Technique

Political actors claim to act in line with the public's interest in some cases to get a vote from them. Bodine says that Castillo needs to change his image in the eyes of the public by saying,

The opposition will try to show you like an elite, an oligarchic ruler. What we need to do is reverse this. We will show the people of Bolivia that you are not a company accessor but one of them, "someone from the public. We will show the loveable, warm Castillo to people.

Then, the following dialogue shows Castillo giving promises he cannot keep solving people's problems.

I am here to tell you that there is a crisis in Bolivia. A large crisis: Social, economic and political. This is a socio-economic crisis. We need action not just words. This is a corruption crisis. A corruption that gradually gets out of control. I am here to fight against corruption. We can save Bolivia from this crisis as we fight side by side.

As Figure 1 shows, events are organized where Castillo can be with people to show he is someone from the people.

Figure 1. Events to show Castillo is someone from the public.

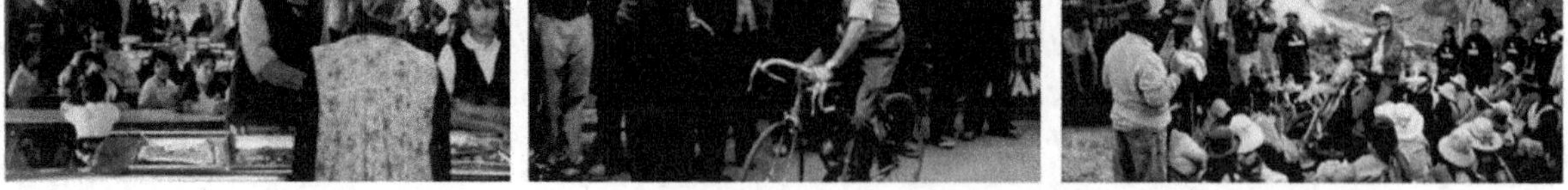

Events for Public Opinion Technique

Events for the public opinion technique represent the desire to attract the attention of an individual or a group. For example, numerous corporate public shows such as posing naked, jumping from the Niagara Waterfalls inside a barrel, and organizing fake street shows were recorded throughout history (Horton, 2008). These events are used to be on the agenda and to be remembered by the public. In terms of spin doctors, spin doctors plan events for the political actors to attract the attention of society. The events for the public opinion technique are preferred by spin doctors for events with large masses such as speeches and ceremonies (Günay, 2015, p. 72).

Figure 2. An event by Castillo for public opinion.

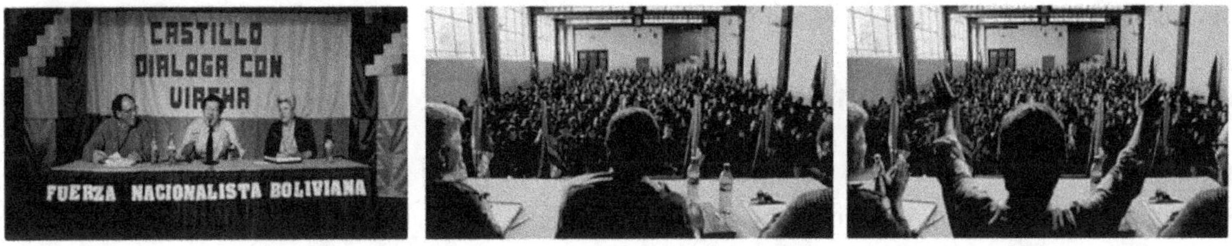

As Figure 2 shows, Castillo is speaking in from of a huge crowd and the following dialogue shows that he is talking about a crisis created by Bodine to attract the attention of the public and get media coverage. *"Today I am here because of this. To fight the crisis, to overcome the crisis, to tell we have a plan. So, I am asking all of you to join me in this fight. For Bolivia. With Castillo."*

Staging Fake Events Technique

Staging fake events technique is identified in the political communication field and the roots of this technique are based on the media logic theory proposed by Atlheide and Snow in 1979. According to this theory, media is considered for interpreting and handling social relationships. The elements of the communication style adopted by the media consist of stylistic formats such as organizing and presenting used news materials, highlights in the prepared news and the language selection (Mazzoleni, 2015). Political actors who are aware of this influence of media put efforts to be included in the media. Spin doctors organize sensational events to positively contribute to the images of the political actors they are working for.

Figure 3. Fake events organized by Bodine for Castillo to win the election.

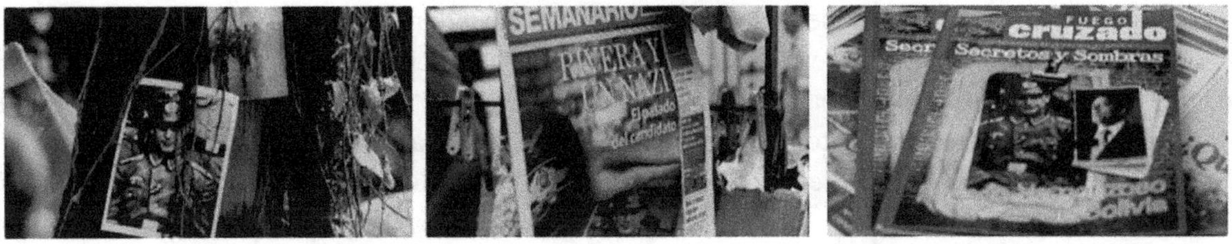

Figure 3 shows that Bodine ensures fake news that will create a negative perception about Rivera, the opponent of Castillo is disseminated. The following dialogue can show this:

Rivero has a photo with Klaus Barbie. Nazi war criminals and murdered thousands of people. We don't say they are connected; we say nothing. We don't have our fingerprint on it, this is just a rumor around the world. There are disturbing images, Rivero is in uniforms and there is a Nazi war criminal behind in the dark. I don't know if there is any connection.

"When Lyndon Johnson was a congress candidate, he asked the campaign manager to put about a rumor that the opponent is sleeping with pigs. The manager said no one will believe that. Johnson said, I know but I just want to listen to him controverting this." In this scene of the movie, we can see how easily Bodine can create fake news by twisting the truth for Castillo to win the election. The fact that the public can be directed to believe in fake news is presented.

Justification of Lies Technique

Politicians might sometimes give promises about things that will never happen and try to convince the public. As the campaign bus is stopped by the public by throwing rocks, Castillo gets off the bus and blends in with the people. The public says they do not want constitutional reform and they want a referendum so that the government will not make a move with IMF without asking the public. Castillo answers, *"I learned from Rozada's mistakes. I am not going to call IMF without a referendum because if you opt for democracy, you will be the voice of the people. I promise you if I win the election*

Figure 4. The scene where Castillo walks inside the people.

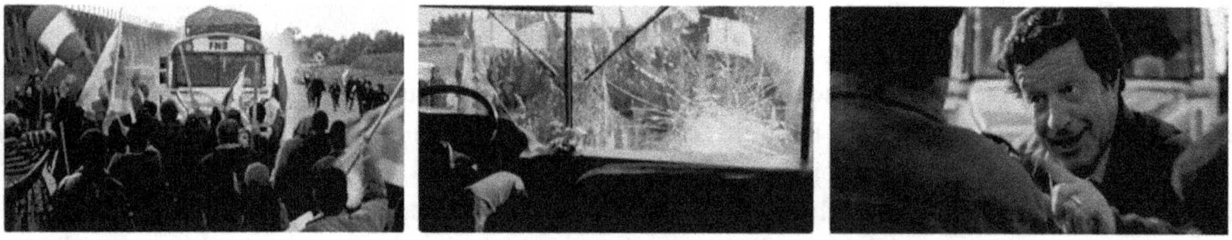

This scene where Castillo promises to meet the demands requested by the public from him just to be elected shows the audience that political actor can easily legitimize lies for their own interests.

Confession With Denial Technique

The confession with denial technique includes a certain and clear denial when the statement is first heard but no denial elements when a more detailed analysis is made (Michael, 2007, p. 71). While the things said here are true for their lexical meanings, this can be referred to as "eluding" i.e. deceiving. Confession with denial technique mostly aims to explain the core or to choose any point among evasive answers of the journalist or critic to avoid detailed answers rather than a misleading impression (Günay, 2015, p. 68).

Figure 5. The scene where Castillo is on a talk show.

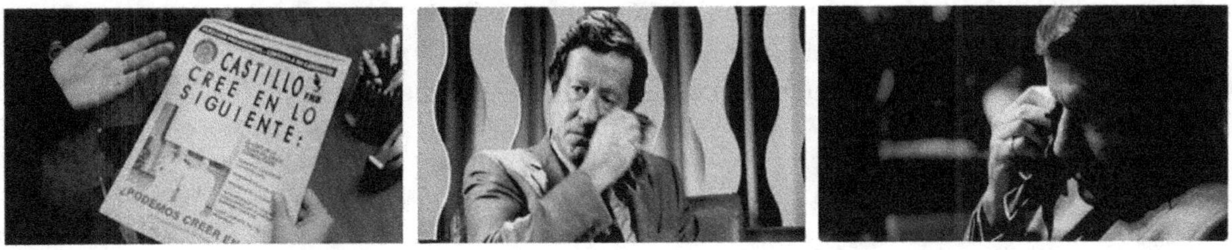

Pat Candy, the campaign manager of Rivella, distributed flyers about Castillo that do not reflect the truth and ensuring the fake news is disseminated. *"The flyer says Castillo is a member of a cult. The flyer says the cult leaders can teach the members how to fly and read minds. Castillo believes in such things. Well, how are we going to believe him?"* Then, Bodine says Castillo that she knows he does not want to talk about it but he needs to be on a talk show to talk about it. Castillo appears on the talk show and focuses on different points without mentioning this event. Castillo said his family is involved in politics and this is not right and he made a statement to completely cover up the real event.

The movie ends with Castillo who started twenty points behind winning the election by using the effective strategies of Bodine. We can see that Castillo does not keep his promise to call for the IMF in the final scene of the movie. The spin doctor tactics considered in the movie show that the politicians give promises they cannot keep misleading the public and defame their opponents easily with fake news.

FUTURE RESEARCH DIRECTIONS

This study was limited to the spin doctor tactics in the analyzed movie "Our Brand Is Crisis". Today, it is known that politicians use social media more actively. Researchers can examine spin doctor tactics in politicians' posts on social media in future studies.

CONCLUSION

Today, there is a process where politicians easily live to win an election and the masses easily believe in these lies. In the era of post-truth, the truth no longer matters. The politicians try to cover up the truth, legitimize lies and organize untrue events. This study focused on the ways of presenting the spin doctor tactics in with content analysis and attempted systematic inference according to identified criteria. Within this framework, Our Brand Is Crisis movie exampled selected with purposeful sampling method was analyzed with media impact technique, opponent definition technique, someone from the public technique, events for public opinion technique, staging fake events technique, justification of lies technique and confession with denial technique. Accordingly, the convenience of Our Brand Is Crisis movie for spin doctor tactics was evaluated. In this movie, Castillo started the presidential elections twenty-eight points back winning the election with Bodine's effective spin doctor techniques. The movie is analyzed with sample scenes that show how individuals can guide the ideas and thoughts of individuals with untrue news and change the agenda just to win an election. As a result, we can see that Bodine who is seen as a spin doctor organized fake events to have a positive contribution to Castillo's images, how easily the truth is distorted to trick the public for Castillo to win the election and how the people were led to believe in a fake event. The sample scenes from the movie shows how lies can easily be justified as Castillo tells lies to be elected and politicians can easily lie for their interest.

REFERENCES

Alpay, Y. (2017). *The Politics of Lies: Legitimating Lies, Trivializing Truth, and Fraudulent Reasoning Techniques* [Yalanın Siyaseti: Yalanın Meşrulaştırılması, Hakikatin Önemsizleştirilmesi ve Hileli Akıl Yürütme Teknikleri]. Destek Yayınları.

Bezembinder, C. (2018). *Is Post-Truth Politics Really Post-Truth?* (Unpublished Master Thesis). Leiden: Leiden University Faculty of Humanities Institute for Philosophy.

Delal, Ö., & Abanoz, E. (2021). Information Sharing and Misinformation about Covid-19 on Social Media in the Context of New Media Literacy [Yeni Medya Okuryazarlığı Bağlamında Sosyal Medyada Covid-19 ile İlgili Bilgi Paylaşımı ve Misenformasyon]. In F. Ünal Çolak & O. Yıldırım (Eds.), *Pandemic, Research and Discussions in the Digital World* [Dijital Dünyada Pandemi, Araştırmalar ve Tartışmalar] (pp. 265–296). Literatürk Academia.

Erdoğan, İ. (2006). *Media and Ethics: A Critical Introduction* [Medya ve Etik: Eleştirel Bir Giriş]. İletişim Kuram ve Araştırma Dergisi.

Foa, M. (2006). The Invisible Threat: How Spin Doctors Bypass Media Ethics Rules? [Görünmez Tehlike: Spin doktorları Medya ve Etik Kurallarını Nasıl Atlarlar?]. İletişim Kuram ve Araştırma Dergisi, 23.

Görgün, A. (2006). A New Communication Trend in Turkey: Spin Doctor [Türkiye'de Yeni Bir iletişim Eğilimi: Spin Doctor]. *21. Yüzyılda Halkla İlişkilerde Yeni Yönelimler, Sorunlar ve Çözümler Sempozyumu.*

Günay, N. (2015). *The Role of Spin Doctors in Persuasion Process of Public Relations* [Halkla İlişkiler Çalışmalarında İkna Açısından Döngü Yönetiminin (Spin Doctors) Rolü] [Unpublished Master Thesis]. Ege Üniversitesi Sosyal Bilimler Enstitüsü.

Gurtan, K. (1982). *Statistics and Research Methods* [İstatistik ve Araştırma Metodları]. İstanbul Üniversitesi Yayınları.

Güven, A. (2020). Post-Truth as the Loss of the Truth: A Conceptualization Attempt [Hakikatin Yitimi Olarak Post-Truth: Bir Kavramsallaştırma Denemesi]. *İnsan ve İnsan, 7*(23), 20-36.

Harsin, J. (2018). Post-Truth and Critical Communication. In *Oxford Research Encyclopedia of Communication.* Oxford University Press. doi:10.1093/acrefore/9780190228613.013.757

Horton, J. L. (2008). *Publicity Stunts, What Are They? Why Do Them?* http://online pr.com/Holding/PRStuntsarticle.pdf

Hsieh, H. F., & Shannon, S. E. (2005). Three Approaches to Qualitative Content Analysis. *Qualitative Health Research, 15*(9), 1277–1288. doi:10.1177/1049732305276687 PMID:16204405

İnal, U. (2016). An Investigation into Film 'Good Night and Good Luck' within Theories of Journalism ['Good Night and Good Luck' Filminin Gazetecilik Kuramları Çerçevesinde İncelenmesi]. *Middle Black Sea Journal of Communication Studies, 1*(2), 87–96.

Ker Dinçer, M., & Başok, N. (2014). Public Relations Spin Doctor Management Public Relations Practitioners are also not Spin Doctors [Halkla İlişkiler Döngü Yönetimi, Halkla İlişkiler Uygulamacıları da Döngü Uzmanı Değildir]. In What Public Relations Is Not [Halkla İlişkiler Ne Değildir?] (pp. 297-328). Say Yayınları.

Keyes, R. (2017). *The Post-Truth Era: Dishonesty and Deception in Contemporary Life* [Hakikat Sonrası Çağ: Günümüz Dünyasında Yalancılık ve Aldatma] (D. Özçetin, Trans.). Delidolu Yayınları.

Kocabay Şener, N. (2019). Post-Truth If You Want Lies, Let Me Lies [Post-Hakikat (Post-Truth) Yalanlar İstiyorsan Yalanlar Söyleyeyim]. In M. N. Erdem & N. Kocabay Şener (Eds.), *Communication in the Age of Posts* [Postlar Çağında İletişim] (pp. 383–416). Literatürk Academia.

Kundakçı, E. (2011). Politics, Media and Spin Doctor [Siyaset, Medya ve Spin Doctor]. In M. Ü. Erzen (Ed.), *Politics with its Historical, Cultural and Social Paradigms* [Tarihi, Kültürel ve Sosyal Paradigmaları ile Siyaset] (pp. 275–328). Der Yayınları.

Lilleker, D. G. (2013). *Siyasal İletişim: Temel Kavramlar* [Political Communication: Basic Concepts]. Kaknüs Yayınları.

Mavioğlu, E. (2012). *Turkey is in a Deserted State in Terms of Journalism* [Türkiye, Habercilik Açısından Çölleşmiş Bir Durumda]. http://www.yurtsuz.net/News.aspx?newsid=1355#.UXsEjrXIZF4

Mazzoleni, G. (2015). *Media Logic.* http://www.communicationencyclopedia.com/public/tocnode?id=g9781405131995_yr2013_chunk_g978140513199518_ss40-1

Michael, L. A. (2007). *The Principles of Existence & Beyond.* Lulu Enterprises.

Nel, F. (2005). *Writing For the Media.* Oxford University Press.

Oktay, M. (2002). *Public Relations in Politics* [Politikada Halkla İlişkiler]. Derin Yayınları.

Oxford Learner's Dictionaries. (2016). https://www.oxfordlearnersdictionaries.com/definition/english/post-truth?q=post-truth

Özgen, E., & Bayraktar, N. (2016). Public Relation is under the Threat of Spin Doctoring [Spin Doctor Kavramının Tehdidi Altında Halkla İlişkiler]. *Marmara İletişim Dergisi, 0*(21), 1–17.

Safire, W. (1996). *The Spinner Spun.* https://www.nytimes.com/1996/12/22/magazine/the-spinner-spun.html

Seıtel, F. P. (1998). *The Practice of Public Relation* (7th ed.). Prentice Hall.

Şen, O. (2021). Robot Journalism [Robot Gazetecilik]. In M. Şahin & E. İlhan (Eds.), *Specialization Areas in Journalism* [Gazetecilikte Uzmanlaşma Alanları] (pp. 57–76). Pelikan Yayınları.

Shabo, M. E. (2008). *Techniques of Propaganda and Persuasion.* Prestwick House.

The Economist. (2016). *The Post-Truth World: Yes, I'd Lie to You.* https://www.economist. com/briefing/2016/09/10/yes-id-lie-to-you

Uluk, M. (2018). *New Media and Fake News in the Post-Truth Age* [Hakikat Sonrası Çağda Yeni Medya ve Yalan Haber]. Dorlion Yayınları.

Wılcox Dennis, L., Ault Philip, H., Agee Warren, K., & Cameron Glen, T. (2000). *Public Relations Strategies and Tactics* (6th ed.). Longman.

Yılmaz, G. E. (2014). The Power without Responsibility in Political Communication: Spin Doctor [Siyasal İletişimde Sorumluluğu Olmayan Güç: Spin Doctor]. Düşünen Siyaset, 197-222.

Zabcı, F. (2021). Truth, Rhetoric and Politics [Hakikat, Retorik ve Siyaset]. In B. Özçelik (Ed.), *Post-truth Politics, Philosophy, Media, International Relations* [Hakikat Sonrası Siyaset, Felsefe, Medya, Uluslararası İlişkiler] (pp. 13–29). Nika Yayınevi.

ADDITIONAL READING

Bernays, E. L. (1923). *Crystallizing public opinion.* Liveright.

Budd, J. (1997). Watch out for the spin. *Public Relations Quarterly*, *42*(2), 4–6.

Schmitz, A., & Karam, F. (2013). The Spın Doctors of News Sources. *Brazılıan Journalısm Research*, *9*(1), 96–113. doi:10.25200/BJR.v9n1.2013.562

KEY TERMS AND DEFINITIONS

Content Analysis: It is one of the essential social science research methods. Generally, themes are determined and used to identify and analyze the parts among these themes whose content is considered essential.

Post-Truth: It is used to describe an era in which the importance of truth is lost.

Public Relations: Strategic communication tries to provide mutual communication and understanding between the institution and the target group.

Spin: Spin is to distort the facts until they come out.

Spin Doctor: They are experts who aim to deceive the target audience instead of communicating honestly.

Section 3

The Possibilities of Narrative in Conflict Resolution

Chapter 12
You're Not the Problem!
There's Always an Exception – Comparison of Narrative Therapy and Solution-Focused Brief Therapy

Aysu Gül Şanli
Ondokuz Mayıs University, Turkey

Doğan Güneş Temli
https://orcid.org/0000-0002-9786-0052
Ondokuz Mayıs University, Turkey

Eren Trabzon
Ondokuz Mayıs University, Turkey

Bozkurt Koç
https://orcid.org/0000-0002-6295-8009
Ondokuz Mayıs University, Turkey

ABSTRACT

In this study, narrative therapy and solution-focused brief therapy, which are the postmodern psychotherapy methods, are compared in terms of similarities and differences. In the study, primarily theoretical information about narrative therapy and solution-focused short-term therapy, which differs from traditional psychotherapy methods, the techniques used, and information about therapeutic application processes are given. Then, narrative therapy and solution-focused short-term therapies are compared in terms of similarities and differences. As a result, although narrative therapy, which is a postmodernist and social constructivist psychotherapy method, and solution-focused short-term therapy, which is a postmodern, inductive, and constructivist psychotherapy approach, have great similarities in terms of both theoretical and therapeutic processes; they also seem to have some differences.

DOI: 10.4018/978-1-7998-9251-9.ch012

INTRODUCTION

In addition to the problem-oriented approaches used in the field of social sciences, postmodernist and contemporary approaches that focus on the positive and strong aspects of the individual have also begun to take their place in the field. The effects of these approaches were also seen in psychotherapies in a short time. Narrative therapy, developed by Michael White and David Epston, and solution-focused brief therapy (SFBT), developed by Steve de Shazer and Insoo Kim Berg, are the main examples showing the reflections of postmodernism in psychotherapies. Based on the assumption that there is no single truth and that reality can be socially constructed through human interaction, solution-focused brief therapy and narrative therapy have offered a different view from most traditional approaches, arguing that the client is the expert of his/her own life (Corey, 2015). Within the scope of this study, these two therapy approaches are evaluated in terms of their similarities and differences.

Narrative Therapy

People give meaning to their experiences simply by "storytelling" their lives, and they realize their stories through their knowledge of them. Stories that enable us to give meaning to the events in our lives determine the nature of our experiences and our action patterns. Some of these stories provide protection for mental health, while others cause pathological effects (White, & Epston, 1990; Morgan, 2000). The narrative approach also offers a therapy method that emphasizes the importance of language in shaping individuals' realities (Shapiro, & Ross, 2002). An eclectic approach, narrative therapy benefits from storytelling, metaphors, and verbal tools (Gladding, 2019; Riley, & Malchiodi, 2003).

Narrative therapy first emerged in the field of family therapy in Australia and New Zealand, led by White and Epston in the late 1980s (Besley, 2002). Unlike traditional therapy approaches, narrative therapy offers a postmodern and constructivist approach and is based on social constructivism (Parry, & Doan, 1994; Shapiro, & Ross, 2002; Abels, & Abels, 2001). In this approach, stories about the problems of individuals are rewritten with the cooperation of the therapist and the client. In narrative therapy, exceptions and meanings are emphasized rather than problems (Gladding, 2019).

Although narrative therapy is a therapy approach that continues to evolve, it makes significant contributions to the field and is accepted by many theorists. Michael White and David Epston's book, Narrative Means to Therapeutic Ends (1990), is the primary source for the practice of narrative therapy (Abels, & Abels, 2001). The success of narrative therapy both in different client groups (immigrants, families, medical patient groups, etc.) and in the treatment process of various problems (post-traumatic stress disorder, eating disorders, diabetes, multiple sclerosis, brain injuries, psychosomatic disorders, etc.) shows that this model is quite effective in short-term therapies (Williams-Reade, Freitas, & Lawson, 2014). Unlike existing therapy approaches, narrative psychology places self-experience at the foundation of inquiry and therapy (Vassilieva, 2016). Narrative therapy is an approach that puts individuals at the center of their own lives and does not blame them. It sees problems as separate from people and assumes that people have many competencies in solving problems (Morgan, 2000).

Four important developments in the field of family therapy contributed to the development of narrative therapy. The first is that sight is set on clients' strengths and problem-solving resources rather than their problems or weaknesses. The second is that clients are seen not as objects, but as a partner who has an equal relationship with the therapist. The third is that more attention is paid to the meanings that family members place on events than concepts such as impulse, defense mechanisms and intrapsychic

tension. The last development is that the self-stories of the clients are taken in the center during the therapy process (Polkinghorne, 2004).
Morgan (2000) summarizes the basic assumptions of narrative therapy as follows:

- The problem is the problem, the individuals are not the problem.
- Individuals are experts in their own lives.
- Individuals can be lead authors of their own life stories.
- When individuals consult a therapist, they will have made an important attempt to lessen the impact of the problem in their lives and relationships.
- Problems are constructed in cultural contexts. These contexts include race, class, sexual orientation, gender, and disadvantaged power relations.
- Individuals generally make negative inferences about their lives and relationships based on the problems they have experienced. These negative inferences cause individuals to see themselves as inadequate. This feeling of inadequacy makes it difficult for them to use their potential related to their knowledge, competence, skills and abilities.
- Individuals' skills, competencies and knowledge can be made available to help them overcome their problems.
- The lives of individuals are not made up of problems. In other words, problems do not correspond to the whole of individuals' lives or relationships.
- It is the therapist's responsibility to provide an environment of curiosity, respect and transparency.

White and Epston (1990) also summarize the key elements for therapeutic practice as follows:

- Discovering relevant aspects of lived experience and developing different perspectives on this issue.
- Investigating the connections of events and relationships over time
- Discovering implicit meanings with exploratory speech
- Identifying these influences that affect the "ownership/authorship" of stories and emphasizing the person as a participant in the story and with the power to rewrite it
- Identifying dominant and subjugated discourses and dominant arrangements of privilege and power in a person's narratives
- Using different 'languages' to describe the experience and create new stories
- Mapping the impact of the problem on the person's life and relationships
- Creating the conditions in which the subject of the story becomes the privileged writer
- Externalizing the problem
- Recognizing unique results

In the literature, it is seen that narrative therapy is constructed to include four basic processes (Williams-Reade, Freitas, & Lawson, 2014):

1. With deconstruction, the personal meanings that clients attribute to the problems in their problem-saturated stories are revealed.

2. With externalization, both the client and the therapist are provided to define the problem separately from the individual, thus enabling the client to use his/her strengths-characteristics in the therapy process.
3. With mapping, the effects of the troubles experienced by the client or other problems related to the trouble on the client and this/her family members are determined.
4. With the re-authoring of the story, a new narrative includes unique outcomes and preferred by the client is developed and rewritten.

Deconstruction

According to narrative therapy, individuals can resist cultural objectification when they learn to detach from their problems (White, & Epston, 1990). At this stage, the therapist enables the client to discover the external factors that support their personal experience and coping efforts (Williams-Reade, Freitas, & Lawson, 2014).

Externalization

Individuals often believe that the problems in their lives are caused by themselves, others, or their relationships with others. Such a point of view causes problems to intensify instead of being solved, and the problems that are trying to be solved become more complex. Talks of externalization objectify the problem (White, 2007). It also enables clients to leave the dominant stories that shape their lives and relationships (White, & Epston, 1990). Metaphors are used to externalize problems (White, 2007).

Mapping the Effects

This stage includes the evaluation of the effects of the problems experienced in various areas (home, workplace, school, peer contexts, family relationships, one's relationship with oneself, friendships, individual's identity, goals, hopes, dreams, aspirations and values, future expectations and dreams, etc.) on the client. This questioning of the effects of the problems also helps to externalization of the problems (White, 2007). In this process, the effects of the problem are primarily investigated. These effects are then evaluated together with the client. Clients are asked mapping questions and the client begins to produce alternative stories (Williams-Reade, Freitas, & Lawson, 2014).

Re-authoring

At this stage, clients incorporate important events and experiences that are not included in their dominant stories but can positively shape their stories in their stories. These events and experiences are considered "unique outcomes" or "exceptions". The therapist also helps clients to develop alternative stories by asking questions to them. When clients adopt these alternative stories and start to include them in their lives, they develop new and alternative solutions to problems (White, 2007). Through the questions at this stage, the clients are provided to transfer their past experiences of problem solving to the solution of present and future problems (Williams-Reade, Freitas, & Lawson, 2014).

Narrative therapy aims to transform the stories people have about themselves and about other important people in their lives. The narrative approach emphasizes that our core beliefs are structured into stories or narratives that connect events, experiences, behaviors and emotions (Dallos, 2006).

Solution-focused Brief Therapy

Solution-Focused Brief Therapy Approach (SFBT), an inductive, constructivist and postmodern approach to psychotherapy, focuses on the client's own strength and the therapeutic cooperation between the client and the counselor (de Shazer, & Berg, 1997). SFBT was introduced in the Center for Family Therapy, founded in the late 1970s by Steve de Shazer, Insoo Kim Berg and their team (de Shazer et al., 1986; de Shazer et al., 2007; Connie, & Metcalf, 2009). For solution focused brief therapy, the books "Brief Therapy: Focused Problem Resolution" (Weakland, Fisch, Watzlawick, & Bodin, 1974) and "Brief Therapy: Two's Company" (de Shazer, 1975), are the main sources (de Shazer et al., 1986). Today, it is used with many models such as psychodynamic or cognitive behavioral therapy (Ratner, George, & Iveson, 2012).

The SFBT approach basically starts from the view that the problem and the solution are independent of each other. Facts, phenomenons, or circumstances are not the reason why a person states a situation as a problem; the person constructs the problem himself/herself and has the necessary resources for the solution. The communication between the client and the counselor in the therapy process is aimed at finding and shaping "past, present and future" solutions (Sparrer, 2012). In this approach that values people, it is thought that the stories that clients bring to therapy contain many solutions. The therapist listens to past stories with an accepting, understanding and constructive point of view and focuses on possible solutions (Güner, 2014). In the SFBT approach, clients can see what their lives will be like when the problem disappears (Proudlock, 2017).

The SFBT approach suggests that instead of looking to the past, it is necessary to focus on the present and the future (Proudlock, 2017). At the same time, the SFBT approach helps clients to develop a desired vision of the future where the problem is solved, to find exceptions, to discover and strengthen their strengths (Bavelas, de Jong, Franklin, Froerer, Gingerick, & Kim, 2013).

The SFBT can be used in different situations (such as depression, anxiety, attention deficit/hyperactivity disorder, trauma, attachment problems, substance abuse, drug use, suicide and risk of self-harm), when working with different individuals and groups (Lethem, 2002; Lutz, 2013). According to this approach, the best way to solve problems is for individuals to discover what they do when they are not having problems. In the therapy process, it is aimed to show clients that there are exceptions to problems and that the individual has solutions (Corey, 2015; Nichols, & Davis, 2012). At the same time, in solution-focused therapy, a large part of the conversation is conducted on self-efficacy and locus of control problems (Beyebach, Morejon, Palenzuela, & Rodriguez-Arias, 1996). While traditional therapy approaches focus on mental mechanisms such as "beliefs, personal characteristics, attitudes, values, thoughts, feelings, weaknesses and strengths"; solution-focused therapists do not make assumptions about these mental mechanisms and do not try to change them (McKergow, & Korman, 2009).

At the center of therapy is the client's future rather than their problems (Iveson, 2002), and therefore the solution-focused therapy process takes a short time (Nichols, & Davis, 2012). It is seen that the SFBT can be applied to most of the difficulties faced by clients (Trepper, Dolan, McCollum, & Nelson, 2006).

There are a number of principles that serve as a guide and base the approach for the implementation of the SFBT; "If it's not broken, don't fix it, the solution is not directly related to the problem, if it works, do more, if it doesn't work, do something different, it's not always a problem, there are always exceptions, look for previous solutions, the future can be built and discussed" (de Shazer et al., 2007; de Shazer, & Dolan, 2012). The main features of the technique are summarized as follows:

- Focuses on strengths, resources, solutions and the future rather than solving the problem.
- The therapeutic focus should be on the client's desired future rather than past problems or current conflicts. The first meeting serves the functions of alliance and solution building.
- The client is seen as stuck with the problem
- It's not always a problem. There are exceptions.
- Process is client-centred: Goals and interventions emerge from client's preferences, resources and feedback
- The client is a specialist and a teacher; the counselor follows the client's lead. The therapist helps clients to find alternatives to existing undesirable behavior patterns.
- Clients are seen as resourceful, having the ability to improve their lives, and already have resolution behaviors.
- Counseling skills are re-adapted for each client.
- Assuming no necessary relationship between problems and solutions: Many solutions are adaptable to most problems regardless of the problem's history, origins or presumed causes
- Effective solutions primarily derive from the client's strengths, resources, feedback and other contributions (Murphy, 2015; Murphy, 1994; Bavelas et al., 2013).

THERAPEUTIC TECHNIQUES

Defining the Problem: Therapy begins with a description of the client's problem. For example, "How do you hope I can help you?".

Goal Setting

After listening to and accepting clients' explanations of their problems and what they are trying to do about them, the next step is to set clear and concrete goals. Solution-focused therapists clarify and embody vague goals by asking questions such as "How will you do this?", "How will you know you have solved your problems?".

Discovering Exceptions

Investigating exceptions (times that clients are not experiencing problems) invites clients to realize that some potential solutions may already be in their hand. At this stage, the therapist asks exceptional questions, such as "When did the problem not arise recently?", "What difference does it make when there is no problem?".

Scaling Question

An emerging technique to help therapists and clients to talk about ambiguous issues such as depression and communication where tangible changes are difficult to describe.

Praise

By using expressions such as "Wow! How did you do this?", attention is drawn to the fact that the clients have already achieved something. At the same time, clients are helped to identify their achievements and increase their self-confidence (Nichols, & Davis, 2012).

While applying these techniques, therapists display a positive, collaborative, solution-oriented stance; looking for previous solutions and exceptions; uses instructions, compliments, questions and comments (Molnar, & de Shazer, 1987; de Shazer et al., 2007; Groot, 2002). During the therapy process, questions are asked about coping, seeking solutions, establishing relationships, and progressing (Kelly, Kim & Franklin, 2008). Through the continuous process of listening, assimilating, connecting and responding, the therapist and client construct new meanings with the solution. (Bavelas et al., 2013). De Shazer and Berg (1997) summarized the main points of the SFBT process as "asking the miraculous question in the first interview, asking the client to rate something on a "0-10" or "1-10" scale at least once in the first interview and in the subsequent interviews, taking a break at some point during the interview, giving some compliments to the client by the therapist after the break, often with a suggestion or homework (also called an experiment)".

NARRATIVE THERAPY AND SOLUTION-FOCUSED BRIEF THERAPY

Similarities Between Narrative Therapy and Solution-Focused Brief Therapy

Influenced by postmodernism, narrative therapy and SFBT focused on the positive and strong aspects of the individual and carried this perspective to the therapy process. These two approaches, the first reflections of which are in the field of family therapy, argue that the client is the expert of his/her own life (Corey, 2015). In these therapies, therapists create a change in their clients' experiences by helping them reshape their perspectives on events (Nichols, & Davis, 2012). SFBT emphasizes that change can be achieved consistently and continuously, and there is no need for long therapy sessions for this change (Arslan, & Gümüşçağlayan, 2018). In the narrative therapy process, the experience of change takes a short time too, and it is seen that the change is possible when the individual differentiates the meanings in his/her own story and realizes the mistakes (Akkuş, Kütük, & Samar, 2020).

In narrative therapy, exceptions and meanings are emphasized rather than problems (Gladding, 2019). The SFBT also helps clients to develop a vision for the future where the problem is solved, realize their strengths and find exceptions (Bavelas, De Jong, Franklin, Froerer, Gingerick, & Kim, 2013). At the same time, in this process, it is aimed to show that the individual has his/her own solutions for the problem (Corey, 2015; Nichols, & Davis, 2012). In this client-centered approach, the therapist only acts as a supportive guide (Groot, 2002; Berg & Miller, 1992). Narrative therapy, which focuses on the client, like the SFBT, sees the problems separately from people and assumes that people have many competencies in solving problems (Morgan, 2000). Similarly in the therapy process, the therapist's job is to provide supportive guidance. At the same time, the fact that the therapist does not position himself/herself as an expert or an authority is seen as one of the common points with SFBT (Akkuş, Kütük, & Samar, 2020).

Some techniques used in SFBT and narrative therapy also show similarities. The "Miracle Question Technique", which is based on the assumption that a miracle occurs and the client's problems are solved, is a technique frequently used in SFBT (de Shazer et al., 2007). In narrative therapy, the exceptions where the problem does not arise and meaningful questions that show the positive outcomes of these situations for the individual and his environment are used (Akkuş, Kütük, & Samar, 2020). These techniques used in both approaches support clients' problem-solving skills. Another similarity is the provision of change by referring to the strengths of the individual. This is tried to be achieved with coping questions in SFBT (Arslan, & Gümüşçağlayan, 2018). In narrative therapy, on the other hand, this is achieved by bringing up the individual's self-reflective stories and raising awareness about thought distortions (Porter, 2006). Questions are used as an important tool in order to better understand the client's experience and to determine the solution steps, both in SFBT and narrative therapy (Erçevik, 2021).

The main goal of therapy models is to provide the client with maximum benefit and not harm. Studies in the literature provide important information about the benefits of therapy models. In this context, studies such as online aggression (Wiretna, Saputra, Muarifah, & Barida, 2020), individuals who have committed crimes in prison (Lindforss, & Magnusson, 1997), children with emotional and behavioral problems (Selekman, 1997; Corcoran, 2006), students at risk in the school environment (Kim, & Franklin, 2009; Rhodes, & Ajmal, 1995; Newsome, 2005), parents (Zimmerman, Jacobsen, MacIntyre, & Watson, 1996), comparison of different approaches (Cepeda, & Davenport, 2006; Langdridge, 2006), career counseling (Burwell, & Chen, 2006), and family therapy (Beyebach et al., 2000), in which the SFBT approach is used in the literature, reveal the effectiveness of the technique (Smith, 2010). There are studies in the literature that show the effectiveness of narrative therapy, such as the SFBT. Related studies have shown that narrative therapy gives effective results in areas such as depression, anxiety, self-esteem, resilience (Akkuş, Kütük, & Samar, 2020), severe pathologies (Combs, & Freedman, 2012), substance abuse (Man-Kwong, 2004), pathological problems in children (Carlson, 2001), and group therapy (Ricks et al., 2014). Williams-Reade and colleagueset state that these two similar approaches, which are effective in different client groups and problems, can be used together in therapies (Williams-Reade, Freitas, & Lawson, 2014).

Differences Between Narrative Therapy and Solution-Focused Brief Therapy

Although the basic starting points and some techniques of the SFBT and narrative therapy are similar, there are also points where they differ. Subjectivity is emphasized in narrative therapy, while subjective experience is emphasized in SFBT. In subjective experiences, the client experiences a problem, but this problem affects the client by being in a position other than the client. There are exceptional cases where this problem does not affect life (Wolter, DiLollo, & Apel, 2006). The concept of subjectivity is examined in situational, environmental and cultural contexts (Murdock, 2013). At this point, it can be said that SFBT is effective in the process leading to the outcome. Narrative therapy, on the other hand, provides a more general framework for the client and examines a process from cause to result. In this technique, past experiences form the center of dominant stories and sources are mostly sought in past experiences. Therefore, the therapist primarily focuses on the past and then turns to the present and the future (Erçevik, 2021). However, unlike the traditional therapy models, SFBT offers a perspective that stays away from the past in the relations and dynamics between the present and the future (Groot, 2002).

However, the goal of narrative therapy is broader and more attitudinal, while the SFBT provides the ability to divert attention from failures to current achievements for activating behavioral solutions. For this purpose, narrative therapy uses the externalization technique (Nichols, & Davis, 2012).

In SFBT, the therapist's view of the client and the therapy process is completely solution-oriented. The therapy process provides the client with coping strategies and offers the opportunity to reach practical solutions (Arslan & Gümüşçağlayan, 2018). De Shazer (1985), emphasizes that in the theoretical background of SFBT, it is not necessary to focus and analyze the problem in order to solve the problems brought by the clients (Lipchik, 1994). (Lipchik, 1994). But, the basis of narrative therapy is to address the problems in the stories people create for themselves. In this context, in narrative therapy, an start-up and process-oriented perspective is presented instead of the result-oriented perspective of SFBT (Semmler, & Williams, 2000). Narrative therapy is more problem-oriented than solution-oriented. Contrary to the superficiality in the SFBT, the details of the problem and different contexts are addressed in narrative therapy, allowing the process to proceed in a more in-depth manner (Shapiro, & Ross, 2002). In this context, the fact that narrative therapy goes into details instead of ignoring the problems suggests that it may be a more effective technique than the SFBT.

CONCLUSION

In this study, narrative therapy and solution-focused short-term therapy methods, which differ from traditional psychotherapy methods, are compared in terms of similarities and differences. It is seen that these two approaches, which are influenced by postmodernism, are similar in certain aspects. These two approaches focused on the positive and strong aspects of the individual and carried this perspective to the therapy process. Both approaches argue that individuals are experts in their own lives and aim to create a change in their experiences by helping clients reshape their perspectives on events. While in narrative therapy, problems are mostly evaluated through exceptions and meanings; in solution-focused brief therapy, individuals are helped to realize their strengths and find exceptions. It is aimed to show that the individual has solutions for his/her own problems. Both therapies view problems as separate from people and assume that people have many competencies in solving problems. One of the common points of these two therapy approaches is that the therapist offers supportive guidance and does not position himself/herself as an expert or authority. These two methods also show similarities in terms of using some techniques that support clients' problem-solving skills. Another similarity is to enabling change by referring to the strengths of the individual. At the same time, in these two therapies, questions are used as an important tool in order to better understand the client's experience and to determine the solution steps.

Although these two therapy methods are similar in terms of their basic starting points and some of the techniques they use, there are also points where they differ. While subjective experience is emphasized in solution-focused brief therapy, subjectivity is emphasized in narrative therapy. At this point, it can be said that solution-focused brief therapy is effective in the process leading to the result; on the other hand, narrative therapy evaluates a process that leads from cause to result by providing a more general framework for the client. In addition, while solution-focused brief therapy allows attention to be diverted from failures to current successes; the purpose of narrative therapy is broader and more attitudinal. In solution-focused brief therapy, it is emphasized that, it is not necessary to focus on the problem in order to solve the problems brought by the clients; in narrative therapy, on the other hand, it is directed to the problems in the stories that people create for themselves. In this context, in narrative therapy, an istart-up and process-oriented perspective is presented instead of the result-oriented perspective of solution-focused brief therapy. Narrative therapy is more problem-oriented than solution-oriented. Contrary to the superficiality in solution-focused brief therapy, the details of the problem and different contexts are addressed in narrative therapy, allowing the process to progress in a more in-depth manner. In this context, the fact that narrative therapy goes into details instead of ignoring the problems suggests that narrative approach may be a more effective technique than solution-focused brief therapy.

As a result, the evaluations reveal that both therapy methods differ from traditional methods in terms of the philosophical foundations they are based on, the theoretical background and the therapy methods they use. At the same time, it is seen in the literature that these two similar therapy methods, whose effects on different client groups and different problems have been proven, can be used together in therapies.

REFERENCES

Abels, P., & Abels, S. L. (2001). *Understanding narrative therapy: A guidebook for the social worker.* Springer Publishing Company.

Akkuş, K., Kütük, B., & Samar, B. Ş. (2020). Narrative therapy: Philosophical and theoretical foundations, therapy techniques and efficacy [Öyküsel terapi: Felsefi ve kuramsal temelleri, terapi teknikleri ve etkinliği]. *Akdeniz İnsani Bilimler Dergisi, 10*, 27–37. doi:10.13114/MJH.2020.515

Arslan, Ü., & Gümüşçağlayan, G. (2018). Solution focused brief therapy: A brief overview [Çözüm odaklı kısa süreli terapiye kısa bir bakış]. *Mehmet Akif Ersoy Üniversitesi Eğitim Fakültesi Dergisi*, (47), 491–507. doi:10.21764/maeuefd.396228

Bavelas, J., De Jong, P., Franklin, C., Froerer, A., Gingerick, W., & Kim, J. (2013). Solution focused therapy treatment manual for working with individuals (2nd ed.). Solution Focused Brief Therapy Association.

Besley, A. C. (2002). Foucault and the turn to narrative therapy. *British Journal of Guidance & Counselling, 30*(2), 125–143. doi:10.1080/03069880220128010

Beyebach, M., Morejon, A. R., Palenzuela, D. L., & Rodriguez-Arias, J. L. (1996). Research on the process of solution-focused therapy. In S. D. Miller, M. A. Hubble, & B. L. Duncan (Eds.), *Handbook of solution-focused brief therapy* (pp. 299–334). Jossey-Bass Publishers.

Beyebach, M., Rodríguez-Sánchez, M. S., Arribas de Miguel, J., De Vega, M. H., Hernández, C., & Rodríguez-Morejón, A. (2000). Outcome of solution-focused therapy at a university family therapy center. *Journal of Systemic Therapies, 19*(1), 116–128. doi:10.1521/jsyt.2000.19.1.116

Burwell, R., & Chen, C. P. (2006). Applying the principles and techniques of solution-focused therapy to career counselling. *Counselling Psychology Quarterly, 19*(2), 189–203. doi:10.1080/09515070600917761

Carlson, R. (2001). Therapeutic use of story in therapy with children. *Guidance & Counseling, 16*(3), 92–99.

Cepeda, L. M., & Davenport, D. S. (2006). Person-centered therapy and solution-focused brief therapy: An integration of present and future awareness. *Psychotherapy (Chicago, Ill.), 43*(1), 1–12. doi:10.1037/0033-3204.43.1.1 PMID:22121955

Combs, G., & Freedman, J. (2012). Narrative, poststructuralism, and social justice: Current practices in narrative therapy. *The Counseling Psychologist, 40*(7), 1033–1060. doi:10.1177/0011000012460662

Connie, E., & Metcalf, L. (2009). *The art of solution focused therapy*. Springer Publishing Company.

Corcoran, J. (2006). A comparison group study of solution-focused therapy versus "treatment-as-usual" for behavior problems in children. *Journal of Social Service Research, 33*(1), 69–81. doi:10.1300/J079v33n01_07

Corey, G. (2015). *Theory and practice of counseling and psychotherapy*. Nelson Education.

Dallos, R. (2006). *Attachment narrative therapy*. McGraw-Hill Education.

de Shazer, S. (1975). Brief therapy: Two's company. *Family Process, 14*(1), 79–93. doi:10.1111/j.1545-5300.1975.00079.x

de Shazer, S. (1985). *Keys to solution in brief therapy*. Norton.

de Shazer, S., & Berg, I. K. (1997). 'What works?' Remarks on research aspects of solution-focused brief therapy. *Journal of Family Therapy, 19*(2), 121–124. doi:10.1111/1467-6427.00043

de Shazer, S., Berg, I. K., Lipchik, E. V. E., Nunnally, E., Molnar, A., Gingerich, W., & Weiner-Davis, M. (1986). Brief therapy: Focused solution development. *Family Process, 25*(2), 207–221. doi:10.1111/j.1545-5300.1986.00207.x PMID:3732502

de Shazer, S., & Dolan, Y. (2012). *More than miracles: The state of the art of solution-focused brief therapy*. Routledge. doi:10.4324/9780203836484

de Shazer, S., Dolan, Y. M., Korman, H., Trepper, T., McCollum, E., & Berg, I. K. (2007). *More than miracles: The state of the art of solution-focused brief therapy*. Haworth Press.

Erçevik, A. (2021). A comparative study regarding solution-focused brief counseling and narrative counseling approaches [Çözüm odaklı kısa süreli psikolojik danışma ve öyküsel psikolojik danışma yaklaşımlarına dair karşılaştırmalı bir inceleme]. *Humanistic Perspective, 3*(2), 400–419. doi:10.47793/hp.942378

Gladding, S. T. (2019). Family therapy: History, theory and practice (7th ed.). Pearson.

Groot, D. S. (2002). *Shifting gears: An integration of solution-focused therapy and experiential therapy in couples counselling* (Master's thesis, University of Manitoba). Retrieved from https://mspace.lib.umanitoba.ca/xmlui/handle/1993/22624

Güner, O. (2014). *The solution is hidden in me* [Çözüm bende saklı]. Eflatun.

Iveson, C. (2002). Solution-focused brief therapy. *Advances in Psychiatric Treatment, 8*(2), 149–157. doi:10.1192/apt.8.2.149

Kelly, M. S., Kelly, M. S., Kim, J. S., & Franklin, C. (2008). *Solution focused brief therapy in schools: A 360 degree view of research and practice*. Oxford University Press. doi:10.1093/acprof:oso/9780195366297.001.0001

Kim, J. S., & Franklin, C. (2009). Solution-focused brief therapy in schools: A review of the outcome literature. *Children and Youth Services Review*, *31*(4), 464–470. doi:10.1016/j.childyouth.2008.10.002

Langdridge, D. (2006). Solution focused therapy A way forward for brief existential therapy? *Journal of the Society for Existential Analysis*, *17*(2), 359–370.

Lethem, J. (2002). Brief solution focused therapy. *Child and Adolescent Mental Health*, *7*(4), 189–192. doi:10.1111/1475-3588.00033 PMID:33158321

Lindforss, L., & Magnusson, D. (1997). Solution-focused therapy in prison. *Contemporary Family Therapy*, *19*(1), 89–103. doi:10.1023/A:1026114501186

Lipchik, E. (1994). The rush to be brief. *The Family Therapy Networker*, *18*(2), 35–39.

Lutz, A. B. (2013). *Learning solution-focused therapy: An illustrated guide*. American Psychiatric Pub. doi:10.1176/appi.books.9781615370986

Man-Kwong, H. (2004). Overcoming craving: The use of narrative practices in breaking drug habits. *International Journal of Narrative Therapy & Community Work*, (1), 17–24. doi:10.3316/informit.228689124056043

McKergow, M., & Korman, H. (2009). Inbetween-neither inside nor outside: The radical simplicity of solution-focused brief therapy. *Journal of Systemic Therapies*, *28*(2), 34–49. doi:10.1521/jsyt.2009.28.2.34

Molnar, A., & de Shazer, S. (1987). Solution-focused therapy: Toward the identification of therapeutic tasks. *Journal of Marital and Family Therapy*, *13*(4), 349–358. doi:10.1111/j.1752-0606.1987.tb00716.x

Morgan, A. (2000). *What is narrative therapy? An easy-to-read introduction*. Dulwich Centre Publications.

Murdock, N. L. (2013). Narrative therapy [Anlatımsal terapi]. In F. Akkoyun (Ed.), *Psikolojik danışma ve psikoterapi kuramları: Olgu sunumu yaklaşımıyla* (pp. 490–513). Nobel Yayıncılık.

Murphy, J. J. (1994). Working with what works: A solution-focused approach to school behavior problems. *The School Counselor*, *42*, 59–65.

Murphy, J. J. (2015). *Solution-focused counseling in schools*. John Wiley & Sons.

Newsome, W. S. (2005). The impact of solution-focused brief therapy with at-risk junior high school students. *Children & Schools*, *27*(2), 83–90. doi:10.1093/cs/27.2.83

Nichols, M. P., & Davis, S. D. (2012). *Family therapy: Concepts and methods*. Pearson.

Parry, A., & Doan, R. E. (1994). *Story re-visions: Narrative therapy in the postmodern world*. The Guilford Press.

Polkinghorne, D. E. (2004). Narrative therapy and postmodernism. In L. E. Angus & J. McLeod (Eds.), *The handbook of narrative and psychotherapy: Practice, theory and research* (pp. 53–67). Sage.

Porter, L. (2006). Narrative therapy: An introduction for counsellors. *Journal of Family Studies*, *12*(2), 294–310.

Proudlock, S. (2017). *The solution focused way: Incorporating solution focused therapy tools and techniques into your everyday work*. Routledge. doi:10.4324/9781315145433

Ratner, H., George, E., & Iveson, C. (2012). *Solution focused brief therapy: 100 key points and techniques*. Routledge. doi:10.4324/9780203116562

Rhodes, J., & Ajmal, Y. (1995). *Solution focused thinking in schools: behaviour, reading and organisation*. BT Press.

Ricks, L., Kitchens, S., Goodrich, T., & Hancock, E. (2014). My story: The use of narrative therapy in individual and group counseling. *Journal of Creativity in Mental Health*, *9*(1), 99–110. doi:10.1080/15401383.2013.870947

Riley, S., & Malchiodi, C. A. (2003). Solution-focused and narrative approaches. In C. A. Malchiodi (Ed.), *Handbook of art therapy* (pp. 82–92). The Guilford Press.

Selekman, M. D. (1997). *Solution-focused therapy with children: Harnessing family strengths for systemic change*. Guilford Press.

Semmler, P. L., & Williams, C. B. (2000). Narrative Therapy: A Storied Context for Multicultural Counseling. *Journal of Multicultural Counseling and Development*, *28*(1), 51–62. doi:10.1002/j.2161-1912.2000.tb00227.x

Shapiro, J., & Ross, V. (2002). Applications of narrative theory and therapy to the practice of family medicine. *Family Medicine*, *34*(2), 96–100. PMID:11874032

Smith, S. (2010). A preliminary analysis of narratives on the impact of training in solution-focused therapy expressed by students having completed a 6-month training course. *Journal of Psychiatric and Mental Health Nursing*, *17*(2), 105–110. doi:10.1111/j.1365-2850.2009.01492.x PMID:20465754

Sparrer, I. (2012). *Introduction to the solution-oriented approach and systemic structural alignment* [Çözüm odaklı yaklaşıma ve sistemik yapısal dizime giriş]. Pan Yayıncılık.

Trepper, T. S., Dolan, Y., McCollum, E. E., & Nelson, T. (2006). Steve De Shazer and the future of solution-focused therapy. *Journal of Marital and Family Therapy*, *32*(2), 133–139. doi:10.1111/j.1752-0606.2006.tb01595.x PMID:16676891

Vassilieva, J. (2016). *Narrative psychology: Identity, transformation and ethics*. Springer. doi:10.1057/978-1-137-49195-4

Weakland, J. H., Fisch, R., Watzlawick, P., & Bodin, A. M. (1974). Brief therapy: Focused problem resolution. *Family Process*, *13*(2), 141–168. doi:10.1111/j.1545-5300.1974.00141.x

White, M. (2007). *Maps of narrative practice*. W. W. Norton & Company.

White, M., & Epston, D. (1990). *Narrative means to therapeutic ends*. W.W. Norton & Company.

Williams-Reade, J., Freitas, C., & Lawson, L. (2014). Narrative-informed medical family therapy: Using narrative therapy practices in brief medical encounters. *Families, Systems & Health, 32*(4), 416–425. Advance online publication. doi:10.1037/fsh0000082 PMID:25329755

Wiretna, C. D., Saputra, W. N. E., Muarifah, A., & Barida, M. (2020). Effectiveness of solution-focused brief counseling to reduce online aggression of student. *Universal Journal of Educational Research, 8*(3), 1092–1099. doi:10.13189/ujer.2020.080344

Wolter, J. A., DiLollo, A., & Apel, K. (2006). A narrative therapy approach to counseling: A model for working with adolescents and adults with language-literacy deficits. *Language, Speech, and Hearing Services in Schools, 37*(3), 168–177. doi:10.1044/0161-1461(2006/019) PMID:16837440

Zimmerman, T. S., Jacobsen, R. B., MacIntyre, M., & Watson, C. (1996). Solution-focused parenting groups: An empirical study. *Journal of Systemic Therapies, 15*(4), 12–25. doi:10.1521/jsyt.1996.15.4.12

ADDITIONAL READING

de Shazer, S. (1985). *Keys to solution in brief therapy.* Norton.

de Shazer, S., & Berg, I. K. (1997). 'What works?' Remarks on research aspects of solution-focused brief therapy. *Journal of Family Therapy, 19*(2), 121–124. doi:10.1111/1467-6427.00043

de Shazer, S., Berg, I. K., Lipchik, E. V. E., Nunnally, E., Molnar, A., Gingerich, W., & Weiner-Davis, M. (1986). Brief therapy: Focused solution development. *Family Process, 25*(2), 207–221. doi:10.1111/j.1545-5300.1986.00207.x PMID:3732502

de Shazer, S., & Dolan, Y. (2012). *More than miracles: The state of the art of solution-focused brief therapy.* Routledge. doi:10.4324/9780203836484

Metcalf, L. (2017). *Solution focused narrative therapy.* Springer Publishing Company. doi:10.1891/9780826131775

Milner, J., O' Byrne, P., & Campling, J. (2017). *Brief counselling: Narratives and solutions.* Macmillan International Higher Education.

White, M. (2007). *Maps of narrative practice.* W. W. Norton & Company.

White, M., & Epston, D. (1990). *Narrative means to therapeutic ends.* Norton & Company.

KEY TERMS AND DEFINITIONS

Deconstruction: A narrative therapy process in which the personal meanings that clients attribute to the problems in their problem-saturated stories are revealed.

Externalization: A narrative therapy process in which both the client and the therapist are provided to define the problem separately from the individual.

Mapping: A narrative therapy process in which the effects of the troubles experienced by the client or other problems related to the trouble on the client and his/her family members are determined.

Metaphor: A form of speech in which a word or phrase is applied to another word or idea that it does not actually denote in order to convey a meaning difficult to convey otherwise.

Praise: A SFBT technique which attention is drawn to the fact that the clients have already achieved something.

Re-Authoring: A narrative therapy process in which a new narrative includes unique outcomes and preferred by the client is developed and rewritten.

Scaling Questions: An emerging technique that helps therapists and clients to talk about ambiguous issues such as depression and communication where tangible changes are difficult to describe.

Chapter 13
Therapeutic Storytelling:
How Can We Use Stories More Effectively?

Gamze Mukba
Van Yüzüncü Yıl University, Turkey

ABSTRACT

Therapeutic storytelling aims to find the psychological difficulties experienced by the individual through creative narratives, uses problem-solving skills, and offers alternative ways based on narrative therapy. In therapeutic storytelling, questions about the meaning attributed to the story, the hero and metaphors that can be asked to the client, and the circular question forms of systemic interventions related to others important to the person are similar. In both forms of these interventions, subjective reality is reconstructed, and so, therapeutic storytelling can be used eclectically with systemic interventions. In this chapter, a sample intervention template for systemic-based therapeutic storytelling has been offered. Moreover, an exemplary hypothetical case of the systemic-based storytelling intervention pattern is presented. As a result, instead of focusing directly on the client's own life story, using storytelling intervention in a less threatening environment for the client through other stories may activate the client to gain insight and different viewpoints.

INTRODUCTION

People tend to disregard unpleasant thoughts, beliefs, and unsatisfactory story elements in their life experiences while turning into the stories they narrate and tell in their biographies. People may also fill in the gaps in their biographies with prominent elements. It is possible to discover unprecedented sections of the story discourses that people dominate, question numerous possible experiences in life stories, and reinterpret interpersonal relationships through narrative therapy. Substantial life experiences of people may be scrutinized within the context of narrative therapy, and through hypothetical/probable life experiences and reorganization of interpersonal relationships, people may ensure that they release emotions over which they have control in their lives and that they allow them to see that their troubles as separate from their own (Denborough, 2014; White & Epston, 1990).

DOI: 10.4018/978-1-7998-9251-9.ch013

Narrative therapy is an intervention strategy that assists children and adults in discovering their strengths as well as establishing a new perspective on their distresses (Serneels, 2013). White and Epston (1990, pp.55-61) cited the unique results in the restructuring of people's stories about the experiences that constitute significant turning points in their lives, and through 'the unique results', new meanings may be attributed to the distresses in the individual's story, as if they were structures that strengthen them. It was stated that individuals might reassess their concerns and interactions with others, according to three basic structures: unique results in the past, unique results in the present, and unique results in the future. The unique results of the past and their effects on people's concerns on their present life may be detected with a historical review. The unique results at present, however, are related to the individual's attribution of new meanings to his/her lived experiences in light of new information and empowerment. Unique results for the future, the existence of future intentions and hope, provide a perspective on the distressing situation that the individual have been experiencing, and the possibility of different experiences in the future. It is possible for an individual to acquire alternative perspectives with many possibilities in his actions, choices, and similar concerns regarding the future actions.

Individuals reflect on their subsequent experiences by narrating their earlier experiences, much as they do in the narrative of unique events in the framework of the past, present, and future. The stories of individuals and the meanings they ascribe to the stories evolve throughout time in this way. As individuals participate in a reflective story process, their stories are frequently reconstructed, re-storified, and altered. In this context, the individual may use storying to consider his own story from different perspectives. The psychological counselor may ask individuals what they heard from their stories and how they interpret it, may not think from that point of view, may create a change in that story by incorporating some narrative aspects, and narrate the newly generated story in a different way (Connelly & Clandinin, 1990). The nature of each individual's story is related to a reality in itself. In this case, the situation underlying narrative therapy is related to storytelling.

BACKGROUND

Our lives are full of stories. Every day, we come across a variety of stories. We reiterate stories we hear from friends and acquaintances to others. We make up stories about our adventures. We watch stories on television and in the movies and read stories in novels and fairy tales. We used to listen to fairy stories and cultural myths as children, and we now pass this on to our children. Many of these stories are about others and their adventures; they are about how they deal with challenges and how they make successful choices come to the fore. Stories that may overcome significant barriers or execute socially important and worthwhile outcomes are compelling (McKee, 2003; Polkinghorne, 2013). Stories that stand out in storytelling attempt to strike a balance between the subjective expectations and the subjective reality of individuals. A skilled storyteller portrays what it means to cope with the expectations of struggling with the hero's sorrow, the hero's inner struggle, the meaning of making difficult decisions and acting despite risks, and ultimately the discovery of subjective reality. Since the dawn of time, all great stories have addressed the basic tension between subjective anticipation and subjective reality, from the ancient Greeks to Shakespeare (McKee, 2003).

According to the researchers, Jung's concepts such as archetypes, the individual's subconscious, and conscious inner journey, and the concept of the collective subconscious (Aguilera et al., 2020) are all related to therapeutic storytelling, as Milton Erikson's use of his clients' metaphors, discussing the client's language and therapeutic stories in his interviews (Larkin, 1988). The decision-making journey of the individuals in the adventure of the story with notions such as the collective unconscious and being consciously or subconsciously influenced by the choices of others may be a reflection of the stories they have acquired. As emphasized by the researchers, on the other hand, the metaphorical language used by the client in the interview session, as mentioned by Milton Erikson, and using the magic of the language with hypnosis refers to the therapeutic state of being a storyteller (Larkin, 1988). It can be stated that expressing the conscious or unconscious life adventures of individuals as a new story with their reflection in another story is meaningful in terms of their treatment processes, and in this context, re-expressing a metaphorical story in visual and auditory contexts may attract individuals to the story. Therefore, therapeutic storytelling is a sort of therapeutic intervention in a post-modern paradigm that aims to address the psychological discomfort experienced by the individual through creative stories, is instructive, and is sensed in the picture like the visuals in the movie (Divinyi, 1995).

THERAPEUTIC STORYTELLING

Therapeutic storytelling, like the roles of good narrators and listeners in a play staged in the theater, refers to a therapeutic intervention that allows a person to freely express their repressed and traumatic sentiments, and the healing process begins with the distressing of the story (Badham, 2020). Similarly, Long (2013) stated that therapeutic storytelling is a relaxing and innovative technique in which problem-solving skills are put to work through metaphors, present alternative ways for people to cope with concerns they experience, reflect on their inner world, and act out the process unconsciously. As a result, in therapy, stories serve as a framework through which the client may reflect on their life story and make sense of everything. Identification may be the most potent acting mechanism here, with the client putting himself in the shoes of the story's protagonists and attempting to imitate what the fictitious hero is doing. The client may reflect and identify with the projection to discover a solution to their conflicts if the story develops and contains enough implicit messages (Bhattacharyya, 2006).

The Benefits of Therapeutic Storytelling

Therapeutic storytelling is beneficial for the client. The interactional processes of the characters are brought to the fore through this intervention; and through interactional processes, the individual may be kept from being caught in the past, focusing on the present, and looking to the future with hope (Badham, 2020). Indeed, the concept of White and Epstone's (1990) unique outcomes in narrative therapy emphasizes the following: unique results for the past, unique results for the present, and unique results for the future. In addition to re-interpreting the elements of the past in the individual's story, it may make sense of its unique results for the present and convey its potential story of new configurations for the future. In some cases, stories may also serve as a warning to the individual about potential risks. For instance, the lesson that it is perilous for an individual to interact and communicate with other people comes to the fore in the story of 'Little Red Riding Hood' (Polkinghorne, 2013, p.31).

This intervention contains beneficial aspects that come to the fore when working with children particularly, just as it does among adults. The intervention of storytelling ensures that children's natural reluctance to change is overcome, that they hear excellent and meaningful ideas, and that they are reminded of the need to take action in the face of change (Carlson & Arthur, 1999; Iglesias & Iglesias,

2016). Healing resources of a child's subconscious are mobilized to provide insight through storytelling (Carlson & Arthur, 1999). Instead of being a passive participant in the therapeutic process, therapeutic storytelling empowers the child to actively participate in the solution (Cook et al., 2004). After listening to a well-selected therapeutic story, various images of the unpleasant experience are formed in the child's mind: old/previous picture, new picture, and future picture. Different visuals may be shaped in a child's head through a story that allows creativity and empathy (Sunderland, 2017). Researchers have discovered that by altering the visuals in the story, anxiety and maladaptive thoughts of the clients can be reduced, while compatible thoughts and positive self-perception may be increased (Cook et al., 2004; Iglesias & Iglesias, 2016).

Stories about others provide us with ideas about how to deal with similar adversity we face and that which the protagonist faces. The stories also include narratives that depict how an objective is reached unethically but that these activities were ultimately wrong at the end of the story. Stories presents society's values by demonstrating which acts are acceptable and which are not (McLean & Tuite, 2016; Polkinghorne, 2013). Stories are retained in memory by offering informative possibilities regarding certain situations. Lessons are gained from what is spoken at the end of the stories without experiencing any traumatic circumstance in our lives (Polkinghorne, 2013; Russo et al., 2006). Therefore, it can be stated that the client may express his feelings and thoughts in a less intimidating environment while listening to concerns and coping with resources in a story that is relevant to the client's own.

Individuals will identify with the main character in a therapeutic story if it is chosen in accordance with the relevant context being studied, such as the client's distress and coping resources. By doing so, the child will embark on the same journey as the character. The individual may distress with the character's setbacks and struggles, yet they will also be able to appreciate the courage of the character in refusing to give up and move forward. In this context, the individual will no longer feel as much anguish and difficulties because these feelings are also in doubt for the person in the story. An excellent therapeutic story that will bring hope to the individual can be a great source of emotional support for the individual. This can be deduced from the individual request to 'tell it again' (Sunderland, 2017, p.17).

Therapeutic storytelling has been shown to be particularly beneficial in the treatment of traumatized individuals. The amygdala, as it is known, is responsible for the activity of the sympathetic nervous system and is generally associated with negative emotions and physical arousals, defined as fear or anxiety. It may be argued that people who do not have a high level of psychological well-being or who feel extreme fear and anxiety have more intense amygdala reactions. For instance, an individual who has experienced a traumatic situation (such as a sudden loss, for instance, a close relative who committed suicide) may have significant anxiety-based emotions, driving the individual to focus and protect himself rather than engage in interpersonal social interaction. Within the context of studies performed, therapeutic stories that carry the individual to the experiences of others' distress may generally inspire compassion in the listener, and in this context, therapeutic stories may also serve as compassion training, and thus, there may be positive changes in the amygdala reactions of the story listener (Spencer-Thomas, 2020). In addition to the listening process of the stories, therapeutic storytelling may take the form of story writing. With the presence of the self, a therapeutic relationship is built through making conversation, sharing emotions, witnessing joyful and sad moments, and ultimately writing and rewriting life narratives. In essence, healing is the process of making sense of the life story and making peace with it, the ability to achieve freedom despite one's life experiences, and being the author of one's own life story. In some ways, storytelling is the process of writing or listening (Gu, 2018).

Therapeutic storytelling has been demonstrated to be an intervention approach in effectively treating many psychiatric disorders in various studies. Therapeutic storytelling intervention aids to improve the psychological well-being of cancer patients (Quiroga et al., 2016; Laing et al., 2019) and contributes to the individual's recovery after trauma-related brain tissue damage. It has also been indicated that it is very effective in the formation of meaningful insight into the inner world of individuals (D'Cruz et al., 2020). Furthermore, such an intervention strategy has been suggested for a variety of psychological issues, including eating disorders (Lodge-Guttery, 2004), children's irritability, and in-school maladaptive behavior disorders (Burrows, 2013). An experiment was undertaken in another study (Rolbiecki et al., 2019), to assess the efficiency of digital storytelling techniques on family members mourning together. Within the scope of storytelling, researchers discovered that activities such as writing about the script and verbally expressing the story contribute to the regulation of family members' emotions and thoughts, and they concluded that this method allows family members the opportunity to express their feelings about the mourning phenomenon with confidence (Rolbiecki et al., 2019). Similarly, in a doctoral dissertation study (Mukba, 2020), it was indicated that children who experienced grief revealed their unfinished emotions and thoughts related to the phenomenon of that grief through the intervention of systemic-based therapeutic storytelling and found that they reconstructed their stories in contextual relationships such as family, past, present and future.

Best Practices of Therapeutic Storytelling

According to the current literature, there are a variety of therapeutic narrative intervention approaches that can be performed with both children and adults. The relevant literature is examined, and the best practices are described below.

Reynolds and Bove (2016) highlighted a technique related to the mutual storytelling process that can be utilized especially with children. According to the researcher's findings, mutual storytelling is a powerful tool for developing new answers through metaphors, solutions, problem selection, power, and new ways of observing oneself and others. In this context, what the client and psychological counselor narrated about the story interact and adapt to each other. With this aspect, it can be claimed that it becomes a flexible technique through the client's engagement in the interaction, and the client and counselor's creativity and problem-solving talents come to the fore. It comprises mutual storytelling of the child and counselor. Reynolds and Bove (2016, p.2) stated that two stages related to this technique came to the fore, and consultants might use these stages to build this application. *Activity 1*

'In cooperation with the child, the psychological counselor begins to narrate the story related to the child's distress': Names actual or imaginary characters, provides details of how events happened, makes definitions, measures how the main character reacts both throughout the problem scenario and after it ends, describes how the child feels and defines the terms for it.

Activity 2

'The counselor works with the child to rewrite another version of the story that was staged in the previous activity and generate a better solution'. To encourage the child, the counselor takes the following steps: The counselor introduces a fantasy supporting or a magical character into the story, then repeats the problem scenario; however, this time asks for a solution from the fantasy character. Meanwhile, while asking for remedy from the fantasy character, the child and counselor are expected to find a solution, then the counselor animates the new options in the story to use the solution, plays the new options, finishes the story with a better ending, and finally, explains the child's feelings, beliefs, and other positive results that emerged after the problems were resolved.

'Storytelling technique through family drawing and systemic approach' was developed via benefitting projective drawing and storytelling techniques; in this technique, interpretation of the child's actual world is targeted in a psychological counseling session (Roosa, 1981, pp.270-271). This technique is also useful in terms of understanding the family dynamics of the child and observing whether or not the child may cope with problems effectively. The researcher indicated that this activity was efficient in establishing rapport with the child and exposing information that would otherwise be non-voluntary or beyond the child's conscious awareness. Making inferences, for instance, is possible about the symbolic content through the child's drawings. It may even involve using dolls or puppets to make assumptions based on the child's thoughts about the principal characters depicted in the picture. Before using this strategy, family members are pooled to gather information if any notable changes in the family occurred (for example, the death of a family member or a divorce in the family).

- **Step 1:** The child is given a blank sheet, a pencil, and paints and instructed to use the drawing paper in the vertical direction. The directives are as follows: 'I would like you to draw your family and yourself'. There may be some certain changes in the family structure through divorce and separation, and it is at issue here to see whom the child includes in his family drawing.
- **Step 2:** In the second stage, the child is instructed to draw a picture of how the family members behave to him/her. In addition, the child may be questioned about what happened before this event, how each family member reacted, and how the story ended. The following questions may be asked with the researchers' suggestions; 'Which one is the strongest?', 'Who tried what in coping?'. When necessary, the child may underline specific shapes in the drawing and react by emphasizing those shapes.
- **Step 3:** After the child has completed the family story, the counselor may inquire if there is any major missing family member who has not been drawn, and if the child wishes to draw it (for instance, one of the divorced parents). This drawing may often be a separated parent paying visits to the child. The counselor may then photocopy the original drawing that depicted the child's family members and generate individual cut-figures and cut-names for each family member.
- **Step 4:** In the following stage, the child is then instructed about how family members might have a story after they get through the crisis together using pieces of paper or objects that symbolize the family members (for instance, cut figures). At this point, the child may make the family members talk by placing them in double and triple positions on a paper. It is expected that during these stages, the child's favorable relationship patterns with family members will be enhanced, and the child will begin noticing their power sources.

All stages of the five-step storytelling technique created by Cook et al. (2004, pp.245-246), which can be used with children experiencing various psychological difficulties such as aggression, are given below. In line with the five-step storytelling technique;

- **The first step is to introduce the main characters:** 'The age, gender, size and physical properties of the character should resemble the client's characteristics. The child's abilities and strengths may also be mentioned'.

- **The second step is to bring up the issue:** 'The hero here experiences difficulties similar to those what the client does. Exaggerated expressions and humor may also be used to reduce the seriousness and hardship of the situation'.
- **The third step is to have a speak with a wise figure:** 'At this point, the hero's parents or the hero himself make a wish to meet a wise person who can assist him in solving the problem. The wise person or object, an unusual being, etc., may offer unconditional acceptance and love to the child, as well as demonstrate new ways of thinking and acting that may be beneficial. The wise person always brings new thoughts to the worried family members and individuals'.
- **The fourth step is to create a new perspective: '**The wise person encourages the hero to take action and new ways of thinking so that the hero of the story may see different outcomes. In the fourth step, a portrait is drawn that the main character learns through current experiences.'
- **The fifth step is to summarize what was noticed:** 'At the end of the story, the hero considers alternative situations and comes to a certain conclusion. It is emphasized that this story may be used when necessary'.

According to the emotional world of the child, Sunderland (2017, pp.22-27) drew attention to the following steps in therapeutic storytelling; first, defining the child's emotional distress or related situation is necessary; in the second step, however, it is necessary to create characters, a place, a situation that contains a metaphorical context related to the distress or subject. In the created situation, the 'current main character' must be experiencing the same emotional problem or emotional theme as the child. The main character should be employing maladaptive coping resources or similar to those used by the child. These maladaptive coping resources are demonstrated that they are self-destructive and/or detrimental to others, or the character is on a maladaptive path. The eventual failure of maladaptive coping resources is shown, resulting in some internal or external crisis in the character's life. Then the child's path from crisis to the solution is depicted metaphorically. It is critical to avoid making a quick transition from crisis to solution; in other words, 'fast improvements' shall be avoided. A journey or a link between the problem and the solution must be included in the story created. Otherwise, the story may lose its credibility and may no longer resemble real life. The third stage, however, is the completion of the transition to the next stage. Something or someone may appear in this subsequent transition stage to assist the character in changing his/her ways or employing more adaptive coping resources and innovative solutions in the essential section of the adventure that leads to a solution. In such a setting, the main character will be able to adjust to new behaviors successfully, use better coping mechanisms, and feel better. There are some points to consider during the indicated stages. It is critical to put the situation the child is worried about in a different context. A child who wets the bed, for instance, may feel ashamed; in such a case, the counselor may tell the child about a hedgehog having a leak in the forest. In the context selection, things, places, and characters that the child likes may be used as objects in the form of Disneyland, chocolate, chips, rainbows, fireworks, and castles. Another factor to consider during the aforementioned stages is to determine correctly the 'emotional theme' of the child's distress. A direction to the child such as 'what is your feeling right now, let the items you draw in this picture sense those feelings, too' may assist the child in determining the emotional theme of the distress experienced.

Regarding therapeutic storytelling practices, Slivinske and Slivinske (2014, pp.3-4) emphasized the storytelling intervention of gradual self-disclosure, especially about the safe self-expression of clients who have difficulties in expressing themselves. Within the scope of gradual self-disclosure storytelling, the client is asked to answer simple questions about the characters in the story in the first step.

Clients are also asked to describe their characters in the first step to gain insight into their own lives. However, in the second stage, the clients are asked whether any family members or friends who may have had comparable experiences to the narrative heroes in the story have had similar experiences, too. The clients may be able to open up themselves slightly as a result of this. In the third stage, the clients are asked questions about the similarities between the hero's life in the story and their own lives. In the fourth stage, the clients are requested to end their story, and they are given instructions to talk while expressing the ending of their story, write the ending of their story, or draw the ending of the story. The instruction given in the fourth stage allows the clients in the 'self-disclosure storytelling intervention' to expose themselves at the highest level.

Mager (2019) stated that therapeutic storytelling intervention may be performed with elderly individuals and have a favorable impact on their indomitability levels. Mager (2019, p.26) also indicated that the following steps can be taken into consideration while designing a group storytelling intervention with older people:

- Activity 1: 'Tell us a story about individuals who overcome difficulties.'
- Activity 2: 'What story comes to your mind when you think of home?'
- Activity 3: 'Tell us a story about a significant relationship you have'.
- Activity 4: 'Tell us a story about a time when a transformation impacted your life.'
- Activity 5: 'Tell us a story about how a health concern affects your self-confidence.'

A storytelling intervention for refugees has been advocated, with one-hour sessions per week that can be held in a few weeks through questions and activities involving their surroundings around them (Moore, 2017, pp.47-50). Within the scope of storytelling, it is also indicated that young immigrants may generate their own content through their social media, written expressions, drawings (comic style), sound recordings, photographs, and videos. Researchers emphasized that the sessions may be tailored particularly to facilitate recovery (healing) through personal narrative and interpersonal relationships, but they will take place in a peer group setting with a flexible format. The format of the intervention begins with audio recordings of storytelling sessions, then moves into written and comic book illustrations, photography, and video. During each session, participants are asked to share their personal journey to the world throughout each session. Participants are asked to describe their current and future journeys. They are also asked to describe the journey that depicts where they hope to be in the future; in other words, 'tomorrow'. Words such as resilience, perseverance, competence, relationships, and hope are terms that go hand-in-hand with those employed in activities that are fundamental to the empowerment and healing process. In the 'comic hero sessions', however, the participants are asked to draw the stories of their journeys in the form of comics. Drawings are revealed through the templates provided and side-by-side group discussions. The comic is given to the participants in the room, and they are asked to respond to the following questions: What is a hero? What are the things that make you strong? How do you continue to endure in the face of difficulties? How do you build trust in others and help them along your journey? The resilience talks in discussion instill bravery in participants by demonstrating that they have successfully conquered adversity in their life events. Problem-solving, competency, and self-sufficiency become more prominent at this stage. It is hoped that the participants would feel like real-life heroes. During the 'photo sessions', participants are urged to use existing photographs from their cameras and social media profiles to put in their own stories. Photographs from participants' distant and recent pasts can be reproduced, and when they touch the pictures in their hands, they are able to reveal various, personal transmissions with the image, which prompt discussion about their sentiments about the image's context, content, and significance. The images could be related to the participants' countries of origin or to the phenomenon of migration. At this stage, participants are asked the following questions: 'How old are you and where are you from?', 'How did you get here?', 'What have you learned from your journey?', 'How can you manage to be so mentally strong?'. In 'video sessions', however, participants may opt to discuss their new roles in their new home country and their final goods related to newly acquired skills with peers or strangers. Final products may create a sense of mastery, competence, and self-esteem; participants not only cherish their experiences, but they also feel successful after learning something new, devoting themselves to a task, taking individual ownership, and creating concrete deliverables.

Eclectic Use of Therapeutic Storytelling

Apart from using creative drawings, colors, and pictures in storytelling, eclectic uses of other self-awareness-based post-modern interventions may also be discussed as a subject. In addition to creative painting practices (Sakaki et al., 2007), verbal transfers, puppet-object use, and art therapy (Desmond et al., 2015) in the use of therapeutic storytelling, researchers in this field emphasized that the use of mindfulness-based storytelling technique, which combines self-awareness practices regarding the past and future by focusing on the present moment, is effective in determining the various possible choices in the individual's life (Vargas Delgado, 2019). In eclectic therapeutic story techniques, researchers stated that individuals create a balance between their past and future lives through focusing on that moment, acceptance of a person's story may actualize, individual's feelings about interpersonal relationships may keep a straight face (expressed), emotion proficiency may be realized, and individuals may give meaning to their lives and have hope in a belief dimension (Vargas Delgado, 2019).

There are some similarities between storytelling and systemic therapy perspective. According to general systems theory, there are a variety of alternative problem-solving skills in interactive circumstances involving the individual's own and related contexts, and these solutions are linked to reflective thinking. In reflective thinking, the language and conscious responses come to the fore (Polkinghorne, 2013). Phipps and Vorster (2011) stated that the internalized perspective that reflects the individual's intrinsic processes in narrative therapy spreads to interpersonal interaction studies and the language used in interpersonal contexts, as in systemic interventions. In other words, as in systemic interventions, the intrinsic processes acquired through stories in narrative therapy evolve into new stories towards interpersonal contexts. Reactions of individuals to what happens around them are not simple behavioral reactions; responses to complex processes are quite what happens within themselves and in the contexts around them. When individuals think reflectively, they search for many unique possibilities and ways to achieve the goal they wish to achieve. The interaction with different contexts in this system is related to the interpersonal contexts in the narrative approach. New approaches to achieving life goals and giving different meanings to new situations are questioned in the narrative approach. Along with many diverse stories from different cultures, gaining new perspectives of individuals on many states, immerse themselves into new experiences, and restructure their story come to the fore (Polkinghorne, 2013).

Within the scope of systemic intervention, questions about emphasizing circular transactional and interpersonal relationships (Brown, 1997), conveying distress used in narrative therapy, actioning, and as well as awareness, life, and power/social processes (Çelik, 2017) all show similarities. For instance, in terms of narrative therapy, while there are mindfulness-oriented questions including 'What do such mindfulness mean to you regarding what you want from life?', and 'What do all these developments mean to you about what suits you behaviorally?'; and with regard to defining the distress question such as 'What can you say about what you want to do as a result of this anxiety you experience?' (Çelik, 2017, pp.40, 43); in systemic intervention (Brown, 1997, pp.112-113), for instance, there may be such a question 'In which state is distress most noticeable?' in terms of revealing the difference between the states. In the direction of expressing the difference between varying contexts of a person, while there can be a question such as 'When you think of your mind and heart, which part of you wish to stay in a relationship? Which part wish to leave the relationship?', there may also be a question such as 'What happened after telling him/her to go to the room?' On the emotional side, the following exemplary questions such as 'When you think about the times when you felt anger towards him/her for a long time, how can these feelings be reflected in your interpersonal relationships?' may be asked. It was concluded that both systemic intervention and storytelling intervention under narrative therapy are postmodern interventions, and it may be argued that they all converge on restructuring the individual's subjective reality, intrinsic feelings, and interpersonal contexts. In this context, the eclectic use of systemic intervention and storytelling intervention may be effective, and there may be an emphasis on contexts in stories through circular questions.

When individuals encounter various traumatic events, and some distress occurs with their somatic sensations and emotions, supportive and developmental interventions come to the fore regarding their emotions and somatic sensations (Ford & Blaustein, 2013). While working with the somatic sensations of the client, psychological counselor may allow the client to transition from a way of thinking of 'either, or' about somatic distress to a 'both, and'. While doing this, they may approach it as 'both physical and psychological distress' instead of 'either physical' or 'psychological' distress and may support the redefinition of distress through including the family in the process of making sense of distress (Watson & McDaniel, 2000, pp.1068-1069). In this context, the study of somatic sensation in the face of traumatic phenomena may allow the clients to reconstruct their stories in the somatic context, as well as to transition into a systemically contextual 'both, and' mentality.

While narrating their stories, clients may employ a range of puppets, seashells, stones, miniatures such as animals and humans, and objects such as sand. In this context, they may symbolize significant contextual individuals, difficulties, and strengths in the process of rebuilding their stories (Kronick et al., 2018). This condition denotes the sequencing studies in systemic intervention. Through sequencing studies, clients will gain insight into patterns of relationships that they have either ignored or recently discovered regarding positions between themselves and others, as well as patterns that are significant to them. The vicarious picture of the clients' interpersonal relationships will come to the fore in this environment, and the clients will then be able to take steps towards transformation. These sequence studies may be used to generate a picture of today's story as well as a hypothetical future version (Cohen, 2006; McQuillin & Welford, 2013).

A Sample Intervention Template for Therapeutic Storytelling

An intervention for systemic-based storytelling, as stated previously, is proposed based on the eclectic use of therapeutic storytelling via a post-modern-based systemic therapy intervention being significant in terms of restoring the client's interpersonal interactions and multiple settings. Various studies in the literature were reviewed while developing this intervention proposal (Burns, 2016; Cook et al., 2004; McQuillin & Welford 2013; Mukba et al., 2019; Sunderland, 2017; Watson & McDaniel, 2000), and an exemplary intervention template in this context was constructed. An example of this intervention proposal is presented below.

Figure 1. A sample intervention template for systemic-based therapeutic storytelling

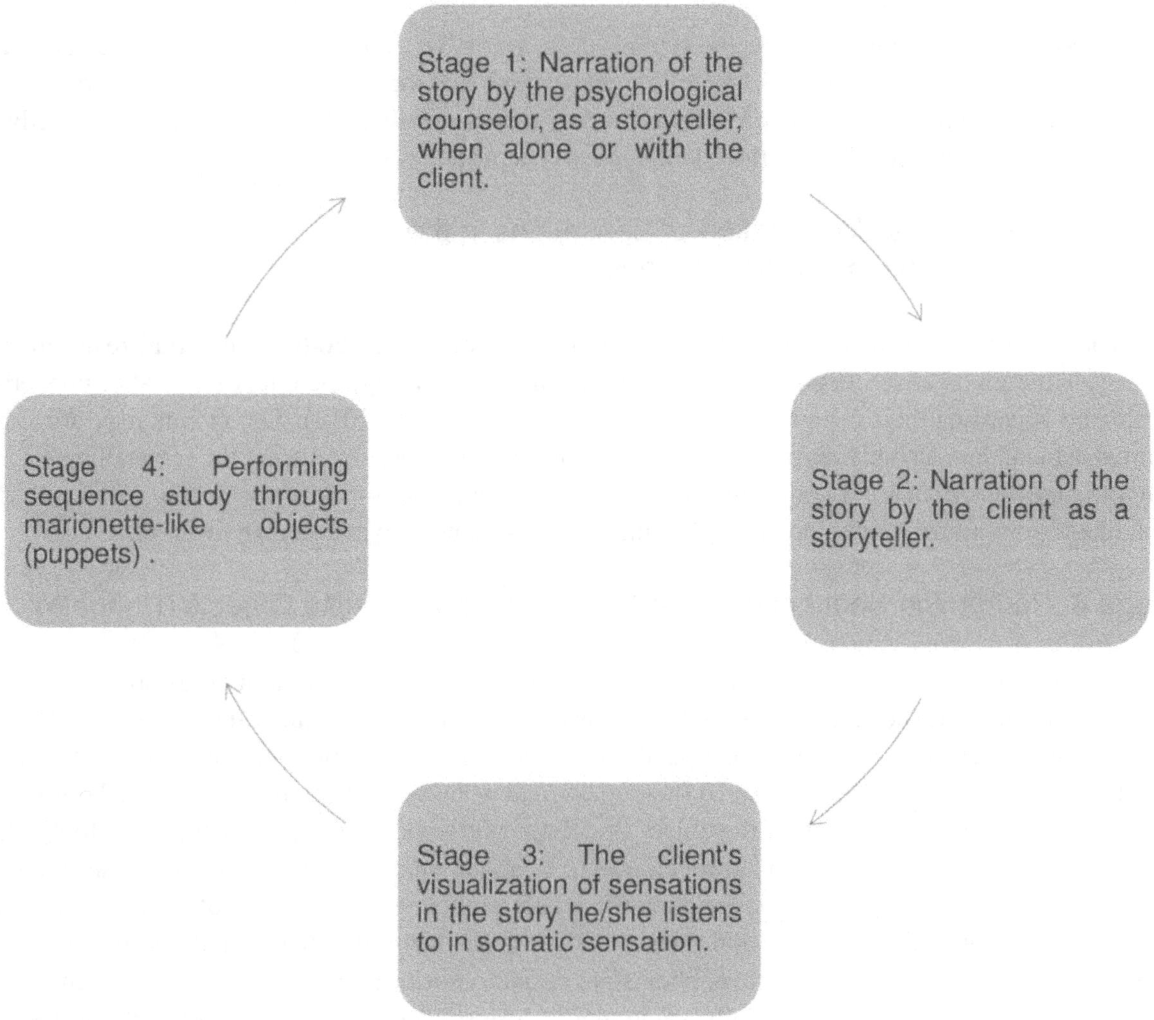

Stage 1: Narration of the Story by the Psychological Counselor, as a Storyteller, When Alone or With the Client

The psychological counselor may begin this stage by establishing a primary hero who is similar to the physical and personality characteristics of the client (Cook et al. 2004; Mukba et al., 2019). Characters and storylines within stories that are interesting to the clients may help them develop a more consistent worldview (Kress et al. 2010). In this context, while the psychological counselors may build a fascinating main hero, they may also develop a wise person in the story based on the client's belief system and power resources, from which the hero in the story may acquire new perspectives. While creating a story pattern, support may also be acquired from the strengths and resources of the client. Art materials such as drawings and paints may also be used in the story pattern if the client prefers. In this way, it is feasible to externalize various contexts in the client's story.

Stage 2: Narration of the Story by the Client, as a Storyteller

In the second stage, the client may be asked to generate a story related to his/her distresses. If the client wishes, drawings may also be used while telling the story so that the client's distresses are externalized. The fact that the counselor presents a curious listener attitude while a client tells a story (Connelly & Clandinin, 1990) will contribute to the client's role as a storyteller.

Stage 3: The Client's Visualization of Sensations in the Story He/She Listens to in Somatic Sensation

In physical interventions including somatic sensations, it is critical to embody and externalize the client's distress. Through creative interventions such as drawing and painting, the client's verbal or nonverbal sentiments regarding their distresses may be expressed (Kim et al., 2018). The clients may draw and paint on a blank human body drawing what they feel in somatic sensation during the storytelling stages. Circular questions such as 'If your injury told you something, what would it say?', and 'What would it look like if your injury resembled an object/animal?' may be used to externalize the client.

Stage 4: Performing Sequence Study Through Marionette-like Objects (Puppets)

At this stage, the goal is to expose the emotional-social contexts of clients through the existing sequences of their own story and the emotional-social contexts they want beyond for the future sequences. Vicarious individuals selected figuratively and positioned according to the emotional-social distance by the clients remain silent for a while and stand motionless, and whatever sensations each selected object has can be positioned by the location of the object associated with those feelings (Cohen, 2006; McQuillin and Welford 2013). In the next step, however, questions about what emotions the client senses for each object in the visual sequence in that position may be asked. Sequence study is a type of activity that allows individuals to view their vulnerable and powerful sides in the form of concrete and visual representation (Bezerra et al., 2018). At this stage, clients are asked to position objects symbolizing themselves, and people with whom they feel socially-emotionally close or distant, their sentiments, the distress in their stories, and the power sources in their stories. For the future sequences, possible positioning for the future story may also be developed. It is also possible that the clients will be asked what emotions these sequences evoke in their senses.

Hypothetical Sample Case

An exemplary hypothetical/presumptive case of the systemic-based storytelling intervention pattern is presented above.

Case

Client-A is a 20-year-old female university student studying medicine in the Eastern Anatolia Region of Turkey. Despite residing in a separate city from her family, she was unable to fully adapt to the individualization process during her two years of the study period. On the one hand, she has desires to participate in various social events with her friends, on the other hand, she has conflicts that her duty as a student is only to study and go out when necessary, based on the values that her family instilled in her and her understanding of loyalty. In terms of the moral values, she learned from her family, she claims that attending university is a big step for her; and that she should take every action carefully, not divert her attention away from her studies, and communicate with her friends and environment only to meet her basic needs, such as going to the market, attending classes, and doing common homework. The conflict between her ambition to be independent on the one hand and her desire to remain faithful to family ties on the other drove her to seek professional help.

Hypothetical Intervention

Stage 1: Narration of the Story by the Counsellor, as a Storyteller, When Alone or With the Client

After the psychological counselor got the story of Client A. about the situation that brought her to counseling, the process of acquiring information about the power sources and various contexts that Client A. had with these situations took place. The counselor realized that the brave-self in Client A. gives strength to her and understood that it is related to premonitions that may call the right decisions in a situation that she may overcome in situations she is in dilemma. For instance, when it snows on a winter day, and when her roommate in the dorm says 'let us play snowball outside' towards the evening, her brave-self says 'you can do it, you will have fun with your friends for a maximum of 15 minutes, you have not played with the snowball for a long time!'. She stated that she had a happy day because she listened to her inner voice and communicated with her friends. The psychological counselor told the following story to Client A.;

Once upon a time, there was a beautiful and intelligent sultan daughter of a king and queen. This sultan girl was the only one of her family, and her family raised her by their own royal rules. The rules in this royal family were very clear and strict. Since her family inherited these rules from their ancestors, they did not allow any flexibility or change. They were saying that since we were able to obey these rules, our sultan daughter will not also find it difficult, that's how we saw it from our ancestors. Sultan daughter would love her parents very much. However, she would like to ride a horse in the outer world, explore new places, and get acquainted with others, but she had intrinsic conflicts that opposing the values her family instilled her meant not being a good Sultan and a daughter. One day, a new decision was taken in the dynasty for this Sultan girl to learn other languages and take on a new task in the palace dynasty. The Sultan was allowed to study in another palace for a while. Even the king and queen had a hard time making this decision. The Sultan, who was curious about the world outside and wanted to spend time with her peers, was hopeful and saying that 'maybe I would have a chance, that I would see different experiences'. While the Sultan was on her way, guards took a break. The Sultan sat in the shade of a nearby tree while the guards rested by the waterfront. The stiff and long branches of the tree spread to the right and left, and it had lush green leaves. The left branch of the tree began to speak. The left branch said; 'I was thoughtful like you once, I would not mind going beyond what I was taught, I would only let the birds that live here that I know to land on my branch, but the right branch was so brave and taught me new things'. The Sultan listened to the branch in surprise. Then, the right branch began to speak; 'yes, I am braver, but I also learned from the left branch, from it I learned not to break away from my values and roots. I learned to balance what I learned from my roots about being both brave and cautious. I always let migratory birds land on my branch. My roots were angry with me and afraid that a migratory bird would peck and drag me away. Even the left branch blushed at me. Then later we talked, understood each other, stopped fighting and made up. There was a time when a migratory bird was actually going to peck at me, when the cautious branch gathered such strength and flung its leaves towards it that the bird flew away and never came back. Not every migratory bird is the same, just as not every native bird is the same... You see, right?' Sultan girl started to make inferences and asked; 'So you both got angry, then you made up and accepted each other and took care of each other?' Both branches said 'Yes'. Sultan girl, with a big smile; 'you taught me something new too, thank you'. She said goodbye and continued on their way with the guards....

After listening to the story, Client A. said that this story allowed her to gain a new insight on what she had to thinks, and that she would consider thinking about it for a week. She Stated that the side of weak insight is also a gain, and then she left the meeting with thoughts of how she could accept herself with her whole being while writing a new story. She also emphasized the feeling of hope.

Stage 2: Narration of the Story by the Client, as a Storyteller

The psychological counselor suggested that the client may tell a story that she would generate by herself, and that she could convey it with visuals if she so desired. The story generated by the Client A. herself was as follows;

One day, there was a lonely girl, she was about 20 years old. This girl traveled from another city for a new educational journey, but she had strong ties with her family. Although she was living in the city physically where she pursued an education at university, she was not living there spiritually. This situation tired her a lot, and she began to feel a burden. According to her family, the duty of a girl was supposed to be only a good daughter, not to communicate with her environment much and only to study her lessons. Besides, this 20-year-old girl got into a beautiful faculty department by working so hard, that is, her student role, she also had a brave self that thought she deserved to have fun and could sometimes make autonomic decisions. The girl began to hear the voice of this intrinsic self, increasingly. Initially, she thought hearing this seemed betrayal to her family, then she began to think this way; the value self that was inherited to her from her family was also precious. But she realized that if she only listened to the voice of her family values, she would not be happy and her student role would weaken and fail. This time the two selves inside of her began to speak. The brave side said that at the age of 20, 'you can extend your fields of action by expanding your values that deserve to have fun and not upset your family'. This time, the value-self understood it and said, 'you are in a different place now, maybe you will not be a student again, so there may be times and places where you can be free and brave without ignoring me'. The girl was very happy because she realized that there could also be a 'both, and' in her life, not an 'either, or'...

The most meaningful part of the story, according to Client A., was accepting and reconciling her both value self and brave self. She stated that she would feel peaceful and happy. Her drawings also included a strong arm for the brave side and a chest for the value side, both of which indicated that they were her possessions.

Stage 3: The Client's Visualization of Sensations in the Story He/She Listens to in Somatic Sensation

The psychological counselor asked Client A. if she felt any sensation in her body regarding these stories and stated that she could picture her somatic sensations in an empty body drawing for both stories, separately. Client A. stated that the story she was narrated resulted in a sensation in her throat and indicated that she felt a tickling-like sadness in her throat. She painted the throat yellow color and associated it with sadness; and when she painted and spoke with that sense, this sensation was just faded away and did not upset her much. Regarding the story she narrated, she felt a sense of peace in her heart and painted it with the color blue, which she associated with peace.

Stage 4: Performing Sequence Study Through Marionette-like Objects (Puppets)

The counselor noted that the client used the miniatures in the interview room to create a hypothetical sequence for the future with a current sequence relevant to her life story. Client A. positioned her family value-self and brave-self side by side in her present story. She sequenced feelings of anxiety and peace, her faculty friends, and the department she studied closer to her yet on the opposite side. She moved her family members back a little so that she could see them. She said that such sequencing made her feel happy, and it inspired her to attempt new things. She used large and small stones in the interview room as items representing persons and emotions in the present array. In the future sequence, Client A. placed her friends and a few hobbies she wishes to do, such as swimming, next to her. She put her profession ahead of herself with a little distance. She placed her family behind her and said, 'They will always be behind me, I know they are my supporters, I can see them whenever I want'. 'Yet I will stand in my own way and move on' she continued. She indicated that this practice provided her strength and hope, that she discovered her own self, and that she progressed well in the path of self-discovery. Client A. also used large and small stones for the future sequence, choosing huge stones for her future employment and hobbies, and claiming that it gave her a sense of independence. She emphasized that she chose a stone that she felt was strong enough for the family she had placed behind her, and that she could feel their power inside her. Client A. further mentioned that the future sequence made her feel free and comfortable.

After all these stages, when Client A. was asked what experiences she gained from this adventure in this intervention process, Client A. replied, 'I discovered states where I could both sense my family and rediscover myself. A hypothetical response might be 'I am clearer about the steps I can take now and, in the future'. Through the hypothetical case, it can be interpreted that Client A. reconciles the viewpoints of 'I can feel my family' and 'I can be an individual' in the hypothetical state and may reconstruct his story from the conflict between 'either I must be loyal to my family' 'or 'I must behave freely and individually'.

FUTURE RESEARCH DIRECTIONS

Externalizing the clients' various contexts through story and systemic interventions will enable them to realize that reconstructing the parts of their story that they consider to be dominant, while realizing that the parts of their story they consider to be weak or negative are the strengths that have them today. Researchers can reveal the application findings of this model in future studies.

CONCLUSION

To summarize, the clients may reposition the people who are significant to them, and their existing distresses through the use of storytelling through eclectic contextual/systemic treatments, therefore, restructures their aspirations, hopes, and beliefs, and thus their story (Carr, 2009; Gammer, 2009; Mukba et al., 2019).

REFERENCES

Aguilera, L., Reed, K., & Goulding, J. (2020). Experiences of engaging in therapeutic storytelling. *Mental Health Review (Brighton)*, *25*(1), 47–61. doi:10.1108/MHRJ-11-2018-0036

Badham, C. (2020). Tales from the east end: Dialogic and confessional storytelling as therapy (?) in the plays of Philip Ridley. In W. C. Boles (Ed.), *After in-yer-face theatre* (pp. 185–200). Palgrave Macmillan. doi:10.1007/978-3-030-39427-1_12

Bezerra, M. S. M., de Souza, I. P., de Souza, S. P. S., & da Silva Barbosa, M. A. R. (2018). Experience of a young woman's cancer and the family care constellation. *Cienc Cuid Saude*, *17*(2), 1–8. doi:10.4025/cienccuidsaude.v17i2.42185

Bhattacharyya, A. (2006). Historical backdrop. In K. N. Dwivedi (Ed.), *The therapeutic use of stories* (pp. 1–18). Routledge.

Brown, J. (1997). Circular questioning: An introductory guide. *Australian and New Zealand Journal of Family Therapy*, *18*(2), 109–114. doi:10.1002/j.1467-8438.1997.tb00276.x

Burns, G. W. (2016). *Çocuklar ve ergenler için 101 tedavi edici öykü* [101 healing stories for kids and teens] (N. Cihanşümül Maral, Trans.). Nobel Yaşam. (Original work published 2001)

Burrows, L. (2013). Transforming 'The Red Beast' within through mindfulness and therapeutic storytelling: A case study. *Australian Journal of Guidance & Counselling*, *23*(2), 172–184. doi:10.1017/jgc.2013.17

Carlson, R., & Arthur, N. (1999). Play therapy and the therapeutic use of story. *Canadian Journal of Counselling*, *33*(3), 212–226.

Carr, A. (2009). The effectiveness of family therapy and systemic interventions for child-focused problems. *Journal of Family Therapy*, *31*(1), 3–45. doi:10.1111/j.1467-6427.2008.00451.x

Çelik, H. (2017). Psikoterapide yeni soluk: Öyküsel terapi. *E-Kafkas Eğitim Araştırmaları Dergisi, 4*(1), 34–50.

Cohen, D. B. (2006). "Family constellations": An innovative systemic phenomenological group process from Germany. *The Family Journal (Alexandria, Va.), 14*(3), 226–233. doi:10.1177/1066480706287279

Connelly, F. M., & Clandinin, D. J. (1990). Stories of experience and narrative inquiry. *Educational Researcher, 19*(5), 2–14. doi:10.3102/0013189X019005002

Cook, J. W., Taylor, L. A., & Silverman, P. (2004). The application of therapeutic storytelling techniques with preadolescent children: A clinical description with illustrative case study. *Cognitive and Behavioral Practice, 11*(2), 243–248. doi:10.1016/S1077-7229(04)80035-X

D'Cruz, K., Douglas, J., & Serry, T. (2020). Narrative storytelling as both an advocacy tool and a therapeutic process: Perspectives of adult storytellers with acquired brain injury. *Neuropsychological Rehabilitation, 30*(8), 1409–1429. doi:10.1080/09602011.2019.1586733 PMID:30822228

Denborough, D. (2014). *Retelling the stories of our lives: Everyday narrative therapy to draw inspiration and transform experience*. W. W. Norton.

Desmond, K. J., Kindsvatter, A., Stahl, S., & Smith, H. (2015). Using creative techniques with children who have experienced trauma. *Journal of Creativity in Mental Health, 10*(4), 439–455. doi:10.1080/15401383.2015.1040938

Divinyi, J. (1995). Storytelling: An enjoyable and effective therapeutic tool. *Contemporary Family Therapy, 17*(1), 27–37. doi:10.1007/BF02249302

Ford, J. D., & Blaustein, M. E. (2013). Systemic self-regulation: A framework for trauma-informed services in residential juvenile justice programs. *Journal of Family Violence, 28*(7), 665–677. doi:10.100710896-013-9538-5

Gammer, C. (2009). *The child's voice in family therapy. A systemic perspective*. W. W. Norton & Company.

Gu, Y. (2018). Narrative, life writing, and healing: The therapeutic functions of storytelling. *Neohelicon, 45*(2), 479–489. doi:10.100711059-018-0459-4

Iglesias, A., & Iglesias, A. (2016). Hypnotic mediated therapeutic storytelling with over-involved children. *Contemporary Hypnosis & Integrative Therapy, 31*(1), 6–12.

Kim, K. S., Loring, S., & Kwekkeboom, K. (2018). Use of art-making intervention for pain and quality of life among cancer patients a systematic review. *Journal of Holistic Nursing, 36*(4), 341–353. doi:10.1177/0898010117726633 PMID:28836473

Kress, V. E., Adamson, N. A., & Yensel, J. (2010). The use of therapeutic stories in counseling child and adolescent sexual abuse survivors. *Journal of Creativity in Mental Health, 5*(3), 243–259. doi:10.1080/15401383.2010.507657

Kronick, R., Rousseau, C., & Cleveland, J. (2018). Refugee children's sandplay narratives in immigration detention in Canada. *European Child & Adolescent Psychiatry, 27*(4), 423–437. doi:10.100700787-017-1012-0 PMID:28643110

Laing, C. M., Moules, N. J., Sinclair, S., & Estefan, A. (2019). Digital storytelling as a psychosocial tool for adult cancer survivors. *Oncology Nursing Forum*, *46*(2), 147–154. doi:10.1188/19.ONF.147-154 PMID:30767963

Larkin, D. M., & Zabourek, R. P. (1988). Therapeutic storytelling and metaphors. *Holistic Nursing Practice*, *2*(3), 45–53. doi:10.1097/00004650-198802030-00009 PMID:3366805

Lodge-Guttery, C. (2004). *The impact of narrative storytelling on cognitive re-composition in individuals struggling with eating disorders* (Order No. 3138725) [Unpublished doctoral dissertation]. University of Oklahoma, Norman, Oklahoma, United States. ProQuest Dissertations & Theses Global.

Long, N. (2013). *Therapeutic storytelling in a pupil referral unit: The story of intersubjectivity* [Unpublished doctoral dissertation]. The University of Manchester, Manchester, UK.

Mager, B. (2019). Storytelling contributes to resilience in older adults. *Activities, Adaptation and Aging*, *43*(1), 23–36. doi:10.1080/01924788.2018.1448669

McKee, R. (2003). Storytelling that moves people. A conversation with screenwriting coach Robert McKee. *Harvard Business Review*, *81*(6), 51–55. PMID:12800716

McLean, L., & Tuite, E. (2016). Stories and their value: Exploring the role of storytelling in social care practice. *Scottish Journal of Residential Child Care*, *15*(2), 29–45.

McQuillin, J., & Welford, E. (2013). How many people are gathered here? Group work and family constellation theory. *Transactional Analysis Journal*, *43*(4), 352–365. doi:10.1177/0362153713519743

Moore, T. (2017). Strengths-based narrative storytelling as therapeutic intervention for refugees in Greece. *World Federation of Occupational Therapists Bulletin*, *73*(1), 45–51. doi:10.1080/14473828.2017.1298557

Mukba, G. (2020). *Yas olgusu yaşayan çocukların yaşantılarının sistemik müdahale içeren hikâye anlatıcılığı tekniği ile incelenmesi: Vaka çalışması* [Unpublished doctoral dissertation]. Çukurova University, Adana, Turkey.

Mukba, G., Sanberk, İ., & Akbaş, T. (2019). An eclectic intervention involving systemic intervention with storytelling. *Psikiyatride Güncel Yaklasimlar*, *11*(3), 386–401. doi:10.18863/pgy.452521

Phipps, W. D., & Vorster, C. (2011). Narrative therapy: A return to the intrapsychic perspective? *Journal of Family Psychotherapy*, *22*(2), 128–147. doi:10.1080/08975353.2011.578036

Polkinghorne, D. E. (2013). Narrative identity and psychotherapy. In C. A. Ingemark (Ed.), *Therapeutic uses of storytelling* (pp. 21–41). Nordic Academic Press.

Quiroga, A., Jimenez, J. V., Beltran, G. A., Casas, V., & Lopez, B. N. (2016). A narrative approach to addressing pain in hospitalised paediatric patients: Handicraft and digital interventions. *International Journal of Narrative Therapy & Community Work*, *4*, 77–85.

Reynolds, J., & Bove, K. B. (2016, February 27). *The power of mutual storytelling in play therapy* [Workshop presentation]. Colorado Association for Play Therapy.

Rolbiecki, A. J., Washington, K. T., & Bitsicas, K. (2019). Digital storytelling as an intervention for bereaved family members. *Omega*, *0*(0), 1–17. doi:10.1177/0030222819825513 PMID:30678536

Roosa, L. W. (1981). The family drawing / storytelling technique: An approach to assessment of family dynamics. *Elementary School Guidance & Counseling*, *15*(3), 269–272.

Russo, M. F., Vernam, J., & Wolbert, A. (2006). Sandplay and storytelling: Social constructivism and cognitive development in child counseling. *The Arts in Psychotherapy*, *33*(3), 229–237. doi:10.1016/j.aip.2006.02.005

Sakaki, T., Ji, Y., & Ramirez, S. Z. (2007). Clinical application of color inkblots in therapeutic storytelling. *The Arts in Psychotherapy*, *34*(3), 208–215. doi:10.1016/j.aip.2007.01.007

Serneels, A. (2013). Picturing stories: Drawings in narrative family therapy with children. *International Journal of Narrative Therapy & Community Work*, *4*, 21–29.

Slivinske, J., & Slivinske, L. (2014). *Therapeutic storytelling for adolescents and young adults*. Oxford University Press.

Spencer-Thomas, S. (2020). Phoenix rising: The power of storytelling in suicide prevention. In S. Shahtahmasebi & H. A. Omar (Eds.), *The broader view of suicide* (pp. 379–399). Cambridge Scholars Publishing.

Sunderland, M. (2017). *Using story telling as a therapeutic tool with children*. Speechmark Publishing. doi:10.4324/9781315148830

Vargas Delgado, J. J. (2019). Storytelling mindfulness: Storytelling program for meditations. In B. Peña-Acuña (Ed.), *Narrative transmedia* (pp. 1–18). IntechOpen. doi:10.5772/intechopen.86778

Watson, W. H., & McDaniel, S. H. (2000). Relational therapy in medical settings: Working with somatizing patients and their families. *Journal of Clinical Psychology*, *56*(8), 1065–1082. doi:10.1002/1097-4679(200008)56:8<1065::AID-JCLP6>3.0.CO;2-S PMID:10946733

White, M., & Epston, D. (1990). *Narrative means to therapeutic ends*. W.W. Norton.

ADDITIONAL READING

Ghasemian, K., & Estahbanati, M. A. E. (2019). The effectiveness of storytelling on reducing depression in cancer patients. *Humanidades & Inovação*, *6*(9), 278–284.

Jones, P., & Pimenta, S. (2020). *Therapeutic fairy tales: For children and families going through troubling times*. Routledge. doi:10.4324/9780429286087

Mannell, J., Ahmad, L., & Ahmad, A. (2018). Narrative storytelling as mental health support for women experiencing gender-based violence in Afghanistan. *Social Science & Medicine*, *214*, 91–98. doi:10.1016/j.socscimed.2018.08.011 PMID:30165294

Mendoza, K., & Bradley, L. (2021). Using storytelling for counseling with children who have experienced trauma. *Journal of Mental Health Counseling*, *43*(1), 1–18. doi:10.17744/mehc.43.1.01

Murray, S. (2021). The therapeutic use of stories in play therapy. In H. G. Kaduson & C. E. Schaefer (Eds.), *Play therapy with children: Modalities for change* (pp. 93–106). American Psychological Association. doi:10.1037/0000217-007

Quiñones, J. V. M., Gamarra, M. M., & Lobera, I. J. (2019). Storytelling as a therapeutic tool for family support in bulimia nervosa. In *Anorexia and bulimia nervosa*. IntechOpen. doi:10.5772/intechopen.86195

Sullivan, M. A. (2021). The use of storytelling with grief reactions in children during the COVID-19 pandemic. *Journal of Psychosocial Nursing and Mental Health Services*, *59*(2), 13–15. doi:10.3928/02793695-20201015-02 PMID:33095265

KEY TERMS AND DEFINITIONS

Eclectic Intervention: It is the realization of multiple applications by bringing multiple theoretical perspectives together.

Hypothetical Case: The concrete presentation of a phenomenon for an application model in stages.

Power Supplies: The presence of harmonious forces in the individual's life history.

Reconstruction of the Story: It is the subjective reconstitution of life sections within the existing resources in cases where the person's story is blocked.

Sample Intervention Template: An application proposal based on the psychological counseling theories.

Systemic Intervention: The reality in the client's mind is reconstructed through post- modern paradigm techniques according to interaction with the counselor, with the client himself and others that matter.

Therapeutic Storytelling: The expression of the psychological distress experienced by the individual in a relaxing way through creative healing stories that are felt like in the fairytales.

Chapter 14
The Healing Effect of the Story:
Gathering the Narrative Data of Patients Using Story Theory

Güven Soner
Ondokuz Mayis University, Turkey

ABSTRACT

Story theory, an intermediate-level nursing theory, was developed by nursing theorists Smith and Liehr. According to theorists, stories express who people are, where they are, and where they are going. Story theory can be used when one wants to understand what is most important to an individual with a health problem. The purpose of story theory is to reveal and evaluate the story of individuals as a basis for systematic data collection and analysis in the practice and research dimension of the nurse's health promotion process. While mostly qualitative analysis is used in the analysis of the story, quantitative analysis is also used. Liehr and Smith point out that stories should be used more in nursing in order to develop nursing knowledge.

INTRODUCTION

Stories are one of the oldest forms of communication for humanity. Stories found in every culture are used to entertain, educate people, record events, and convey cultural behaviors (Fischer, 2019). People's stories are both understood and shaped (Leight, 2002). An emotional bond is formed between the storyteller and the listener in a well-told story. This turns an ordinary situation into a significant sharing experience (Fischer, 2019). Stories can provide an opportunity to share experiences and allow us to understand the lives of individuals (Alicea-Planas, 2016). Stories enable us to understand how individuals evaluate their health from their perspectives (Lee et al., 2016).

Stories are also indispensable for nursing (Kiser-Larson, 2000). Nurses have been using the story in nursing practice for a long time. Stories play an important role in planning nursing care (Liehr & Smith, 2020). The importance of using the story in nursing is also seen in the experiences of the first modern nurse, Florence Nightingale. Nightingale paid great attention to listening to the wounded soldiers in the

DOI: 10.4018/978-1-7998-9251-9.ch014

Crimean War and became a part of the soldiers' stories by writing letters to the families of the soldiers when necessary (Liehr & Smith, 2020).

Stories and nursing care are interrelated (Kiser-Larson, 2000). Stories allow the nurse to enter the individual's life for a while and observe the individual's experience (Leight, 2002). The use of stories in nursing is an aesthetic and practical way of revealing details about the individual's health story experiences (Wang & Geale, 2015). One of the essential theories in the field of nursing is Story Theory.

STORY THEORY

Story Theory was developed by nursing theorists Patricia R. Liehr and Mary Jane Smith. According to the owners of the theory, the story has a healing power on the individual. In line with this knowledge, theorists have realized the importance of the story that unites nursing research and practice. This situation led to the emergence of the theory (Smith & Liehr, 1999; Liehr & Smith, 2018).

The process of creating Story Theory is based on Liehr and Smith's longstanding and collaborative relationships on similar research topics. The owners of the theory, who studied similar issues in their doctoral theses, talked about the importance of the story on the individual's health at a nursing conference. Thus, a theory about the effect of sharing the individual's story on the healing process has emerged (Liehr & Smith, 2018).

When Story Theory first emerged, it was published as Attentively Embracing Story (Smith & Liehr, 1999). The owners of the theory later simplified the name of the theory between 2003 and 2006 to make the story the focal point. The ontology of Story Theory recognizes that the story is an internal human resource for creating meaning. The epistemology of the story, on the other hand, is based on the understanding that intermediate theory integrates research and practice into a knowledge development method (Liehr & Smith, 2018).

Liehr ve Smith (2018) describes the story as "a narrative happening of connecting with self-in-relation through intentional dialogue to create ease." According to theorists, a story is a narrative of one's current life situation to clarify the present meaning of the past with an eye toward the future. Stories explain where individuals come from, where they are now, and where they are going (Liehr & Smith, 2018, 2020).

The Purpose of Story Theory

The theory is a dynamic process in which the individual who tells the story carefully embraces the story as it unfolds (Smith & Liehr, 2005). Therefore, the purpose of the Story Theory is for the nurse to evaluate the individual's story for systematic data collection and analysis to improve the individual's health (Liehr & Smith, 2018).

Assumptions of Story Theory

Story Theory considers the story of a person as a health story. The theory has three assumptions. These are; "Persons change as they interrelate with their world in a vast array of flowing connected dimensions.", "Persons live an expanded present where past and future events are transformed in the here and now.", "Persons experience meaning as a resonating awareness in the creative unfolding of human potential." (Liehr & Smith, 2018).

Three Concepts of Story Theory

Story Theory consists of three fundamental concepts that are interconnected. These are intentional dialogue, connecting with self-in-relation, and creating ease (Liehr & Smith, 2018).

Intentional Dialogue

Intentional dialogue is the central nurse-person process for collecting the person's story of a health problem that complicates daily life. The nurse approaches the individual's story without judgment and listens with focus—the nurse questions what the individual considers most important in the health problem. As the story progresses, the nurse questions the emergence of the story, focusing on understanding the story from the person's perspective (Liehr & Smith, 2020).

Intentional dialogue has two basic concepts, true presence, and querying emergence. Liehr and Smith describe "true presence" as "the nurse's nonjudgmental rhythmical focusing/ refocusing of energy on the other, which is open to what was, is, and can be" (Liehr & Smith, 2018). True presence is the nurse's activity while sharing the individual's story. The nurse focuses on the individual and the individual's story. The nurse makes the individual feel that the individual's story is worth listening to and shows respect for the individual (Liehr & Smith, 2018, 2020).

Querying emergence is to clarify the ambiguous points of history. Both the nurse and the individual embark on a journey through the story behind the health problem. The nurse tries to understand the individual's story from the eyes of the individual in a concentrated way. The nurse makes no assumptions about the story; Only the person who owns the story knows the story's details (Liehr & Smith, 2018).

Connecting with Self-in-Relation

The second important concept of the theory, connecting with self-in-relation, is "an active engagement in the process of acknowledging self as related to others in a developing story plot that is uncovered through intentional dialogue" (Liehr & Smith, 2020). "Connecting with self-in-relation" has two dimensions, "personal history" and "reflective awareness." Personal history is the unique story about where individuals came from in their lives, where they are now, and where they are going in life. To reach the beginning of the story in the background of the health problem, it is traveled to the past so that the hidden meanings in the depths of the story are tried to be reached (Liehr & Smith, 2018, 2020). Reflective awareness, "the second dimension of the concept, is the opposite of taking life for granted." Reflective awareness includes being in touch with bodily experience, thoughts, and emotions. Reflective awareness allows a thoughtful observation of one's self. This allows physical experiences, thoughts, and emotions to be recognized as authentic and separate entities (Liehr & Smith, 2018).

Creating Ease

The last concept of the theory, creating ease, is "an energizing sense of flow as story moments come together through anchoring to realities and releasing self from limiting story boundaries." (Liehr & Smith, 2020). "Creating ease" has two dimensions, "remembering disjointed story moments" and "flow amid anchoring" (Liehr & Smith, 2018). Liehr & Smith (2018) describe "remembering disjointed story moments" as "connecting events in time through the realization, acceptance, and understanding that comes as health story fragments sort, converge, and come together." While telling the story, the individual recalls disconnected memories. Attention is paid to the meaning of important individual lives. As the connection between the separate moments in the story is established, the individual is liberated from the boundaries he/her had before. The individual feels an "ah-ha" feeling (Liehr & Smith, 2020).

Application of Story Theory

Liehr, one of the owners of the theory, expresses the application of the Story Theory as "a healing art that promotes the transformational and self-transcendent potential of people ."(Liehr, 2000). Studies conducted with Story Theory prove this evaluation. Jolly et al. (2007) created a structure to collect an adolescent's health history using Story Theory. Gobble (2009) used Story Theory as a theoretical framework to provide culturally sensitive nursing care to a woman of Appalachia culture. Brodziak et al. (2017), on the other hand, draw attention to nurses' use of Story Theory in countering the negative consequences of loneliness.

Nurses rely on story sharing to optimize nursing care (Liehr & Smith, 2020). Collecting the individual's narrative data initiates an intentional dialogue with the individual and invites the individual to share the story about a health challenge that complicates daily life. Focusing on a health problem is necessary for the nurse to use story theory. There is a story in the background of the health problem that the individual has, and this story has connections with the individual, his environment, and other people. By discovering these connections, the nurse uncovers the story. As the story unfolds through these connections, an opportunity arises for a solution to the individual's health challenge (Liehr & Smith, 2018).

Complicating Health Challenge

Complicating Health Challenge is any situation in which an extraordinary change in an individual's life causes distress in an individual's daily life. This may be a health problem, or it may be a natural situation such as the child in the family going to university. In addition, it can be mobbing at work or bullying a small child experiences at school. It is the question that the nurse asks the individual "what matters most" in the intentional dialogue (Liehr & Smith, 2018).

Developing Story Plot

The evolving story plot connects the moments in a meaningful way. The nurse invites the individual to reflect on the past by focusing on the critical issues for the current health problem. They are essential to evolving storytelling and understanding the self in the relationship. The story develops as high points, low points, and turning points that occur against the background of the health problem. High points include when things are going well. Low points include times when things aren't going so well. On the other hand, turning points include moments when vital decisions are made in life (Liehr & Smith, 2018).

Liehr and Smith found that the use of the story path was influential in revealing the individual's health story. When using the story path approach, the nurse starts with the line "Story of ..." on a blank sheet of paper. The development of the story will always be about a health issue. The story path begins with questioning the individual's opinion about the current health challenge. Then, how the health challenge emerged in the past is questioned. The final stage of the story path is concluded by asking the individual about their hopes and dreams for the future (Figure 1) (Liehr & Smith, 2020).

Figure 1. Developing the story plot

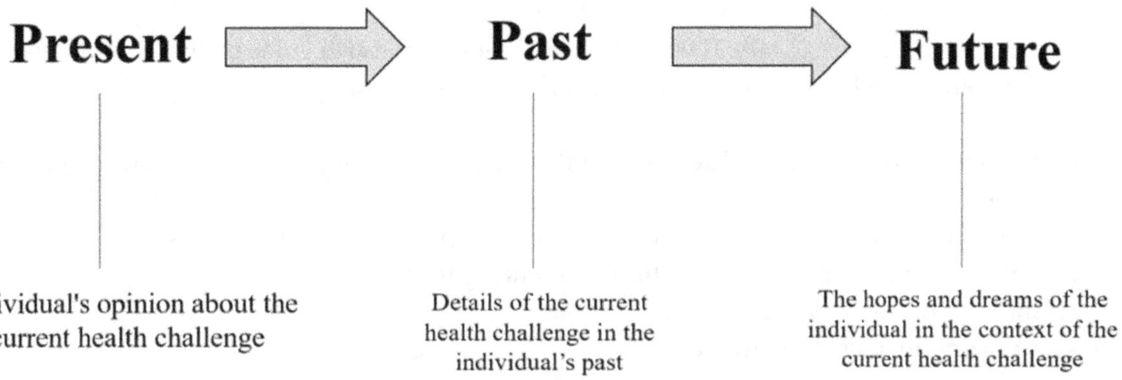

An example of the application of Story Theory is when applying the theory to an interview with a person with diabetes. The following questions can be used.

1. Can you talk about the difficulties you face with diabetes?
2. What is most important to you right now?
3. Do you remember a difficult period you overcame in the past? Can you tell me how you achieved this?
4. What are your hopes and dreams for the future?

Movement Toward Resolving

The movement toward resolving occurs when the individual who shares the story becomes aware of the health experience. The individual takes on the health problem and sees it as manageable. When the individual sees the health problem as manageable, this creates an opportunity to change his thoughts and feelings. Thus, the individual embraces the present moment. There is no final solution for any story, and the resolution does not close when the story sharing ends (Liehr & Smith, 2018).

Analysis of Story Data

The analysis of narrative data is mainly based on qualitative analysis, but quantitative analysis methods are also used. Stories are essential data for qualitative research. For this reason, qualitative research analysis methods are also used in Story Theory data analysis. The phenomenological analysis is used to analyze an experience, and content analysis is used to analyze the main concepts related to the story. Quantitative methods are also used in story data analysis. The frequency and temporal order of the prominent words in the story provide an essential opportunity when making sense of the data (Liehr & Smith, 2018).

Liehr and Smith suggest the Story query method for data analysis. The story inquiry method consists of 5 steps. These are; (a) gathering the story about complicating health challenges, (b) identifying the dimensions of the health challenge, (c) identifying the highs, lows, and turning points of the story, (d) describing the movement toward resolving and (e) synthesizing the findings to address the research question (Liehr & Smith, 2018, 2020).

Story Inquiry Method

The story inquiry method is a Story Theory approach that nurses use to guide patient data collection and analysis. This approach has five steps (Liehr & Smith, 2018). These;

- asking questions about a complicating health challenge using a systematic structure to encourage individual story-sharing
- revealing the background and dimensions of the complicating health challenge
- identifying high points, low points, turning points in the story
- finding movement toward resolving
- synthesizing findings from the story

CONCLUSION

Every person has a free story. There is an essential interaction between the person telling the story and the person listening to the story. Stories can have a healing effect on the health problem. Patient stories have an important place in the practice of the nursing profession, which has a deep-rooted history. Nurses have been listening to patients' stories for a long time. Therefore, they are aware of the importance of stories because each individual's unique story relates to their health.

Story theory offers a systematic approach to listening to the patient's story. Nursing theorists Liehr and Smith's Story Theory emerged over the story's meaning in the field of health. Theorists, who think that the individual's health history is the individual's story, have developed the Story Theory over time.

The story theory enables the nurse to initiate communication with the patient about a health problem. In this communication, a journey is taken from the present to the past regarding the individual's health problem. Finally, the nurse asks the individual about their future hopes and dreams regarding the individual's health problem. In this dialogue with the nurse and the patient, the nurse and the patient try to find a solution to the health problem. As the connections in the story based on the individual's health problem are revealed by the nurse, the solution to the individual's health problem becomes apparent. The use of story theory in nursing can contribute to the nurse's getting to know the patient better, expressing the health problem better, and finding a solution for the health problem.

REFERENCES

Alicea-Planas, J. (2016). Listening to the Narratives of Our Patients as Part of Holistic Nursing Care. *Journal of Holistic Nursing*, *34*(2), 162–166. doi:10.1177/0898010115591396 PMID:26088595

Brodziak, A., Wolinska, A., & Myrta, A. R. (2017). The Story Theory is a Key Element of Many Holistic Nursing Procedures. *Journal of Gerontology & Geriatric Research*, *6*(6). Advance online publication. doi:10.4172/2167-7182.1000454

Fischer, D. (2019). Storytelling as a nursing pedagogy. *The Midwest Quarterly*, *60*(3), 311–319.

Gobble, C. (2009). The Value of Story Theory in Providing Culturally Sensitive Advanced Practice Nursing in Rural Appalachia. *Online Journal of Rural Nursing and Health Care: the Official Journal of the Rural Nurse Organization*, *9*(1), 94–105. doi:10.14574/ojrnhc.v9i1.108

Jolly, K., Weiss, J. A., & Liehr, P. (2007). Understanding Adolescent Voice as a Guide for Nursing Practice and Research. *Issues in Comprehensive Pediatric Nursing*, *30*(1–2), 3–13. doi:10.1080/01460860701366518 PMID:17613138

Kiser-Larson, N. (2000). The Concepts of Caring and Story Viewed from Three Nursing Paradigms. *International Journal for Human Caring*, *4*(2), 26–32. doi:10.20467/1091-5710.4.2.26

Lee, H., Fawcett, J., & DeMarco, R. (2016). Storytelling/narrative theory to address health communication with minority populations. *Applied Nursing Research*, *30*, 58–60. doi:10.1016/j.apnr.2015.09.004 PMID:27091254

Leight, S. B. (2002). Starry night: Using story to inform aesthetic knowing in women's health nursing. *Journal of Advanced Nursing*, *37*(1), 108–114. doi:10.1046/j.1365-2648.2002.02050.x PMID:11784404

Liehr, P. (2000). Using Story Theory to Guide Nursing Practice. *International Journal for Human Caring*, *4*(2), 13–18. doi:10.20467/1091-5710.4.2.13

Liehr, P., & Smith, M. J. (2020). Claiming the Narrative Wave With Story Theory. *Advances in Nursing Science*, *43*(1), 15–27. doi:10.1097/ANS.0000000000000303 PMID:32015246

Liehr, P. R., & Smith, M. J. (2018). Story Theory. In M. J. Smith & P. R. Liehr (Eds.), *Middle Range Theory for Nursing* (pp. 241–264). Springer Publishing Company. doi:10.1891/9780826159922.0011

Smith, M. J., & Liehr, P. (1999). Attentively Embracing Story: A middle-range theory with practice and research implications. *Scholarly Inquiry for Nursing Practice*, *13*(3), 187–210. PMID:10628236

Smith, M. J., & Liehr, P. (2005). Story theory: Advancing nursing practice scholarship. *Holistic Nursing Practice*, *19*(6), 272–276. doi:10.1097/00004650-200511000-00008 PMID:16269946

Wang, C. C., & Geale, S. K. (2015). The power of story: Narrative inquiry as a methodology in nursing research. *International Journal of Nursing Sciences*, *2*(2), 195–198. doi:10.1016/j.ijnss.2015.04.014

ADDITIONAL READING

Doan, W. J., Fick, D. M., Hill, N. L., & Kitko, L. (2018). The Art and Science of Nursing. *Journal of Gerontological Nursing*, *44*(12), 3–5. doi:10.3928/00989134-20181109-01 PMID:30484839

LeBlanc, R. G. (2017). Digital storytelling in social justice nursing education. *Public Health Nursing (Boston, Mass.)*, *34*(4), 395–400. doi:10.1111/phn.12337 PMID:28561376

Leight, S. B. (2002b). Starry night: Using story to inform aesthetic knowing in women's health nursing. *Journal of Advanced Nursing*, *37*(1), 108–114. doi:10.1046/j.1365-2648.2002.02050.x PMID:11784404

Sheilds, L. E. (2016). Narrative Knowing: A Learning Strategy for Understanding the Role of Stories in Nursing Practice. *The Journal of Nursing Education*, *55*(12), 711–714. doi:10.3928/01484834-20161114-09 PMID:27893908

Thoft, D. S., Møller, A. K., & Møller, A. K. K. (2021). Evaluating a digital life story app in a nursing home context – A qualitative study. *Journal of Clinical Nursing*, jocn.15714. Advance online publication. doi:10.1111/jocn.15714 PMID:33590641

Wood, P. J. (2014). Historical imagination, narrative learning and nursing practice: Graduate nursing students' reader-responses to a nurse's storytelling from the past. *Nurse Education in Practice*, *14*(5), 473–478. doi:10.1016/j.nepr.2014.05.001 PMID:24875838

KEY TERMS AND DEFINITIONS

Complicating Health Challenge: Any situation in which an extraordinary change in an individual's life causes distress in an individual's daily life (Liehr & Smith, 2018).

Connecting With Self-in-Relation: An active engagement in acknowledging self as related to others in a developing story plot uncovered through intentional dialogue (Liehr & Smith, 2020).

Creating Ease: An energizing sense of flow as story moments come together through anchoring to realities and releasing self from limiting story boundaries (Liehr & Smith, 2020).

Intentional Dialogue: Intentional dialogue is the central nurse-person process for collecting the person's story of a health problem that complicates daily life (Liehr & Smith, 2020).

Story: A narrative happening of connecting with self-in-relation through intentional dialogue to create ease (Liehr & Smith, 2018).

Story Inquiry Method: A Story Theory approach that nurses use to guide patient data collection and analysis (Liehr & Smith, 2018).

Chapter 15
Parents in the Grip of Parental Guilt:
Narrative Paths to Rediscover a Future

Sabine Vermeire
Interactie-Academie VZW, Belgium

Luc Van den Berge
https://orcid.org/0000-0001-9340-3391
Ghent University, Belgium

Tomas Van Reybrouck
Adentro VZW, Belgium

ABSTRACT

The authors present their work with parents of addicted children, some of whom died as a result of their addiction. Stuck in pain, guilt, shame they often experience a discomforting lack of understanding from those around them. Behind their worries is often the wish that things would go well for their children. Under the pressure of cultural parenting discourses feelings of guilt became 'toxic'. Subsequently any sense of a viable future got lost. In order to restore a sense of a viable future, the authors drew on narrative ideas. They organized a three-day hike with parents. A life review interview was applied to highlight their efforts, involvements, decisions, responses, and 'unique moments'. The interviews were recorded, and as such, the process was documented. Finally, 'outsider witness practices' were installed. The conjecture that this fourfold 'stage setting' could help these parents to entertain new perspectives on the future proved to be promising.

INTRODUCTION

This chapter deals with the question of how isolating experiences that are accompanied with toxic feelings of guilt and shame can be successfully approached from a post-structural narrative point of view.

DOI: 10.4018/978-1-7998-9251-9.ch015

The authors try to make use of the momentum of 'making public' that is inherent in narrative practices and that under certain conditions can re-generate a sense of a liveable future.

BACKGROUND

A Parental Predicament

'When children do not do well, parents go back in time to look for a reason, for a better way they could have protected them. I wish I had...' (Schaubroeck, 2010, authors' translation from Dutch).

Parents who have an addicted child have often come a very long way. They found themselves in previously unimaginable and exhausting situations, full of stress and tension. They heard themselves and their child saying or doing things that clashed with their beliefs, principles and dreams. The constantly changing emotions such as fear, anger, helplessness, guilt and shame suffocate and exhaust them. Their minds are filled with negative thoughts (Van Reybrouck, 2007).

'Five years ago It was unthinkable that I would change the locks on all the doors. After giving her 300 euros to buy drugs so she wouldn't steal, I could no longer look at myself in the mirror.' (Nathalie)

When an adult child struggles with addiction, this problem also has a huge impact on the parents' lives. The addiction problem has often infected the partner relationship as well as their relationship with the other children, and last but not least the relationship with the child that struggles with an addiction. The distance from meaningful others has increased. They no longer experience the concerns of those around them as genuine. Their hope for change is gone and the future seems dark. Their parental identity is under pressure. They ask themselves 'What am I worth as a parent? What have I done wrong?' They confront their counsellor or therapist with a flood of negativity towards the outside world, towards themselves, or their child and often towards the whole idea of counselling. Good moments, uncontaminated parts of their lives, alternative stories have disappeared from sight. They lost any sense of connection with their values and cherished dreams.

Nathalie (50) is the mother of Kirsten (29). She stays at home most of the time and only leaves the house for the daily shopping. She walks quickly and anxiously, hoping that no one will notice her or talk to her. She is always aware of the sound of her phone or doorbell. She changed her phone number. Her daughter's text messages were too stressful to read. Kirsten's drug addiction reached such proportions that Nathalie has lost all hope of recovery. She fears the worst every moment of the day. In an attempt to protect her daughter, she has incurred many debts. The advice of others is numerous and well-intentioned, but it has only made her more quiet. Therapists have tried to make her understand that there is nothing she can do as long as her daughter does not want to be helped. After all, she is a grown woman. Nevertheless, her thoughts are dominated by Kirsten's drug abuse. Together with her daughter she has become a prisoner of addiction.

The problems are subjected to endless analysis, a whole range of possible solutions is tried, but the problems only seem to escalate. Faced with their child's drug addiction, parents often react in a strange and incomprehensible way in the eyes of those around them. They start watching their child very closely, chasing them, spying on them or questioning their friends. Sometimes they beg them on their knees to stop or go to a rehabilitation centre. Other parents talk down on them for hours, scream and even use physical violence to change their child's mind. And still others try to cut off all contact. All these efforts and attempts to stop drug abuse make them very sensitive and vulnerable to the judgements of others.

We live in a world where many ideas and beliefs about parenting circulate. These ideas inform and even constitute parenting practices, and entail many norms and expectations about parenting (Van den Berge, 2013). They act as a mirror in which parents inevitably look at and judge themselves. Moreover, we live in a child-centred age, that considers children as extremely valuable and, by extension, parents and parenting have also become increasingly important.

In fact what this focus on children and children's wellbeing masks is that we live in an age of parenting (see for instance, Van den Berge, 2017). This emphasis on the importance of parents and parenting is inseparable from the belief that children are the product of parenting and that there is a strong causal relationship between parenting and the success or failure of children, as sociologists have pointed out (Lee et al. 2014; Van den Berge, 2014). This 'parental determinism' aligns with the belief that parents influence their children, but not the other way around. It has been remarked that children are default not taken as having an influence on their parents in mainstream developmental psychology. It is only fairly recently that has been acknowledged by some researchers in this field that children are full agents, who can influence deeply the way their parents experience themselves, or behave themselves (Kuczynski & De Mol, 2015).

Applied to parenting and drug addiction, these *social and professional discourses* lead to the often unquestioned conviction that parents, especially mothers, are guilty of their child's addiction. Parents often will also blame themselves, but also 'parent blaming' by others always lurks around the corner. Qualifications such as "a symbiotic relationship", "spoiling parent", "emotionally unstable parent" can easily become seen as the sole explanation for the child's addictive behaviour. What sociologists have named the parenting culture, with its perfectionism and high standards (Lee et al., 2014) can easily feed back into the parental self-understanding under the form of guilt and shame. The idea that parents, if they do the right thing, can produce 'good' children, adds to the pressure, and leads to the self-tormenting of parents: 'What have I done wrong?' Parents become ever more silent, when they feel that their acquaintances and their environment also look with condemning eyes. There is the shame for their child's behavior and what they do to others. The shame sometimes takes enormous proportions when they discover feelings of hate towards their child and sometimes they wish their child was death. These parents tend to make themselves invisible, or to isolate themselves.

The worries and pain of these parents mostly go unnoticed. Their child is an adult, so they are not invited into their child's care, counselling or therapy unless the professional thinks it may be helpful to the child's treatment. Especially in addiction care, the definition of the problem, who will be involved in solving the problem and how much time is needed to bring about change are considered the prerogative of the professional and so the parents are often excluded (Madigan & Epston, 1998; Van Reybrouck, 2007). As their experiences and stories are not taken seriously they feel sidelined by their child as well as by professional care.

Nathalie's daughter repeatedly yelled at her: 'You have no rights towards me! Stay away from me; you just make things worse!'

People are relational beings through and through (Gergen, 1999, 2009). And in order to experience parenthood as a worthwhile journey, it is necessary for parents to perceive that they matter to their child and that what they do makes sense (Vermeire, 2012). Parents with an addicted child easily lose sight of the fact that they matter. Family, friends and professionals offer advice, full of concern. They contribute both general 'expert knowledge' and their own personal local knowledge. Many of their ideas and advice tie in with the idea of 'letting go'. The reasoning is that the child is an adult and help is only possible if the addict himself wants to be helped. Often, the parent hears this as criticism and as advice to stop interfering, to stop worrying. Which proves to be a mission impossible.

Some Proviso's

From a post-structural, narrative point of view, there are some proviso's when engaging in therapeutic conversations with these parents.

1. Instead of addressing problems and problematic feelings immediately, save territories of identity need to be created first (White, 2006b), in order to find or dis-cover less prominent stories that make less destructive identity conclusions more accessible.
2. As counselor or therapists, one does not consider it one's task to examine whether one's clients prove to be guilty or not, but one rather chooses to be curious about how those feelings and thoughts entered the client's life. Although the authors believe they should acknowledge parents' feelings or ideas of guilt and failure they think it is better not try to erase them in an urge to help or to be supportive to the parent. Trying to get rid of problematic feelings too quickly can put therapists and counselors in an expert position and risks to deprive parents from the possibility to explore what values are inherent in these feelings.
3. Although parents, in their isolation, perceive their feelings and problems as private, the authors *choose* to regard them as symptoms of social or collective challenges, the social aspect of which is obscured (Denborough, 2008).
4. The authors believe it to be of great importance to take emotions as guilt and shame as active *responses*, rather than as passive reactions, to continuous intrusive life-events. And they take those responses to be deeply informed by what it is that parents give value to in their lives (White, 2006c). Helping people to live in alignment with what they value, is considered an important step towards regaining a sense of personal agency (White, 2007).

MAIN FOCUS OF THE CHAPTER

The history of the problems is often so long, the negative experiences so penetrating and overwhelming and the degree of despair so great that these parents have lost their sense of hope and no longer see a future for their child and themselves. With our proviso's in mind, we wanted to create more 'powerful' trajectories, that allow subordinate storylines to surface, leading to fewer negative identity conclusions, to less paralyzing feelings of guilt and shame, and to new actions or more constructive responses.

A Pathway to Recover a Future

The authors proceeded as follows. One of the authors has been organising group conversations for several years with parents to an adult child with serious addiction problems or a child who died of an overdose or committed suicide. It was decided to launch an invitation for a three-day group hike in the mountains as a 'strong' trajectory. Two group hikes eventually were organised.

Some parents came as a couple, others as a single parent. For some of them it was the first time in up to twenty years that they left their homes and slept in another bed. A week later, after the journey, they were brought together a second time to conduct biographical interviews in the presence of witnesses. The authors' intentions were to bring together those parents in contexts that offer different, new or forgotten experiences so afterwards 'rich descriptions' could emerge which are versatile, layered, nuanced, differentiated, polyphonic and valuable. The authors wanted to create re-connection with what parents find valuable as well as with the community they belong to so new identity stories become possible and their sense of agency and belonging rewound. The three days walk would offer the opportunity for scaffolding conversations. It would offer plenty points of entry in order to proceed from a problem saturated story to more rich stories and rich descriptions of identity.

Walking Together (1): New and Forgotten Stories

The parents who participate in the walking project take an important step by joining the group. Most of them are isolated both factually and emotionally, so it takes a great effort to get out the door. They are invited to take a literal distance so they can (more easily) take a figurative distance of the problems. Being away from home for three days and walking in a company of people with similar experiences and two companions gives them the opportunity to chat in different formations. Planned group conversations alternate with spontaneous individual conversations on the journey. They talk about their child and the problems but also about the weather, clothes or other subjects of small talk. Serious issues alternate with light-hearted things. At the end of the day there is a group meeting where pictures taken during the day are shared and discussed. The parents gather and talk about their experiences, thoughts, feelings that passed by. By telling and retelling, new stories are written that are different from the stories from home. These are about sometimes small but important alternative actions and initiatives such as getting a helping hand from another parent during the walk when it was difficult to keep going, giving a wink and being answered with a smile, pushing someone when climbing a rock or reaching the top of a hill at the end of the day. Such stories can shed a new light on forgotten capacities, skills, knowledge and values.

A mother was surprised by the collaboration of people in climbing a hill. It was the first time in years that she dared to rely on the help of others.

While walking together and telling each other stories, recognition and acknowledgement of everyone's situation arises. The participants discover that they have all had doubts at times about the meaning of their lives. Stories and lives become linked. Walking acts as a kind of antidote to the feeling of isolation.

In the evening while dinner is served, a mother receives a telephone call of her daughter. Loud and clearly she says to the group: 'This time, I won't answer the call! I won't spoil my evening by listening to her begging for money.' First, the group stays silent. Some parents nod encouragingly. The mother sits down and starts eating.

In this new experience and with the support of other parents, parents can make different choices or take a new stance towards the difficulties. Their sense of personal agency gets enlarged. By going on this weekend, by walking, by supporting each other, they are no longer just a victim of their child or the situation. Neither are they any longer the 'offender' or 'cause of the problems'. They start to see that what they do in the group is meaningful and makes a difference, however small it may seem.

Walking Together (2): New and Forgotten Connections

Identity is a relational, social and public project (Myerhoff, 2007; White, 2007) and stories of identity are continuously created in relations (Winslade, 2002). The journey gives them the opportunity to emerge in different roles and position than as the parent with an addicted child. They can experience what is important for them.

A mother discovers how happy she makes another mother by offering her her walking sticks.

A father makes everyone laugh with his jokes during dinner. Earlier in the day he told what a good biker he was before troubles came in.

A parent offers seats in his car and proposes to drive home together.

They have the same worries, difficulties and dilemma's as 'Do I have to throw him out of the house? Do I still give him money? Should I inform the police?' Sharing these stories creates connection and acknowledgement. The social issues that are inherent in the problems can be discussed. Possibilities are offered to counter some social discourses and hear how people take a stance towards them. At the same time there is space for the differences and everybody's personal experiences, stories and responses. The parents get linked not only in pain and suffering but also in the moments of joy and making fun together. Little sparkles of hope emerge. Hedtke (2014) proposes to conceive of 'hope' as an active verb that refers to a process. Hope then becomes an expression of agency in the face of significant challenges. By having such experiences during the journey, by taking those actions and by weaving those stories hope, as a glimpse of a possible future, emerges.

Scaffolding Conversations: A Biographical Interview, Outsider Witnesses and Documents

Once back home, the thoughts and good intentions parents made during the walk, can disappear very quickly. Once back in daily life, they usually will once again do what is known and familiar to them in their effort to address their predicaments and concerns (White, 2007). The authors don't want them to tumble again in the old familiar conclusions about their lives and relationships. So it kept the authors puzzling how they could create a conversational context about the different experiences and 'scaffold' and 'consolidate' the discoveries and ideas they had during the journey? At the same time they wondered how they could acknowledge the pathways of their life until now, so they could re-find possibilities and support to go on and hold on to those novel ideas?

Annie is a 59 years old mother whose son committed suicide last year. He had been addicted for many years. Until his death she struggled to keep him alive and to keep him away from the drugs. The last three years she took him back into her home, hoping she could offer him a new perspective. From that moment on she became isolated. She joined the walking group and was interviewed one week after the walk in the presence of more than twenty people.

Many of these parents saw a lot of social workers, counselors or therapists passing by. They can almost 'predict' the questions and ideas that will be presented. Instead of having a more traditional counseling conversation with each parent after the journey, it was decided to invite them to a kind of definitional ceremony (White, 2007). The authors wanted to create a context that allowed different questions could to be asked and different subjects to be addressed.

The authors created a special context where the parent is interviewed about his life and life experiences until now (Vermeire, 2011) and these are linked with the experiences of the three days walk. This happened in the presence of other parents, counselors, outsider witnesses and people interested. The whole interview was recorded so they received afterwards a DVD and a letter of the interview with themselves and the witnesses. This special context puts parent and therapist in a unconventional position. The parent is now an interviewee, not a "client", or a "problem case" or a parent with whom is spoken in function of their child. As an interviewer, one is a guest in their world (Anderson & Goolishian, 1992).This meeting offers an opportunity to highlight other sides of their story. The 'life review interview' can be used as a platform from which we look at and think about the different experiences, events and moments.

The Life Review Interview

Bateson (1989) observed: 'Composing a life involves a continual re-imaging of the future and reinterpretation of the past to give meaning to the present.' Many parents the authors spoke to have become trapped in chaotic and frozen stories where experiences remain a sequence of random events (Stern and Doolan, 1999). The stories are fragmentary, they offer neither a sense of control, nor a sense of agency. They rather create confusion. Such stories are also difficult to listen to. They keep revolving around one recurring theme, revealing and stressing feelings of meaninglessness and powerlessness. Stern and Doolan (1999) distinguish these stories from stories of restitution or reparation in which the experience of different life events are transformed into meaningful phenomena that occupy a place in the persons' life.

S: *Annie, when you made the choice to join the three days walk, what did you hope for? What did you hope it could bring you?*

A: *The common things between parents whom experienced terrible things. It can give an alliance. An alliance of trust. It was a chance to go on a walk together and talk together.*

S: *What means 'talking together' for you?*

A: *While talking you recognize things that people experienced. As parents it was a long way and some of us are still on the way. I recognized the efforts to protect your child and at the same time not being able to do so. The enormous powerlessness and disillusion.*

S: *What kind of efforts did you make?*

A: *As a parent, you want the best for your child. You know they are on the wrong track. You try to make them clear it is wrong...*

Some excerpts from the letter one of the authors wrote after the interview:

Annie, your son went living on his own. He studied at that moment. You allowed this, but pretty soon you discovered he was in trouble. It didn't go well. You thought you still had a grip on him.

You were very clear: 'I never gave up on him!' You kept following him! The last two and a half years he came living with you again. You asked: 'Tim, please, go to the doctor. Let them help you out.' He made a lot of debts. You paid them and went to the judge. You wanted to help so he could make a new start. For two years it went rather well. He went to the doctor and took his medicine. But at a certain moment it was over. You saw him gradually decline. This powerlessness was an incredible confrontation. He said: 'As long I don't want it, no one can do anything'. But you still tried to convince him 'gather yourself together!'.

At a certain moment he said: 'Mum, I know what I want.' You never thought he would really take that step of suicide... once you even begged not to do so... but some time later he did it anyway.

S: *How do you stay on your feet as a mother at a time like this?*
A: *(shaking her head) How did I stay on my feet???... My other children supported me by being there and having more contact. The first few months I didn't realise it. I felt I was going downhill. The pain and sorrow became enormous.*
S: *What made that you didn't give up totally?*
A: *I did not want this! I didn't want to decline. I wanted to be there for my other children and grandchildren. There is still a lot of anger in me because of what Tim did.*
S: *Was it in the past imaginable that you, as a mother, could end up in such a story?*
A: *No! At a certain point you are preparing yourself that you, sooner or later, can lose him. But when it actually happens, you cannot prepare for it. There is a big difference between 'knowing it can happen' and the moment it actually happens. You cannot predict it.*
S: *When we go back to the three days walk, was your son with you along the way?*
A: *No, for a little while not. Now and then... but no, not for me. At the end of the three days when we said goodbye, then he came back in my mind.*
S: *This 'for a while not' moment, what did it mean to you?*
A: *Oh! This was positive, really positive. For a while, I can put it aside. It doesn't control my life. It doesn't control all my doings. This was a very good feeling.*
S: *Is this important for you?*
A: *Very important!*
S: *Are these moments rare?*
A: *Yes, indeed! If I had not had the weekend, I would never have felt the difference.*
S: *Annie, are you saying that you don't want it to rule your life 100%?*
A: *Indeed, I don't want this.*
S: *How does this fit into the days ahead and into daily life?*

A: *It's a dilemma but in the meanwhile I know it is possible.*

Looking for a Sense of Coherence

During their lives, many questions kept the parents busy and started to occupy their minds. *How could this happen? Why? Why us? Is it my fault? What do I have to do? What is the meaning of all of this?* Sometimes they found answers, sometimes the answers got frozen and reduced without any context. They became stories coloured by all the negative experiences and negative identity conclusions about themselves, their child and the outside world. Every nuance, subordinated story or sense of personal agency seemed to have disappeared. They offered no perspectives or a future.

In the biographical interview one of the authors re-asks the questions the parents had asked themselves during the previous years and that perhaps were still wandering around in their heads. She listens to their answers and offers questions that can deconstruct their conclusions (Vermeire, 2011; Vermeire & Van Reybrouck, 2012). Narrative practices provide a framework for the ongoing review and questioning of strongly held beliefs that have an impact on the construction of identity.

In this 'scaffolding' process, the therapists strive towards the restoration of 'a sense of coherence'[1], in the sense that the events, experiences and responses the therapists bring into the picture lead to new or at least different answers. Throughout the interview, the different experiences and stories acquire meaning in the course of life as it was until now, are connected to the present and shed light on possible projects and expectations in the future (White, 2007). Subordinated storylines can be developed and what happened can be somewhat understandable, brings in a sense of personal agency and becomes more meaningful. The initiatives and unique outcomes on the three days walk form a base and offer plenty points of entry for rich story development. The therapists try to reconnect them with what is valuable for them in life, the important persons in life and their community. The authors devised three kinds of questions:

1. **Questions seeking an understandable coherence:** *How could this happen? What is really the problem? Who is guilty? What are the reasons? Am I really evil? Am I a bad parent?* Making sense of things does not boil down to searching the truth. The aim is rather rich story development. It is about the circumstances in which they live and how they interpret them. Stories are conceived as sequences of events linked over time, not necessarily in a linear or logical trajectory (Deleuze, 1990), but in series that lends coherence to whom we are becoming (Winslade, 2014).
2. **Questions that arouse a sense of personal agency, by developing subordinated storylines:** *How did I act? Did it make any difference? Were my efforts meaningful? Was I still supportive? What did I mean after all for my child? What helped me to go on? Who or what is still important for me?* A sense of personal agency, according to White (2006b, p150) is 'the sense of self that is associated with the perception that one is able to have some effect on the shape of one's own life; a sense that one is able to intervene in one's own life as an agent; a sense of what one values and as an agent of one' own intentions, and a sense that the world is at least minimally responsive to the fact of one's existence'. White believes that the restoration and/or development of this sense of personal agency can be a powerful antidote to the kind of highly invalidating conclusions about one's identity that these parents suffer from.
3. **Questions that create hope, a perspective for the future and give meaning:** *How can I go on with my life despite all the problems? How can my life still be meaningful? Does it make any sense to still have dreams? Is there still a future? How can I stay connected with others, the community*

and society? We try to detect which ideas, values and expectations are important for these parents in the many stories full of involvement; and which dreams did not become infected by their life course yet or which hope they have not yet given up.

The biographical interview takes about an hour and a half. Bit by bit the stories told change from problem-saturated stories to stories that restore a sense of personal and relational agency and a sense of coherence.

The Outsider Witnesses as Sources of Reconnection and Rich Description

The interview, with its different experiences and its creation/discovering of new stories and meanings, doesn't take place inside a dyadic cocoon (the interviewer-parent). As the authors conceive of identity as a relational, social and public project (Myerhoff, 2007), they take it has to be negotiated and acknowledged by many others involved.

Eric is a parent who took part in the three-day walk. He has a son with a severe addiction. He was one of the first to speak as a witness after Annie's interview.

S: *Where were you drawn to while listening to the story of Annie?*
E: *I was triggered by how she lost her son. It brought me to the point that my son is still alive but this isn't my child any more. Don't misunderstand me… he is still my child but I have no longer a grip on him. He is someone different so I lost him also in a certain way.*
S: *Is this connecting with the things Annie said about 'you can never, as a parent, imagine beforehand you can lose a child in such a way'?*
E: *Yes, I know already for ten years that once this fact will come. Sooner or later. It will come. There will be someone at my door in a police uniform… The moment you open that door, you will know what happened.*
S: *Annie said: 'you can know it with your head but…'*
E: *Yes, I know there is a big difference between knowing, feeling and what it 's going to do with you. It is not possible to prepare oneself. You will never be ready.*
…
S: *Is there something in Annie's story you take with you?*
E: *The confidence and the trust that those three days gave. I will think also about the 'for-a-while-not moment'. It was the first time in years I didn't have my son in my luggage. Otherwise you carry always a kind of soup pot in your backpack. You stir the soup, you turn around in it, but the pot is round and you can keep turning around. And now, for once, I didn't.*

The parent who was interviewed can listen to the outsider witnesses from a distance. Ideas, feelings and beliefs can be reviewed from a different position. The retelling has the potential to be highly resonant for the people whose lives are at the center of the definitional ceremony. This resonance contributes significantly to the development of rich stories, to stronger familiarity with what one accords value to in life, and to the erosion and displacement of various negative conclusions about one's life and identity (White, 2007, p189). Winslade (2012) refers to the importance and key principle to join people together in mutual support, rather than assume that people need to deal with isolation. At the same time parents' 'wisdom' can be shared and the social issues in the problems (Denborough, 2008) can become collective issues.

Frank, also as a parent of a daughter with a drug addiction tells how he was taken by the story of powerlessness during the interview of Annie. It brought him to his rage towards the politics of tolerance on drugs in our country and how they as parents are forced to accept this ways of organizing things by 'experts'. This conversation brought him back to his refusal to accept and linked him with the other parents.

Documenting the Story and the Ideas About the Future

The interviews are filmed. At the end the parents receive a DVD with the interview of their life story and the interviews of the witnesses. Approximately a week later they receive a letter from the interviewer with a written account of everything told in the definitional ceremony. After such an interview it can be difficult for the interviewed parent to remember certain words, sentences or statements. Words in a letter don't fade away in the same way as in a conversation but exist through space and time (White & Epston, 1990). The parents can re-read, re-view and re-listen. By reflecting on their words, they can feel and understand what they say over and over again, so that it will stick longer. They can share the material with others if they wish to, and receive other reflections of listeners. It allows them to revisit what they themselves or others told.

An Ongoing Conversation and Traces to a Future

Drawing on Andersen (1992) who pointed out the importance of 'ongoing conversations', the authors asked and received permission from the different parents to use the DVD and the letters in workshops and trainings or in conversations with other parents. After presenting their story, the authors ask trainees or other parents to write a letter to them using the outsider witness structure. This means that Annie still gets reflections and rich descriptions on her story. It's also a way to spread the parents' local knowledge and wisdom (Epston & White, 1992). A few months after the walk and the biographical interviews parents themselves report they take a different stance in their life: they became more gentle and mild towards their child, themselves and other parents; they enjoy more the little things in life; put things more in perspective. Annie for instance became member of a walking club. All these are little sparkles of hope for the future.

SOLUTIONS AND RECOMMENDATIONS

Isolating experiences demand openness, safe spaces where stories can be shared and witnessed, but moreover where people can write new histories together, regaining a sense of agency, and a sense of belonging and coherence, and accordingly a sense of a future, not only through interaction, but also by acting together.

FUTURE RESEARCH DIRECTIONS

The authors hope foremost to inspire other narrative and systemic therapists to relentlessly scrutinize post-structural ways of therapeutically dealing with isolating experiences. And of course they also welcome academic research into this part of the clinical field, dealing with interpersonal phenomena of extreme isolation and despair. Especially research into the role of witnessing others and audiences is welcomed.

CONCLUSION

In this small clinical project, parents of adult children who struggle with severe addiction, and who suffer from toxic feelings of guilt and shame, were engaged in a three days hike, and a recorded life review interview in the presence of outsider witnesses. The whole process was documented. The authors engaged with the following questions which were only preliminary answered.

1. How can therapists support parents in extremely difficult circumstances, where classical science-based parenting support, advises from an expert point of view, disregarding the fact that parents remain parents after the child has become an adult?
2. Is it helpful to engage parents in collective activities such as a three day hiking tour?
3. What therapeutic approaches to "going public" are feasible within existing ethical standards and can provide an antidote to the strong isolating forces of toxic feelings of shame and guilt? How 'public' can one go?
4. Is there an idea of wholeness (the sum is more than its parts) at work in bringing together novel approaches to therapy, namely: walking together; being interviewed in front of an audience; being witness to the interviewing of the witnesses; having the whole process documented in detail on film and on paper; receiving still afterwards reflections from others; and so on, or do they just add up?

Regarding the first question, one of the authors suggested elsewhere a different approach to parenting support, in which a counselor not only listens to parents' stories, but 'the meeting with a parent counselor will itself become a story, with a diachronic structure, that leads to changes in the self-understanding of those involved in the encounter' (Van den Berge, 2016, 268). Although not explicitly mentioned, the idea that narratives are developed during the walking and staying about event leading to changes in self-understanding is certainly 'at work' in the authors' approach, albeit not so much in an interaction with a parent counsellor, but rather with a group of mostly parents.

As to the second question, in classical therapy there is (at least at first glance) not much action. Perhaps the therapist offers their client a glass of water, or at the end of the session a payment is due. The authors noticed however that while walking, there seems to be much more 'communication', in the sense Wasserman & Fisher-Yoshida refer to as a 'reflexive cycle in which actions create meanings and meanings, in turn, shape actions' (2017, 13). An instance is when hikers help each other down a slippery slope into the forest. The presented approach is different from Darmody's (2019) who developed a Narrative Walks program that is designed in such a way that it serves as a group therapy for people who are not willing to engage in more traditional therapy forms.

As regards question 3, isolating forces are first the fact that the child is no longer seen as a child in society, as they reached at least in a juridical sense adulthood, which means the 'right' to parenting support, and maybe even the right to worry becomes less self-evident, and is sometimes even directly denied. This adds up with the fact that guilt as well as shame are feelings that rather inhibit the social sharing of emotions, instead of promoting it (De Mol & Rimé, 2017). By bringing people together who share analogous experiences, and who need not to be ashamed for each other because of what they feel or experience or do, the threshold is lowered to actually share stories. The life review interviewing method can help, in any degree of detail wanted, to unravel events and emotions. Outsider witnesses with whom some of the stories resonate can further add to the detoxification of painful emotions, and can even help parents to see that for instance feelings of guilt often hide very powerful intentions, hopes and values, from which the parent seemed to have become estranged. These not often heard parents' stories can become inspiring and supporting to many other parents when the recorded material can be used in training programs or during conferences and can influence and resonate in ever widening circles. It would be worthwhile to investigate in a qualitative study how this does affect parents' sense of self-esteem and self-worth.

Finally, regarding the fourth question, it can be remarked that the presented therapeutic design looks a bit like a postmodernist *bricolage*, where different objects are put together into an object that displays no obvious connection between its constituting parts. The authors impression was that parents anyway experienced a growing sense of coherence, but to answer the question an intricate qualitative research design would be required.

ACKNOWLEDGMENT

We would like to express our gratitude to the parents who allowed the authors and many others to meet them in vulnerable circumstances, and to all those who helped and assisted in a practical way to make this project possible.

REFERENCES

Andersen, T. (1992). Reflections on reflecting with families. In S. McNamee & K. J. Gergen (Eds.), *Therapy as Social Constructionism* (pp. 54–68). Sage.

Antonovsky, A. (1987). *Unraveling the mystery of health*. Jossey-Bass.

Bateson, M. C. (1989). *Composing a life*. Atlantic Monthly Press.

Carey, M., Walthers, S., & Russell, S. (2009). The absent but implicit: A map to support therapeutic enquiry. *Family Process*, *48*(3), 319–331. doi:10.1111/j.1545-5300.2009.01285.x PMID:19702920

Darmody, C. (2019). Narrative walks. *International Journal of Narrative Therapy and Community Work*, (1), 52–60.

De Mol, J., & Buysse, A. (2008). Understandings of children's influence in parental-child relationships: A Q-methodological study. *Journal of Social and Personal Relationships*, *25*(2), 359–379. doi:10.1177/0265407507087963

De Mol, J., & Rimé, B. (2017). Depression in young people: the family as a source of change and a place for sharing emotions with others or how my depression can also become my friend [Depressie bij jongeren: het gezin als bron van verandering en een plaats voor het delen van emoties met anderen of hoe mijn depressie ook mijn vriend kan worden]. In S. Vermeire & J. Sermijn (Eds.), *Wegen naar herverbinding. Narratieve, collaboratieve en dialogische praktijken*. Interactie-Academie VZW.

Denborough, D. (2008). Responding to trauma / responding to social issues. In *Collective Narrative Practice*. Dulwich Centre Publications.

Epston, D., & White, M. (1992). Consulting your consultants: 'The documentation of alternative knowledges. In *Experience, Contradiction, Narrative and Imagination*. Dulwich Centre Publications.

Fredman, G. (2004). *Transforming emotions*. Wurr Publishers Ltd.

Gergen, K. (1999). *An invitation to social construction*. Sage Publications.

Gergen, K. (2009). *Relational being: beyond self and community*. Oxford University Press.

Hedtke, L. (2014). Creating stories of hope: A narrative approach to illness, death and grief. *Australian and New Zealand Journal of Family Therapy*, *35*(1), 4–19. doi:10.1002/anzf.1040

Jenkins, A. (2009). Becoming ethical. A parallel, political journey with men who have abused. Rusell House Publishing Ltd.

Kuczynski, L., & De Mol, J. (2015). Dialectical Models of Socialization. In W. F. Overton & P. C. M. Molenaar (Eds.), Theory and Method. Volume 1 of the Handbook of Child Psychology and Developmental Science (7th ed.). Wiley. doi:10.1002/9781118963418.childpsy109

Lee, E., Bristow, J., Faircloth, C., & MacVarish, J. (2014). *Parenting culture studies*. Palgrave Macmillan. doi:10.1057/9781137304612

Madigan, S., & Epston, D. (1998). From 'Spy-chiatric Gaze' to communities of concern. From professional monologue to dialogue. In D. Epston (Ed.), *Catching up with David Epston: A collection of narrative practice-based papers published between 1991 & 1996* (pp. 127–148). Dulwich Centre Publications.

Madsen, W. C. (2007). *Collaborative Therapy With Multi-Stressed Families* (2nd ed.). The Guilford Press.

Ramaekers, S., & Suissa, J. (2012). *The claims of parenting: reasons, responsibility and society*. Springer. doi:10.1007/978-94-007-2251-4

Schaubroeck, K. (2010). *Een verpletterend gevoel van verantwoordelijkheid. Waarom ouders zich altijd schuldig voelen* [A crushing sense of responsibility. Why parents always feel guilty]. De Geus.

Stern, S., Doolan, M., Staples, E., Szmukler, L., & Eisler, I. (1999). Disruption and reconstruction: Narrative insights into the experience of family members caring for a relative diagnosed with serious mental illness. *Family Process*, *38*(3), 353–369. doi:10.1111/j.1545-5300.1999.00353.x PMID:10526771

Van den Berge, L. (2013). Parenting Support and the Role of Society in Parental Self-Understanding: Furedi's Paranoid Parenting Revisited. *Journal of Philosophy of Education*, *47*(3), 391–406. doi:10.1111/1467-9752.12008

Van den Berge, L. (2016). From fiction to friction: Towards an ethics of hermeneutics in parent counselling. *Ethics and Education*, *11*(3), 259–273. doi:10.1080/17449642.2016.1242041

Van den Berge, L. (2017) *Parenting support revisited: retrieving an ethics of hermeneutics. A philosophical investigation inspired by the viewpoints of Heidegger, Wittgenstein and Taylor* [Doctoral dissertation]. KU Leuven, Belgium.

Van den Berge, L., & Ramaekers, S. (2014). Figures of Disengagement: Charles Taylor, Scientific Parenting and the Paradox of Late Modernity. *Educational Theory*, *64*(6), 607–625. doi:10.1111/edth.12086

Van Reybrouck, T. (2007). *Mijn kind en drugs. Antwoorden voor ouders* [My child and drugs. Answers for parents]. Houtekiet.

Vermeire, S. (2011). Narratieve wegen tot herstel, het interview als therapeutische methode [Narrative paths to recovery, the interview as a therapeutic method]. *Systeemtheoretisch Bulletin*, *29*(2), 123–142.

Vermeire, S. (2012). Ouders en schuldgevoelens: een hefboom tot verandering [Parents and guilt: a lever for change]. *Tijdschrift voor ouderschapskennis, 15*(1), 36-49.

Vermeire, S. & Van Reybrouck, T. (2013). Een zoektocht naar sprankeltjes hoop en toekomst [A search for sparkles of hope and a future]. *Tijdschrift voor ouderschapskennis, 16*(1), 59-75.

Walsh, F. (2006). *Strengthening Family Resilience*. The Guilford Press.

White, M. (2006a). Working with people who are suffering the consequences of multiple trauma: a narrative perspective. In Narrative responses to traumatic experience. Adelaide: Dulwich Centre Publications.

White, M. (2006b). Children, Trauma and Subordinate Storyline Development. In D. Denborough (Ed.), *Trauma: Narrative responses to traumatic experience* (pp. 143–165). Dulwich Centre Publications.

White, M. (2006c). Working with Children who have Experienced Significant Trauma. In M. White & A. Morgan (Eds.), *Narrative therapy with children and their families* (pp. 85–97). Dulwich Centre Publications.

White, M. (2007). *Maps of narrative practice*. Norton.

White, M., & Epston, D. (1990). *Narrative Means to Therapeutic Ends*. Norton.

Winslade, J. (2014). *Time travel and narrative practice using Deleuze's time machine.* Presentation at the 3rd European Narrative Conference, Iasi, Romania.

Winslade, J. & Williams, M. (2012). *Safe and Peaceful Schools. Addressing Conflict and Eliminating Violence*. Corwin, a Sage Publications Company.

ADDITIONAL READING

Ackley, J., & Wilson-Menzfeld, G. (2021, September 19). The theatre as therapy for military veterans? Exploring the mechanisms which impact psychosocial well-being and social connections during theatre-based programmes. *Arts & Health*, 1–18. doi:10.1080/17533015.2021.1979608 PMID:34538198

Freedman, J. (2014) Witnessing and positioning: Structuring narrative therapy with families and couples. *The International Journal of Narrative Therapy and Community Work*, *1*, 11-17.

Vermeire, S. (2017) What if ... I were a king? Playing with roles and positions in narrative conversations with children who have experienced trauma. *International Journal of Narrative Therapy and Community Work*, (4), 50-62.

Vermeire, S. (2021). No child is an island: From attachment narratives towards a sense of belonging. *Journal of Family Therapy*, *43*(3), 414–425. doi:10.1111/1467-6427.12312

White, M. (1999) Reflecting teamwork as definitional ceremony revisited. *Gecko: A Journal of Deconstruction and Narrative Ideas in Therapeutic Practice*, *1*, 55-82.

White, M., & Epston, D. (1990). *Narrative means to therapeutic ends*. W.W. Norton.

KEY TERMS AND DEFINITIONS

Biographical Interview: A form of conversation that allows reflection on the various experiences and events in a person's life, enabling a new understanding of these experiences and events and the initiation of new actions.

Documenting: The practice of preserving in written form or by means of recording on tape or film parts of what happened during counselling or therapy.

Identity Conclusions: Self- or other-identity interpretations, which can be very persistent.

Narrative Practice: Ways of doing therapy and counselling that depart from the idea that people interpret their lives, that stories are the preferred way of making sense of one's life, and that different stories allow for different actions which in turn allow for the development of new stories.

Outsider Witnessing Practice: The practice of letting other people be present during therapeutical conversations and asking them in semi-structured ways to retell from their own point of view certain aspects of the telling of the clients.

Sense of Belonging: The feeling of belonging to people who matter to him or her, and also to smaller communities or systems of people whom one knows personally, but also to larger and anonymous communities (for example, the group of parents).

Sense of Coherence: The felt sense that one's life forms a more or less coherent whole or Gestalt, notwithstanding certain discrepancies that one can usually cope with and endures.

Sense of Personal Agency: The sense that one has something to say in the way one's life develops, and that this is in agreement with what one hopes for, or what one values in life.

Subordinate Storylines: Storylines that were forgotten, and do not repeat what is often referred to regretfully as "the story of one's life"; and which, when remembered, especially in the presence of others, allow for alternative story/life developments.

ENDNOTE

1 Antonovsky (1987) was a medical sociologist who conducted research on women who had survived the Holocaust and the Nazi concentration camps. Two thirds of the group did not fare well, but one third managed to live a reasonably good life after this disastrous period. He considered it normal that the health of these women was not good. So he was intrigued by the question "What made that one third say that they managed to live a good life?" Hence, he focused his research on the question "What creates health?". He saw stress and disease as natural aspects of life and abandoned a pathological framework in his search for the causes of illness. In addition to some general sources of support, an important source, namely 'a sense of coherence'. He described it as a global life orientation in which someone has a strong belief that whatever happens is comprehensible, manageable and meaningful. This sense of coherence is an important contributor to health, mental well-being and quality of life. It has a greater impact than individual characteristics (cf. Stern & Doolan, 1999; Walsh, 2006; Eriksson & Lindstrom, 2007).

Chapter 16
Interweaving Narrative Methods Into a Mandala of Transformational Practices

Susan Mossman Riva
https://orcid.org/0000-0002-7231-9251
Creighton University, Switzerland

ABSTRACT

Narrative therapy can be understood as part of a narrative continuum where generative story threads are interwoven into a mandala of transformational practices. Individual and social transformation is elicited by narrative practices that reinforce narrative coherency. Through engagement with narrative methods, phases of narrative practice and inquiry are analyzed, revealing the emergence of narrative concrescence within an integrated narrative framework. Autoethnography, narrative therapy, narrative mediation, narrative conflict resolution, and transformational learning using "transformagram portfolios" can be understood as connected storying practices contained in mediatorship. This holistic approach to narrative methods creates linkages that further the generative potential of narrative practices as illustrated in case studies. By reinforcing narrative coherency in the noosphere, "narrative truth" can be generated and used as a guiding force in a post-truth era.

INTRODUCTION

Narrative therapy can be regarded as a transversal approach that can be applied to different forms of therapeutic interventions and professional practices. When conflicts and illnesses are perceived to be interconnected, narrative therapy and narrative conflict resolution can be practiced together, using an integral approach based on narrative methods aligned with the appropriate practice pathway. Narrative therapy can be imagined as an integral part of an integrated continuum framework. When practitioners working in therapy, naturopathy, mediation, and conflict resolution adhere to a holistic vision, the components of narrative therapy can be adapted and interwoven into specific contexts. Narrative therapy can

DOI: 10.4018/978-1-7998-9251-9.ch016

also be integrated within transformative pedagogies to train future practitioners providing an experiential approach for adult learners.

As narrative therapy recognizes the importance of power relationships, using references from anthropology and the social sciences, it provides an analytical framework for understanding the causes of both illnesses and conflicts. By working with narratives, intrapersonal conflicts as well as illnesses are shown to be interconnected. When these multiple layers of relationships are analyzed, they reveal a form of "linkedness". Generating reflexivity, through the analytic process brings forth narrative coherence and concrescence using a relational lens (Rankin, 2002). This approach spans a continuum ranging from the local and personal to the global and societal. This "glocal" paradigm provides a vision of increased planetary relatedness.

Autoethnography is a powerful performance pedagogy and narrative practice that generates self-transformation (Denzin, 2014, p.80). When it is integrated into the narrative therapy continuum, it can be used to elicit transformational processes within the larger relational matrix. Duoethnography can also be used to create a dialogical space to increase reflexivity. This method can be used in higher education to foster deeper understanding while providing an experiential pedagogy as part of the transformational learning process. "Grounded in social justice, duoethnography has been used purposefully to promote change" (Sawyer and Norris, 2012, p. 3).

This chapter will illustrate how narrative therapy can be used in a transversal manner, eliciting connectivity throughout the therapeutic continuum process. A mandala of narrative practices can be interwoven into an integrated framework that can be adapted to various professional postures while remaining connected to the fundamental concepts and practices developed in narrative therapy.

Case studies will be presented to show how narrative therapy was adapted to multiple contexts to foster transformational processes. Narrative inquiry englobes a large spectrum of methods that can cultivate transformative pathways for individuals, families, and communities. Narrative methods like narrative therapy and narrative conflict resolution engender flyways that lead to wellbeing, constructive problem-solving, and social transformation.

Individual and social transformation will be presented within an integrated framework, showing how narrative approaches are transversal, interconnected, and multilayered. These approaches can be imagined as an interwoven mandala of methods that together elicit generative processes. Mediatorship, is a vessel or container of these transformational processes that use narrative methods as a vehicle for transportation.

In the following sections narrative mediation with political asylum seekers and within intercultural contexts, narrative inquiry research methods, transformative pedagogies, auto/duoethnography, as well as community based participatory research will be recollected to demonstrate how narrative therapy is a foundational practice that can be applied to varying contexts using narrative methods.

Interdisciplinary and relational approaches can be used in conjunction with narrative methods to foster social transformation, especially when they are adapted to meet the needs of scholar practitioners with different professional postures. The core components of narrative therapy will be presented in a way that reveals a form of generative "linkedness" where narrative therapy is nested within an integrated continuum of narrative practices.

The evolving narrative practices that were used throughout the different phases of my lifework can be considered as part of a narrative continuum. Each method and practice can be recognized as part of an integrated framework that constitutes what I refer to as mediatorship. This multilayered container links narrative practice pathways. In this way, mediatorship is a vessel of transportation, a meaning-making container, exploring narrative potential. This chapter offers a cartography of narrative practices where mediatorship has set a course towards a holistic vision and where narrative approaches are integrated into a mandala of interwoven practices that develop mindsight within the noosphere. By focusing our attention on narrative coherency, narrative concrescence is fostered. These narrative processes can transport humanity to more desirable outcomes in a post-truth era.

A CARTOGRAPHY OF NARRATIVE PRACTICES

Michael White and David Epston analyzed narrative practices using a lens that reveals how practices are inevitably political. Their work opened dialogical space where liberating storylines transport participants to more desirable outcomes. Michael White mapped narrative practices in an exploration of narrative potentialities (White, 2007, p. 7). His lifework lays out areas of narrative practice including externalizing conversations, re-authoring conversations, re-membering conversations as well as scaffolding conversations to attain conceptual development that he understood as a foundation for "self-mastery" and "self-regulation" (White, 2007, p. 281).

He referred to Vygostky's ideas about learning and development to assist in the further development of narrative practices, connecting narrative therapy to social collaboration (White, 2007, p. 280). He explained how the foundations of personal agency and responsible action are linked to social collaboration. He also placed an accent on word meaning that he understood to be an essential component of the transformational process.

White saw language and conversations as essential elements of narrative therapy and other narrative practices. He explained how the meaning-making process that the practitioner scaffolds is configured to assist the participant with the goal of initiating change. Social collaborations are the cornerstone of the scaffolding process conceptualized in Vygotsky's proximal zone of learning. This scaffolding is erected so that participants can learn how to participate effectively in the emancipatory processes that are inherent in narrative practices. This orientation underscores the importance of learning processes and relationships.

White referred to learning tasks that allow for the development of reflexivity. "The achievement of the capacity to see the consequences of one's actions, to reflect on specific developments of one's life, and to develop concepts about life and identity by abstracting learnings and realizations about one's life are dependent upon such social collaboration" (White 2007, p. 280). In this sense, narrative therapy is not just a therapeutic endeavor, but also a learning process. By using Vygotsky's theories to explain narrative therapy, White provided a conceptual framework that integrates the importance of learning processes and lifelong learning within therapeutic practice.

When teaching the techniques of narrative therapy and narrative mediation, it is necessary to lead students to discover the art that invents and supports the techniques. "Transforming training back toward education must create space for the art of imagination and provide space for naming the knowledge and the process" (Lederach, 2005, p. 124). Therapists and mediators are artisans of social change (McNamee, Hosking, 2012). When teachers use storytelling to convey important concepts, they align themselves with the generative power inherent in narrative practices. Storytelling is part of the scaffolding process that guides and models learning relationships.

Narrative therapy also has an important relational dimension that links it to social collaboration. This relational dimension in narrative therapy gave rise to narrative mediation and narrative conflict resolution practices. Oftentimes, the insights that individuals have in a therapeutic setting involve reflections about relationships with others as well as the social, cultural, and political aspects that are configuring their narrative. "Mediation can be defined as assisting two or more people to negotiate the relational conditions for going forward in a relationship" (Winslade, 2017, p.88).

Re-membering is a way to participate in the reconstruction of identity. "Re-membering, as defined by Myerhoff, contributes to the development of a "multivoiced" sense of identity and facilitates activity in making sense of one's existence and achieving a sense of coherence through the "ordering" of life" (White 2007, 137). The narrative practitioner plays an important role witnessing definitional stories and can also configure communal spaces of witnessing to enhance the story development process (White 2007, 184). Witnessing encourages rich story development as people identify preferred outcomes. By eliciting the telling of life stories and then the retelling to other audiences, momentum arises from the storying process. White identified phases of expression, image, resonance, and transport (White 2007, 191). When various phases of storying practices are interconnected, they become a vessel of transportation.

Remembering not only allows participants to recall and re-collect life stories, but to re-assemble them in ever more coherent narratives of becomingness. By looking more closely at the contexts where narrative practices are employed, we can begin to see how they can be assembled in integrated frameworks that range from the intrapersonal to the societal, even global. Evolving narrative strands permeate multi-layered story templates. A holistic approach to narrative practices seeks to link multiple methods and relational dimensions in an ever more coherent conceptual vision. Using narrative practices in transformational pedagogies brings narrative therapy even further. Life-o-grams become transform grams through transformational learning pedagogies that have been effectively used in medical anthropology classes and naturopathic certification courses (Riva, 2021).

By defining mediation as "linkedness" the relational aspect of being in-between is reinforced (Riva, 2009). In this way mediation can be understood to relink broken relational bonds. People can move from states of brokenness to "linkedness". This understanding opens a transversal pathway that can facilitate the linkage of phases that move from narrative therapy to phases of narrative mediation and conflict resolution.

Mediatorship is a word that emerged from my autoethnographic process. It is a word container that holds insights gleaned from both autoethnographic practice and narrative mediation practice. Mediatorship can be defined as the function or position of a mediator. When the position of the mediator is in-between, mediatorship acts in a way to facilitate connectivity. Inventing new uses for words brings forth new practice pathways. The creative process involves imagining new words that represent new visions of practice. Vygotsky understood language to be social and mediate in nature. He saw writing as a complex cultural activity. And he was convinced that writing must be taught in a way that renders writing "relevant to life" (Vygotsky, 1978, p. 118). In this way writing can be understood as a form of social mediation that opens new flyways or passageways.

Autoethnographic practice provided a template for narrative transformation. Concepts emerged from the writing process that offered a conceptual framework. Words presented themselves as meaning containers. Writing connected me to a form of living wisdom that revealed important insights. I came to understand that mediatorship facilitates dialogical processes that in turn engender resolution processes and increased narrative coherency. Mediatorship became a guiding metaphor for my exploratory process. "The recognition of the root word "ship" became a guiding force, taking me on a meaning voyage to other words of significance. "Ship" as a suffix means to create form" (Riva 2020, p. XIII). In this way, writing brings forth meaning. Mediatorship has allowed me to formulate my understanding of transformative narrative practices, providing a container for a continuum of practices, as well as offering a conceptual framework.

Storying conceptual insights gives rise to a methodological mandala that generates narrative concrescence through the meaning-making process. Mediatorship provides a vessel for narrative explorations, mapping transformational practices through journeymanship. Interconnectivity is yet another aspect of mediatorship. When various narrative methods and practices are seen to be connected, linkages are reinforced. Connectivity is enkindled through the storying process that acts upon relational matrixes, interweaving story strands in a story mandala. In this way, storying has the potential of mediating and transforming relationships through a continuum of narrative practices. Mediatorship transports and is propelled forward by the generative potentiality encapsulated in narrative practices. Mediatorship connects the different layers and dimensions of our lifeworld with the appropriate narrative practices that can all together, in an interconnected way, elicit transformation. This vessel or ship enhances interconnectivity by holding it together. By scaffolding an integrated framework, narrative practices are reinforced.

Witnessing transformative process also reinforces the transformative potential inherent in individual and social transformation processes. This can happen within the therapeutic space that is configured. But it can also happen when authorship gives birth to readership. Reading our lives enhances the comprehension of our life stories. Analyzing our "textistences" elicits increased narrative agency. We can "develop an appreciation for the richness and potential of our own emerging story" (Randall and McKim, 2008, p. 60). The anthropology of becoming looks at how we are all unfinished. Tapping into narrative potentiality brings forth becomingness, as we actively fill in the contours of our unfinished portraits with determined strokes and bright colors (Biehl & Locke, 2017). We enhance our narrative agency by submitting our life histories to aesthetic readings that can give rise to enriched storylines.

Autoethnography, narrative therapy, narrative mediation, narrative conflict resolution, and community based participatory research that uses narrative inquiry, all draw from narrative modes that locate participants in their lifeworlds. "This is a world of interpretative acts, a world in which every retelling of a story is a new telling, a world in which persons participate with others in the "re-authoring," and thus in the shaping of their lives and relationships (White & Epston 1990, p. 82). Narrative practices are characterized by their inclusion of Michel Foucault's theories on "truths" and power that develop how discourses are inseparable from actions of power. "In considering the constitutive dimension of power, Foucault concludes that power and knowledge are inseparable-so much so that he prefers to place the terms together as power/knowledge or knowledge/power" (White & Epston, 1990, p. 22).

Awareness of the power relations inherent in our storylines allows us to reflexively consider the poetics and politics that constitute us. Gnothi Seauton, "know thyself" is a central concept in the Greek wisdom tradition that underscores the importance of self-knowledge. Gnosis is a Greek noun for knowledge or awareness. The self-knowledge gained through narrative practices contributes to empowerment. This can also be understood as narrative coherency. This coherency is increased when we participate in "generative social fields" or mindwebs, allowing energy and information to emerge within the interactions of many interconnected individuals. This permits individuals to share their experience and wisdom with others in a way that shapes the life course. (Siegel, 2020, p. 453). By building on the power inherent in narrative coherency, we reinforce potential pathways towards social transformation that are generated through higher levels of coherency that foster relational processes that not only increase meaningful connections but positive relational attachment.

Sarah Cobb's work in narrative conflict resolution develops the importance of the aesthetic dimensions of our narratives as well as the political dimensions of our humanness. "The act of constructing people as works of art, as colorful and multilayered *is* the work of the beholder, the witness, and does not demand particular conditions to be present, as though some people deserve to be characterized as complex human beings. But it does demand that we locate and engage specific kinds of conversational partners that do not simply elaborate the narrative of our Other ("they are right") or our own victim narratives ("the Other is terrible"). And without someone to support the emergence of a better-formed story, it is not likely to appear" (Cobb, 2013, p. 284). Cobb connects Hannah Arendt's theory of "natality" to human rights, freedom, and to that which constitutes humanness. "And as long as that person lives, he or she is entitled to freedom, to create plans, to initiate, to respond in his or her own particular way to his or her life conditions" (Cobb, 2013, p. 126). Cobb also poses the question about what constitutes a better storyline. "The better-formed story, as I have described it, provides a set of aesthetic principles for assessing narrative as an ethical project/product" (Cobb, 2013, p. 234). The narrative transformation project is an artistic project calling for new "lines of flight" with new configurations of meaning and the social construction of relationships that are more complex and beautiful. This form of questioning follows Kandinsky's search for what is spiritual in art, and the criteria that defines beauty in artform (Kandinsky, 1977).

The basic blueprint of narrative therapy has engendered narrative conflict resolution practices that give rise to emancipatory processes that act upon social and political dimensions. Therefore, an integral approach to narrative transformation requires the conceptualization of an integrated continuum of narrative practices that contribute to self-realization and even peacebuilding, aiming to reinforce strong institutions that are guided by principles of social justice.

Lederach uses storytelling in an integrated framework for peacebuilding that centers on the redefinition and restoration of broken relationships. "The integrated framework suggests that we are not merely interested in "ending" something that is not desired. We are oriented toward the building of relationships that in their totality form new patterns, processes, and structures" (Lederach, 2020, p. 492). This requires not only the constructive transformation of conflicts, but a visionary approach. We need to have a vision of what we are trying achieve.

Narrative mediation has developed a theoretical approach that aligns narrative practice with democratic values. Engaging in resolution processes allows mediators to participate in the creation of improved democracies. Winslade and Monk refer to Derrida who spoke of *démocratie à l'avenir* or "democracy to come." This reference connects the process of deconstruction to the process of reconstruction, underscoring a dedication to furthering emancipatory processes. After deconstructing our narratives, developing important analytical skills and reflexivity, we are invited to engage in re-authoring or re-storying. Because individual storylines are connected to *master narratives*, we can write *counterstories* in response to political oppression, reclaiming moral agency in the face of marginalization (Nelson, 731). Responding to new forms of conflict requires response-ability. "Narrative mediation is an effort to create a vision of a future in which democracy is improved through professional practice" (Monk & Winslade 2008, p. 287). Professional practices that use narrative methods can thus be understood to participate in the edification of more democratic systems that challenge marginalization using narrative repair.

Not only does narrative mediation facilitate conflict resolution, but it is a professional practice that upholds democratic values. Narrative methods can be used to facilitate emancipatory processes in varying fields of practice. Narrative repair happens when we actively engage in the writing process, manumitting, or writing to set ourselves free from oppression. "It is clear that conflict resolution as a profession has developed the knowledge, skills and experience needed to begin thinking and planning how we might contribute, even in small ways, to building the capacity of people around the world to resolve chronic conflicts" (Cloke, 2017, p. 293). The "glocal" challenges that the people of the world are facing require integrated global capacity building.

Higher education has an important role to play in developing moral imagination and agency. Capacity building involves educational approaches that can effectively prepare students to participate in society. There is a relational imperative that needs to be cultivated in educational relationships to keep students engaged. "From a relational standpoint, we may see this as *enabling participation in a positive flow of coordinated action*. This is to place the focus of education neither on developing the individual, nor enhancing the society, but on relational processes for sustaining and creating flourishing forms of life" (Gergen, 2021, p. 45). Coordinated actions and relational mind arise from narrative approaches that foster transformational processes in higher education. By integrating *appreciative* practices for social change, teachers can enhance relationships and partnerships.

In this chapter, I will draw from case studies, sharing my work as a scholar practitioner, to illustrate how narrative methods were used in different circumstances to facilitate resolution processes and capacity building. I will also illustrate how narrative therapy can be integrated into naturopathic practice and medical anthropology, providing a foundation for integrative medicine.

Firstly, working with the police and the social services gave me the opportunity to us narrative mediation and narrative therapy to improve democracy by providing a pathway to increased social justice. Secondly, as a researcher, I was able to do needs assessment, incorporating narrative inquiry to improve healthcare policy. Using narratives of resilience in documentary films that were part of larger community based participatory research projects cultivated yet another aspect of narrative inquiry. Thirdly, my autoethnographic work reinforced my certitude that autoethnography generates self-transformation. Incorporating auto/duoethnography in curricula furthered this conviction. Finally, developing transformative learning pedagogies has allowed me to scaffold transformational methods for students in the social sciences as well as for naturopathic practitioners. These mediating pedagogies have been designed to elicit social transformation processes. My teaching experience affirms that using pedagogies that value narrative methods enhances the experiential learning process that becomes a passageway. By integrating narrative practices in learning environments, students gain knowledgeability about narrative potentiality that allows them to home *in* to new "lines of flight."

DEVELOPING RESPONSE-ABILITY

I was initiated as a mediator on a helicopter accident site, working for the Valais Police after the worst helicopter accident in Swiss history in 2000. That experience was followed by my work with political asylum seekers in the Social Services, where I headed a mediation service from 2001-2005. In both instances, I developed narrative mediation practices in intercultural contexts that required a holistic approach to the human suffering that I witnessed (Riva 2009). Narrative practices allowed me to define my professional posture while facing complex situations that elicited innovative and transformative responses.

As I also worked closely with a psychiatrist, we developed an intercultural mediation practice that integrated ethno-psychiatry. Our practice evolved to a form of narrative therapy that gave an important place to culture bound syndromes and meaning networks that were developed in the field of medical anthropology. Notably Arthur Kleinman's work provided a referential framework that allowed us to interpret the conflict and illness narratives that were shared in interdisciplinary consultations (Kleinman, 1989). When my mediation service was closed for political reasons, I took my intercultural mediation cases to the academic world, creating a dialogical and analytical space where marginalized voices could be heard and acknowledged. In this way, narrative mediation evolved into narrative inquiry (Riva, 2009).

Needs assessment research in mental health, immigrant health, and LGBT health further developed narrative inquiry methods using the lens of medical anthropology and social psychology. Methods were developed that created dialogical space using professional's narratives (Riva, 2015). Using community based participatory research methods, I went on to make a film on hopeful, healthy aging. Using older women's narratives of resiliency, the film elicited a life course approach to aging and "growing old" (Riva, 2017).

This community based participatory research model was later used to produce a documentary film on the development of mediation practices in Valais, Switzerland in 2022. The documentary film was made to celebrate the 10th anniversary of the Valais Mediation Association (AVDM). Interviews with partners in the field were carried out and then analyzed by the association's committee members. Important themes were integrated within the film, in a visual manner, to highlight the concepts that emerged[1]. A celebratory event was organized with students studying mediation from the University of Geneva and the naturopathic students from the Valais College of Alternative Medicine (CVMA) which further underscores how interdisciplinary and holistic approaches to resolution processes and lifelong learning can be fostered in communities of practice (Wenger, McDermot, Snyder, 2002). Government officials were invited to participate in a round table discussion to advance the creation of a culture of mediation in the canton and reflect upon future legislation, thus integrating the groups and norms creating culture into the transformation process (Hansen, 2020, p. 754).

After working in the field as a researcher, developing narrative inquiry methods, my lifework eventually led to teaching courses in the Department of Cultural and Social Studies at Creighton University. I then applied the transformative pedagogies from my online teaching courses to the naturopathic certification courses in Valais, Switzerland at the CVMA (Riva, 2021). "Transformagram Porfolios" offer a transformative pedagogy that emerged from my autoethnographic practice, writing "Homing In, An Adopted Child's Story Mandala of Connecting, Reunion, and Belonging" (Riva 2020). The insights from my different phases of narrative inquiry dovetailed with my autoethnographic practice, bringing forth a teaching story.

Writing transported me to landscapes of meaning where guiding metaphors accompanied my experiential process. The Holy Grail Way is an important insight that emerged from my autoethnographic process. The Holy G-rail Way is a railway that offers a metaphor or sign post indicating a pathway or walkthrough-a stepwise way through our conflict and illness narratives. The human condition involves confronting our conflicts and illnesses that elicit resolution processes. The Holy Grail is part of the Arthurian legends that provides a formidable storyline where questing is revered. The quest for the Holy Grail is at the heart of the legend. The Holy Grail is a cup or sacred chalice, a vessel filled with consecrate verses or narratives. It is a sacred vessel of verses that transports. The walkthrough is a transformative performance and passageway.

"The Holy Grail was revealed to me as the rail or railway forward and a vessel or container for our quests. Our illnesses as well as our conflicts present an intrinsic potential for our becomingness. We are invited to understand them as metaphors. Illness narratives as well as conflict narratives open space as we speak and write of our sufferings. The story containers hold transformational potentialities. The *viriditas* or greenness of our narratives is brought to fruition through the reflexive process. Newfound meaning resides in the hollow of our wounds, where a road map is hidden, indicating as well as informing the Holy Grail-Way" (Riva, 2020, p. 427).

We move from brokenness to linkedness when we behold. Beholding implies a transformed way of perceiving. By developing narrative coherency, our perceptions are transformed. Transformed perception holds the potential of transporting our storylines as we discover new "lines of flight" or flyways.

Daniel Siegel writes about the importance of narrative coherency with explanations that illustrate how mindsight is developed on what he refers to as the Wheel of Perception. "What such a capacity can do is to allow us to see directly-to sense and conceive and perceive within ourselves-so that our mind's concepts and categories of interrelational life can become a part of the noosphere within which we are all immersed" (Siegel, 2020, p. 493).

Mediatorship sails on the waves of the noosphere or planetary mind that emerges from acknowledging the interrelations connecting all lifeforms. The noosphere is a field of interconnection that extends beyond the self to a body of knowledge that we belong to. Increasing our narrative coherency through practices including autoethnography, allows us to experience narrative integration that brings forth a sense of well-being. "Narrative integration is about making sense of our lives, and the research is clear that it makes sense to make sense" (Siegel, 2020, p. 466). Siegel's research in psychiatry has proven that autoethnographic writing and narrative practices foster brain integration that leads to a heightened sense of well-being. By achieving narrative coherency, our ability to relate, as understood in attachment theory, is enhanced. This capacity to relate in family relationships can also be applied to human-Earth relationships (Berry, 1999).

In the preface of Homing *In*, I refer to Pierre Teilhard Chardin's theory about the noosphere, using his concept as an explanatory model that can explain how my birth sister and I homed *in* to find our birth parents in what might be understood as a convergence, before our maternal grandmother died. "Pierre Teilhard de Chardin uses the term noosphere to describe an evolving sphere dominated by the mind, consciousness, and interpersonal relationships" (Riva, 2020 p. XI)

Engaging in meaning-making process allows us to increase our sense of self while making linkages with other levels of belonging. Having a sense of belonging is an essential component of well-being. In my autoethnographic work, I explore belonging through the lens of the adopted child. Storying kinship fostered insights about belonging on a planetary level. This exploration transported me to question how we might better live in/on Earthship. "The social construction of our relational being includes relations of human kinship and planetary Earthship" (Riva, 2020, p. 341). Creating the Homing *In* website allowed me to embark upon what I refer to as "glovircal pilgrimage." The global and local connected through virtual landscapes[2].

I conclude my autoethnographic work by sharing a vision of living in/on Earthship.

"As I hold the Book of Changes, the I-Ching falls open to "On the Earth, there is water: the image of Holding Together," an offering for this ending. Here hexagram, genogram, life-o-gram, and narrative *transformagram* are intricately laced together. As we behold, we actively transform the image. When seen from space our emerald planet, Earthship takes on the form of chalice, vessel, and sacred container, holding us together" (Riva, 2020, p.433).

My autoethnographic process illustrates how narrative practice is a tool for developing narrative coherency, which in turn allows us to co-construct more desirable relationships. Through the transformational process life-o-grams become "transformagrams".

Hinton and Kirmayer developed the hypothesis of flexibility coining the term transformagrams in the context of psychiatry. "The flexibility hypothesis suggests that, in conveying a sense of change, healing rituals shift sufferers' mode of being-in-the world, including their cognitive, emotional, and physical state or stance, toward openness to new ways of being" (Hinton & Kirmayer, 2017, p. 4). They explain how healing occurs by representing a person's emotions and life problems through symbols. They call the schema that represents the transformation a transformagram. The transformagram is a sequence of images of transformation that work to reinforce a more positive self-image as well as a narrative of self-efficacy (Hinton & Kirmayer, 2017, p. 9).

While writing about life-o-grams, or holographic representations of life history, I discovered the transformagram concept. It gave me a referential framework for the transformational process. Within this framework narrative process is understood to elicit transformation much like other healing methods, including psychoanalysis and rituals. Subsequently, narrative transformation generates flexibility, allowing people to increase their ability to adapt. It became clear to me that autoethnography is a generative practice, with the potential of increasing flexibility.

My autoethnographic process brought me to the understanding that auto/duoethnographic methods can generate transformation, which encouraged me to develop pedagogies that incorporate these narrative practices. Life-o-grams can be transformed through experiential learning pedagogies that I refer to as Transformagram Portfolios. Hence, autoethnography is a practice, method and performative pathway towards increased flexibility. This important realization gave rise to the creation of transformational pedagogies that I have incorporated into my courses, transporting narrative processes to the level of higher education (Riva, 2021). The transformagram pedagogy is a narrative teaching tool that integrates aspects of narrative therapy. This pedagogical tool creates a space where students can *walkthrough* their conflict and illness narratives. This transformative learning process is a passageway (Nicolaides, Eschenbacher, Buergelt, Gilpin-Jackson, Welch, et Misawa 2022).

Remembering the different phases of my inquiry process illustrates narrative generativity. My experience suggests that narrative therapy is part of a much larger continuum of narrative practices, that are enhanced when they are conceived as part of an integrated framework. As we are storied beings, we use words and narratives in our learning and resolution processes. The different narrative practices are part of an integrated continuum that contributes to multi-layered meaning-making processes. Reinforcing the linkages between the different narrative approaches that are relevant within specific contexts, allows for the envisioning of a narrative blueprint to come into sight. This ever more coherent vision increases knowledgeability and conscious awareness in the noosphere.

ANALYZING THE FUNDAMENTAL COMPONENTS AND GUIDING PRINCIPLES OF NARRATIVE PRACTICES

Opening and configuring dialogical space is a fundamental component inherent in narrative approaches ranging from autoethnography to community based participatory research. Another guiding principle is how narrative practices are used for problem-solving. Finding our words dovetails with resolving our problems. This problem-solving dimension can be observed on multiple levels spanning across individual, relational, community, and planetary resolution processes. When the linkages between these different levels are acknowledged, our vision of narrative practice is transformed. Beholding generates a cogent methodological mandala. Integrating symbols that arise from experiential processes elicits "creative mythology" and interpretive practices that can be understood as living myth that transcends mere words (Campbell, 1968, p. 4).

Opening dialogical space requires collaborating, translating, and fostering intercultural and interdisciplinary processes. Listening to stories and finding ways to create space for marginalized voices to be heard and integrated into larger social conversations is yet another fundamental principle. Storying processes often move from narrative therapy to narrative conflict resolution, especially in relation to marginalized groups of people that are seeking social justice. Co-constructing solutions involves creating analytical space to increase reflexivity on both individual and systemic levels. Narrative concrescence happens by generating reflexivity and linkages between the story strands that connect the story layers.

Events elicit the need to configure dialogical space that often connects narrative therapy and narrative conflict resolution through unfolding phases of intervention. There is a snow-balling effect as reflexivity is elicited to improve long-term outcomes and define best practices. Narrative concrescence occurs when linkages are reinforced between dialogical processes, resolution processes, and learning processes.

Crisis intervention, therapy, mediation, and conflict resolution are configured by judicial systems, social and healthcare networks, and public health policy. Conflict resolution can be understood to encapsulate narrative therapy, providing care for the traumatized while resolving the pressing problems at hand. "Serendipity pushes us to demystify theory. Theory is not writing perfectly defined but intangible explanations about social realities. It is about the common sense about how things are connected, how they influence each other, and how they may relate to desired change. Theory is our best speculation about how complex things work" (Lederach, 2005, p. 125).

Developing theories contributes to our understanding of complex situations. This can be illustrated through the case study of the helicopter accident. At first, there was the accident event. The mediation processes that were initiated, offered a dialogical space for the overall resolution process that included mediating, translating, and configuring intercultural and interdisciplinary collaboration in response to the needs of the different people, organizations, and nations involved in the crisis intervention. Narrative mediation on the initial accident site grew to encompass narrative conflict resolution that brought together the different stakeholders.

After the initial response, the crisis intervention team reflected on the intervention. This allowed for a systemic vision to emerge and best practices to be identified. Developing this case study as part of my PhD. thesis, provided an academic space that fostered the co-construction of an analytical framework, through the process of narrative inquiry. Much later, the helicopter accident was presented to students in a course on forensic anthropology, sharing the knowledgeability gained from the accident site intervention. The teaching methods included storying the crisis intervention with the support of photo-elicitation by showing pictures of the accident site and other photos used in the judiciary process.

When working with political asylum seekers, another generative pathway unfolded, eliciting narrative coherence and contributing to the co-construction of innovative professional practices. When working with political asylum seekers in the mediation service in Valais, Switzerland, stories were shared. At times it was necessary to have a cultural mediator or translator to be able to understand the conflict and illness narratives. To resolve these situations, interdisciplinary resolution processes were configured, involving the social services, institutional representatives, as well as a psychiatrist. The mediation service offered a narrative mediation approach that often included narrative therapy in the first phase of the consultation. The narrative approach linked the different phases of the resolution process in an integrated framework.

By co-authoring a master's degree with the psychiatrist, I was collaborating with, we created a reflexive space to analyze our evolving professional collaboration. Our increased narrative coherency subsequently enriched our intercultural and interdisciplinary professional practice. This led to a systemic transformation within the professional network that incorporated our interdisciplinary approach. Narrative mediation acted on the way conflicts and illnesses were addressed by both the psychiatric services and social action services in our canton. Narrative therapy connected and fostered interprofessional practice in an integral approach that put less focus on professional roles.

After the mediation service was terminated for political reasons, engaging in a PhD. allowed the political asylum seeker's case studies to be brought to the academic world through my thesis' publication. This narrative inquiry further developed concepts in relation to narrative therapy, narrative mediation, and narrative conflict resolution. The narrative coherence that I sought to elicit through the conflict and illness narratives expanded to include my personal narrative coherence as a scholar practitioner. Narrative concrescence allowed the process to reach the realm of academia in the pursuit of social justice.

Sharing the stories of political asylum seekers and providing explanatory models to better understand the social and cultural determinants that were configuring their conflict and illness narratives, reinforced the meaning-making process. The illness narratives that were shared in intercultural mediations were understood to enfold conflicts that were linked to social and cultural determinants of health. Listening to conflict narratives allowed me to make connections, identifying linkages between conflict and illness narratives that I confronted in my professional practice.

I began to understand that these culture-bound syndromes were often unique to political asylum seekers who were influenced by political and judicial systems, social services, and rites of passage that applied to their specific legal status. There was also a performative dimension to their conflicts in reference to Victor Turner's anthropology of performance (Turner, 1966). The political asylum seeker's representations, communicated during consultations, can be understood as idioms of distress shaped by cultural concepts of distress that influence help-seeking behaviors (Ventriglio, Ayonrinde, and Bhugra, 2016). By investigating their idioms of distress, a better understanding came forth that contributed to providing more relevant care from professionals in the network. This required new forms of collaboration and coordination within the social and healthcare networks. Narrative therapy offered a therapeutic approach that valued political asylum seeker's networks of meaning, using an interpretive paradigm developed through interdisciplinary research in medical anthropology and psychiatry (Good, 1994). Narrative therapy and narrative mediation dovetailed, offering an integral approach to political asylum seeker's narratives of distress.

When the social services no longer offered mediation services, another dialogical space opened through narrative inquiry, integrating the political asylum seeker's case studies into evolving theories in narrative mediation, medical anthropology, and social psychology. These case studies and professional experiences and their subsequent theoretical analysis, increased reflexivity through academic publications, conferences, and higher education. A methodological mandala arose from the reflexivity gained through analyzing the different case studies. An interdisciplinary mandala of narrative practices came together in an integrated representation informed by the social sciences. This mandala of methods was interwoven with insights gained from the different phases of my training, studies, and practice. Lifelong learning or journeymanship supported my re-searching process, as I sought to find effective practices that increased my response-ability, in turn adding to my knowledgeability.

The Senior Living Lab offered yet another opportunity to develop narrative methods in the context of an interdisciplinary research project on aging. Women at the age of retirement participated as in-tandem research partners in the field. While working together, stories of resilience were shared in conversations. Each life history gave voice to a unique aspect of aging. To give value to these stories of resilience, a film project took form, allowing each participant's life experience to be shared in a documentary film on hopeful, healthy aging. "Older adults connected through embodied narratives of resilience, illustrating their know-how while facing the challenges of healthy aging" (Riva & Verloo, 2017, p. 15).

This community-based participatory research gave voice to important themes at the heart of aging. "The themes that emerged from the narrative content enriched the reflexive space by incorporating individual insights and connecting them to emerging patterns that ran throughout the five narratives documented in the film" (Riva & Verloo, 2017, p. 17). The Avant-Première showing brought together citizens from the canton with experts in a round-table discussion that allowed the larger community to reflect on healthy aging, imagining the joint actions necessary to enact a hopeful future. This provided not only a dialogical space, but a reflexive community learning space. The film is also available online and can be used as a teaching tool[3].

This exploratory research on healthy aging inspired a similar community based participatory research project concerning mediation practices in Valais, Switzerland. When the Valais Association for Mediation (AVDM) decided to make a film to celebrate its 10-year anniversary in 2021, it embarked upon a questioning process that brought forth "narrative truths" in relation to mediation practices. The method developed for the Senior Living Lab provided a blueprint for the narrative inquiry process that reinforced partnerships while identifying words used to describe the practices and key themes articulated by the professionals working in the field. The participatory process served to reinforce the practice of mediation within the judicial system as well as the community's shared understanding.

The narrative phases included interviews organized with key stakeholders that collaborate with the association's members. The experts in the field represented family mediation, penal mediation for minors, mediation services for conflicts within business organizations, and a political representative advocating for the inclusion of mediation within the legal framework. Divorce legislation not only configures legal procedures but influences children's psychological and somatic health. This illustrates how illness and conflict narratives are often interwoven and interconnected. An integrated approach acknowledges that family centered divorce procedures are part of a larger systemic response and can be understood as part of an all-inclusive public health prevention program.

The mediation narratives were analyzed to increase reflexivity, reinforcing the meaning-making process by identifying important themes that provide a storyline for resolution processes. The documentary film serves the greater community by opening dialogical and performative space for a social mediation process, advocating for participatory forms of conflict resolution. The relational linkages reinforced partnerships while increasing the narrative coherency of the entire social justice network. This narrative approach was used by civil society to reinforce democracy with citizen-centered practices that can bring forth new policies. By integrating stakeholder's voices in a documentary film, systemic change is fostered through polyphony.

Partnerships are also reinforced when there is a focus on relationships within the network. This example shows how narrative mediation methods and practices can strengthen collaborations between citizens, business organizations, and governmental institutions, serving democracy while advocating for social justice and human rights. This exemplifies how social narratives are co-authored for social change.

This is especially relevant for the development of new collaborative practices that reinforce systemic approaches to divorce and children's rights in divorce proceedings. Engendering communal mindsight allows for increased narrative coherency that reinforces linkages between political policy, practice, and human rights. Citizen-centered governance also necessitates lifelong learning possibilities for professionals and citizens to be able to enter participatory processes with relevant skill sets and knowledgeability. Participatory governance requires the ability to collaborate and incorporate the multiple voices of citizens expressing their varying needs in a form of community polyphony.

Lines of contention have been revealed under the pressures of increased polarization and inequality that the COVID-19 pandemic laid bare, accelerating divisions within society. Narrative repair can help relink fractured communities, transforming *master narratives* with *counterstories* of social justice. Stories are connective. "Stories create meanings through the relationships of their internal elements, but also through their relationships to one another" (Nelson, 741). Illness and conflict narratives dovetailed following the pandemic, illustrating their interrelatedness. COVID-19 triggered social and political acts of violence like the murder of George Floyd, the insurrection on the Capitol, and the war in Ukraine. During this period, engaging in a medical anthropology project provided an autoethnographic space to reflect and find purpose while documenting the pandemic period[4].

Engaging with stories enriched the connectivity between my lifework and my teaching. Developing courses and curriculums that teach narrative mediation and narrative therapy engendered an introspective process that has ultimately led to the conceptualization of transformational pedagogies that are aligned with narrative practices. These insights were first expressed in adult learning conferences and publications[5]. Scaffolding a teaching method that illustrated "linkedness" and using stories to relay important practice insights, led to the creation of experiential learning pedagogies that modeled and integrated transformational processes, using narrative approaches (Riva, 2019).

INTERWEAVING MANDALAS OF WHOLENESS WITH GENERATIVE NARRATIVE THREADS

This phase in my academic lifework has allowed me to develop a cogent theoretical mandala. The narrative threads that have been integrated into my autoethnographic work further developed my conceptual framework. An important theoretical strand has been the development of transformative pedagogies that use a holistic approach. These teaching methods have proven to generate a kind of wholeness and narrative coherency, acting on the individual with the potential of generating social transformation. Kenneth Gergen refers to this as future forming research (Gergen, 2015).

The Gergens developed a social constructionist theoretical framework that illustrates how storying processes are a relational endeavor, a lived narrative. "Not only do we tell our lives as stories, but there is a significant sense that our relationships with each other are lived out in narrative form" (Gergen & Gergen, 1988, p. 18). Mary Gergen analyzed womanstories and manstories. She concluded that womanstories depend heavily on their affiliative relationships with others. "Their stories highlight the interdependent nature of their involvements and the centrality of emotional well-being to all facets of life much more vividly than men's stories do" (Gergen, 2007, p.75). She refers to life stories as pieces of a dream. The Gergens provide a relational approach to narrative practices and narrative therapy.

Thomas Berry advocates for a new story, in "The Dream of the Earth". "It's all a question of story. We are in trouble just now because we do not have a good story. We are in between stories. The old story, the account of how the world came to be and how we fit into it, is no longer effective. Yet we have not learned a new story" (Berry, 2015, p. 123). Berry's teachings engendered the book and film, Journey of the Universe.[6] The Yale Forum of Religion and Ecology[7] is dedicated to sharing a cosmology story that transforms how we understand our origins and envision our future. Their collaborations have grown to include a film series about the noosphere, featuring Brian Swimme[8].

The film series provides a template for understanding the acceleration of planetary consciousness and awareness that is akin to planetary mind. The storying process engenders a form of planetary narrative coherence. The images presented illustrate humanity's evolutionary process and increasing interconnectivity. This accelerating consciousness can hopefully allow global citizens to find new ways of relating to planetary systems that will generate flourishing human-Earth relationships.

As humanity is currently facing a marked increase in global challenges, narrative approaches can help generate increased awareness that can act on the Anthropocene. Narrative coherency can generate effective resolution processes on a planetary scale.

"The Great Acceleration represents a set of interrelated anthropogenic global trends that are profoundly impacting human and living beings as well as the Earth system as a whole. It is therefore crucial for human- kind—simultaneously the collective agent and patient of the Great Acceleration—to have available broadly shared, scientifically compatible, and globally acceptable paradigms in which to understand this period of immense change. Indeed, in the absence of such global paradigms, it is unclear how we can fully recognize the precarities and prospects of our own species in the 21st century" (Shoshitaishvili, 2021).

Higher education contributes to the development of shared and accepted paradigms that are capable of guiding humanity into the future. Integrating these thought-provoking educational materials into coursework allows students to become more aware of the challenges humanity if facing. The noosphere film series takes core concepts from the social sciences and shows how these evolutionary processes are unfolding at an accelerated rate. The series highlights the importance of storytelling as a vehicle for transmitting knowledgeability. Having understood the importance of storying processes, the producers have created short films that convey important scientific insights. They use multimedia to share the Third Story of the Universe and the formation of the Noosphere. "Worldviews participating in the Third Story logic, are just beginning to develop. Our project puts forward the emergence of the Noosphere as a promising and motivating Third Story vision"[9].

By integrating the film series and the article that presents the Anthropocene and Noosphere paradigms in my courses in anthropology, I give value to narrative forms of learning that contribute to humanity's current resolution process. The Noosphere paradigm illustrates the interconnectedness that spans from individual ways of being in the world to planetary systems that are transforming the face of the Earth.

Pierre Teilhard de Chardin's theory of the noosphere provided an explanatory model for my adoption and reunion story. It is also a concept that Dr. Siegel has used to explain interconnectivity. The noosphere film series provides images that enhance our understanding of the current acceleration, engendering a noosphere paradigm that reinforces our narrative coherency on a planetary scale, developing our collective mindsight, and using story as a connective medium.

The effective tools and components that are present in narrative therapy are thus applied on a global scale in the hopes of finding new "lines of flight" or flyways that can provide a promising Third Story Vision. As more women are participating in the storying process, the evolving storyline highlights our interdependent nature and our quest for physical and emotional well-being. The questing process has been further developed by applying the holistic lens of anthropology alongside narrative therapy to engender glovircal landscapes of meaning.

The courses that have been designed at Creighton University develop anthropological subjects including the social and cultural determinants of health, cultural epidemiology, complementary and alternative medicine, and conflict resolution. Integrative medicine is enkindled by mediating biomedical approaches with traditional world medicines. And conflict resolution methods are taught in a way that gives value to discourses and narrative practices (Cobb, Federman & Castel, 2020). The Transformagram Portfolios that replace traditional final papers use an experiential learning template so that students can gain insights into their conflict and illness narratives while mapping the resources that can support their resolution processes (Riva, 2021). This cartography of resources allows them to identify the social and cultural determinants that influence conflicts and illnesses using the holistic and comparative lens of anthropology, while working with duoethnographic partners.

Student's gain insights through auto/duoethnographic processes that allow them to perceive intricate relational patterns that make up the complexity of our interrelatedness. These narrative practices provide experiential learning templates that foster the lived experience of transformation. Students also discover the potential of autoethnography as they are encouraged to use a method that engenders social justice, telling stories that "write to right" injustices. Teachers can "Create work that not only makes the case for cultural change but also embodies the change it calls into being" (Adams, Jones, and Ellis, 2014, p. 114). The holistic and comparative lens used in anthropology, makes linkages between environmental factors, the cultural and social determinants of health, epidemics and pandemics, as well as the societal challenges that arise from inequality.

The theoretical concepts in medical anthropology provide a backdrop for making sense of global challenges, understanding that a more equal society is more conducive to the psychosocial well-being of whole populations. "Now, facing the evidence of global warming and calamitous climate change, the world is in need of a radical alternative, a clear vision of a future society which is not only environmentally sustainable, but in which the real quality of life is better for the vast majority. Only then will people commit to bringing that society into being" (Wilkinson and Pickett, 2018, p.265). Transformational pedagogies can foster the commitment needed to co-construct a better world. Transformagram Portfolios actively involve students in the imaging process that contributes to constructive social change.

Using the lens of the Ignatian Principles that is part of the Magis Core Curriculum at Creighton University,[10] students grow to accept complexity with gratitude as they learn to identify relational linkages, narrative processes and transgenerational pathways seeking "the good life." A coherent narrative continuum emerges from holistic and appreciative ways of questioning. "Narrative inquiry is a relational research methodology and is guided by relational ethics" (Clandinin, 2013, p. 141).

Narrative therapy is an integral part of the naturopathic practitioner training. Narrative therapy offers a therapeutic approach for naturopaths using holistic questionnaires to determine case analysis and management as well as therapeutic strategies (Micozzi, 2015, p. 307). In this context, the Transformagram Portfolio provides a template for exploring conflict and illness narratives in the context of naturopathy. Practitioners learn from an experiential narrative pedagogy that can be transposed and used as a therapeutic tool with patients. Narrative therapy is also used as a mediating practice that provides a foundation for medical pluralism to burgeon. Patient's narratives and care-seeking strategies are woven together in what emerges as a pathway towards integrative medicine. In the context of naturopathy, narrative therapy offers a therapeutic method that can incorporate different healing traditions. Auto/duoethnography cultivates self-knowledge, congruent with the Greek wisdom tradition "Gnothi Seauton," while reinforcing narrative coherency in reflexive relational approaches, preparing future practitioners.

The challenge of re-storying continuously requires the creative act, giving birth and space to the moral imagination. Homing *in* to autoethnographic process has been a form of journeymanship. John Paul Lederarch describes vocation and voice, "When you find your way to that home, there you will find yourself, the unique gift that God has placed on this earth. You will find the place from which your journey begins and to where it returns when the road is confused and hard. This is the deeper sense of vocation" (Lederach, 2005, p. 166). When we find our voice, we find our way. Narrative methods and Transformagram Portfolios provide methods that allow higher education to cultivate a Culture of Care and a Culture of Encounter (Francis 2015) (Francis 2020) using mediatorship to transport humanity towards a hopeful future.

Life-o-grams become transformagrams in a transformational pedagogy that has therapeutic ends. This is significant because as White and Epston point out, we are simultaneously participating in domains of power and knowledge. As we are intertwined in complex relational matrices, we need to explore our personal motives and the relationships that configure our practices, "We would work to identify the context of ideas in which our practices are situated and explore the history of these ideas. This would enable us to identify more readily the effects, dangers, and limitations of these ideas and of our own practices" (White & Epston, 1990, p. 29). Narrative therapy can benefit from reflexive teaching practices that reinforce the understanding of our motives within the matrix of power/knowledge relationships. Narrative therapy and narrative mediation require reflexive practitioners that are consciously aware of their relationships. When education and training identify the multiple levels and continuums that configure stories, the practice and quality of narrative therapy is reinforced.

CONCLUSION

Interweaving narrative methods gives form to a mandala of therapeutic practices. Within an integrated framework, a continuum of narrative practices comes into sight that spans from autoethnography to Transformagram Portfolios used in the context of higher education and lifelong learning. Developing a holistic vision and approach to narrative practices reinforces the linkages between the relevant approaches that correspond to specific contexts. The case studies that were presented illustrate the different phases of practice that unfolded through time in response to human suffering and global challenges (Wilkinson & Kleinman, 2016). Resolution processes incorporated different narrative practices depending on the circumstances. This enhanced response-ability.

Narrative inquiry offers a research method that is aligned with narrative therapy, narrative mediation, and narrative conflict resolution. Resolution processes that include narrative approaches in community-based participatory methods can also be used to reinforce social transformation. Learning to recognize the emerging patterns and forms of interconnectivity with mindsight reinforces narrative coherency on both individual and societal levels, that in turn reinforce the acceleration of the noosphere.

Autoethnography can be used to increase narrative coherency. Writing Homing *In* and creating my website[11] has allowed me to foster encounters with my readership in glovircal[12] lifeworlds. Online learning communities can incorporate transformational pedagogies that allow students to participate in experiential learning processes using narrative practices to explore the social sciences. "We could argue that all research is designed to move thinking and perhaps practice on, but art, I might suggest (encompassing all forms in its widest sense), takes us to a different 'place' (Turner, 2018, p. 7). Autoethnographic research and practice can incorporate aesthetic dimensions that encapsule the potential to transport, exploring future-forming methods that uplift, while opening spaces that provide new "lines of flight".

Mediatorship is a vessel and meaning-making container that enkindles connectivity. Words can be used as problem-solving tools to imagine more livable flyways in/on Earthship. Even research can use narrative therapy, showing how migrant youth are learning to be freed[13] through emancipatory processes. By cultivating relational processes in education using narrative methods, educators and researchers can contribute to constructive social change. Narrative practices that incorporate hybridity using multimodal methods offer a Third Space, in reference to Dr. Homi K. Bhabha's Third Space Theory. This Third

Space interweaves discourses with symbolic representations in virtual landscapes of meaning. By opening new spaces of relational engagement, "narrative truth" can be co-constructed with the use of images that elicit the Jungian transcendent function (Jung & Shamdasani, 2009).

An integral vision of narrative methods focuses on generative and performative practices that underscore the importance of relationships, partnerships and co-creation. By identifying the different practices and phases in narrative continuums, a holistic vision emerges. This *appreciative* approach recognizes the linkages that exist within integrated frameworks. Systemic coherency arises from a relational way of imagining narrative therapy and practice.

In a post-truth era, narrative methods can elicit narrative coherency that strengthens mindsight while linking together multiple layers of beingness in a cogent storyline. In the process of connecting these different dimensions of beingness, higher forms of narrative concrescence emerge. By recognizing the importance of narrative coherency that fosters wellbeing in storytellers, narrative methods can orient future forming processes and the edification of "the good life", coordinating complexity with radical presence[14] and in so doing, increasing narrative coherency through storytelling.

Stories and storytellers offer "narrative truth" that informs us about the human condition in a more holistic way. In an era where historical truth is contested, narrative methods can cultivate integrated continuums that provide a holistic approach to "telling the truth" in the space of generative conversations. Subsequently, holistic approaches bear witness to "narrative truths" that can potentially generate increased reflexivity in practitioners. By reinforcing linkages that span narrative continuums, constructive social change processes can positively influence what has been described as the post-truth era. Increased narrative coherency can be achieved by generating response-ability through multiple practices including autoethnography, narrative therapy, narrative conflict resolution, and lifelong learning. In this way narrative therapy is not only a holistic and relational approach to therapy but a questing process.

REFERENCES

Adams, T. E., Jones, S. H., & Ellis, C. (2015). *Autoethnography.* Oxford University Press.

Berry, T. (2015). *The Dream of the Earth.* Counterpoint Berkley.

Berry, T. M. (2000). *The Great Work: Our Way into the Future.* Bell Tower.

Biehl, J. G., & Locke, P. A. (Eds.). (2017). *Unfinished: the anthropology of becoming.* Duke University Press. doi:10.1215/9780822372455

Campbell, J. (1976). *The Masks of God: Creative Mythology.* Penguin Books.

Clandinin, J. D. (2013). *Engaging in Narrative Inquiry. Developing Qualitative Inquiry* (Vol. 9). Left Coast Press, Inc.

Cloke, K. (2017). Thinking Locally, Acting Globally, Mediating beyond borders and integrated global capacity building. In A. Georgakopoulos (Ed.), *The Mediation Handbook, Research, Theory, and Practice* (pp. 293–304). Routledge.

Cobb, S. B. (2013). *Speaking of Violence: The Politics and Poetics of Narrative Dynamics in Conflict Resolution. In Explorations in Narrative Psychology*. Oxford University Press. doi:10.1093/acprof:oso/9780199826209.001.0001

Cobb, S. B., Federman, S., & Castel, A. (Eds.). (2020). *Introduction to conflict resolution: discourses and dynamics*. Rowman & Littlefield International.

Denzin, N. K. (2014). *Interpretive Autoethnography* (2nd ed.). SAGE. doi:10.4135/9781506374697

Francis. Laudato si. (2015). 1st ed.). Our Sunday Visitor Pub.

Gergen, K., & Gergen, M. (1988). Advances in Experimental Social Psychology: Vol. 21. *Narrative And The Self As Relationship*. Academic Press Inc.

Gergen, K. J. (2009). *Relational Being: Beyond Self and Community*. Oxford University Press.

Gergen, K. J. (2015). From Mirroring To World-Making: Research As Future Forming. *Journal For The Theory Of Social Behaviour, 45*(3), 287-310. http://works.swarthmore.edu/fac-psychology/797

Gergen, K. J. (2021). *The Relational Imperative, Resources for a World on Edge*. Taos Institute Publications.

Gergen, M. (2007). Life stories: pieces of a dream. In M. Gergen & K. Gergen (Eds.), *Social Construction, A Reader*. Sage Publications.

Good, B. (1994). Medicine, rationality, and experience: an anthropological perspective. In The Lewis Henry Morgan lectures 1990. Cambridge University Press.

Hansen, T. (2020). Critical Conflict Resolution Theory and Practice. In An Introduction to Conflict Resolution, Discourses and Dynamics (pp. 759-777). Academic Press.

Hinton, D., & Kirmayer, L. J. (2017). The Flexibility Hypothesis of Healing. *Culture, Medicine and Psychiatry, 41*(1), 3–34. doi:10.100711013-016-9493-8 PMID:27142641

Jung, C. G., & Shamdasani, S. (2009). *The Red Book = Liber Novus* (1st ed.). W.W. Norton & Co.

Kandinsky, W. (1977). *Concerning the Spiritual in Art*. Dover Publications.

Kleinman, A. (1989). *The Illness Narratives: Suffering, Healing, and the Human Condition*. Basic Books.

Lederach, J. P. (1999). *The journey toward reconciliation*. Herald Press.

Lederach, J. P. (2010) *The Moral Imagination: The Art and Soul of Building Peace*. Oxford University.

Lederach, J. P. (2020) An Integrated Framework for Peacebuilding. In An Introduction to Conflict Resolution, Discourses and Dynamics (pp. 481-491). Academic Press.

McNamee, S., & Hosking, D. M. (2012). *Research and social change: a relational constructionist approach*. Routledge. doi:10.4324/9780203127537

Micozzi, M. S. (2018). *Fundamentals of complementary, alternative, and integrative medicine* (6th ed.). Elsevier.

Nelson, H. L. (2020) Narrative Repair, Reclaiming Moral Agency. In Introduction to Conflict Resolution, Discourses and Dynamics. (pp. 730-757). Roman & Littlefield.

Nicolaides, A., Eschenbacher, S., Buergelt, P. T., Gilpin-Jackson, Y., Welch, M., & Misawa, M. (2022). *The Palgrave Handbook of Learning for Transformation*. doi:10.1007/978-3-030-84694-7

Randall, W. L., & McKim, A. E. (2008). *Reading Our Lives: The Poetics of Growing Old*. Oxford Univ. Press. doi:10.1093/acprof:oso/9780195306873.001.0001

Rankin, J. (2002). What is Narrative? Ricoeur, Bakhtin, and Process Approaches. Concrescence. *The Australasian Journal of Process Thought*, *3*, 1–12. Retrieved June 20, 2020, from http://citeseerx.ist.psu.edu/viewdoc/download;jsessionid=D1CCBE62D6C8DC41942C868A2FA1D76E?doi=10.1.1.452.6099&rep=rep1&type=pdf

Riva, S. (2019). Linkedness: Relational transformation and narrative conflict resolution. In Togetherness and Its Discontents (pp. 497-513). Pensa MultiMedia Editore s.r.l.

Riva, S. K. M. (2015). Creating Dialogical Space In Generative Research Using Professional's Narratives. Nova Perspectiva Sistémica, 33-51.

Riva, S. K. M. (2019). Writing to Transform Relations. In E. Alegre-Agis & S. Fernandez-Garrido (Eds.), *Autoetnografias, Cuerpos Y Emociones (1) Perspectivas metodologicas en la investigacion en salud* (pp. 47–70). Publications URV.

Riva, S. M. (2020). Homing in: An Adopted Child's Story Mandala of Connecting, Reunion, and Belonging. WriteLife Publishing.

Riva, S. M. (2021) From Life-o-grams to Transformagrams: Storying Transformational Processes and Pedagogies. *Interdisciplinary Studies in Education & Society, 23*(89).

Riva-Mossman, S., & Verloo, H. (2017). Explorative healthy aging processes fostering social innovation: Thematizing life course narratives for older adult women participating in a documentary film. *Qualitative Research in Medicine & Healthcare, 1*(1), 14–22. doi:10.4081/qrmh.2017.6199

Riva-Mossman, S. K. (2009). *Conflict Narratives: Mediation Case Studies in an Intercultural Context*. Tilburg University. https://www.taosinstitute.net/Websites/taos/files/Content/5693761/Susi_Riva_-_Conflict_Narratives.pdf

Sawyer, R. D., & Norris, J. (2013). *Duoethnography. Understanding qualitative research*. Oxford University Press.

Shoshitaishvili, B. (2021). From Anthropocene to Noosphere: The Great Acceleration. *Earth's Future, 9*. doi:10.1029/2020EF001917

Siegel, D. J. (2020). *The developing mind: How relationships and the brain interact to shape who we are* (3rd ed.). Guilford Press.

Turner, L. (Ed.). (2018). *International Perspectives on Autoethnographic Research and Practice*. Routledge. doi:10.4324/9781315394787

Turner, V. W. (1995). The ritual process: structure and anti-structure. In The Lewis Henry Morgan lectures 1966. Aldine de Gruyter.

Ventriglio, A., Ayonrinde, O., & Bhugra, D. (2016). Culture-bound syndromes in 21st century. *Psychiatry and Clinical Neurosciences*, *70*(1), 3–6. doi:10.1111/pcn.12359 PMID:26332813

Vygotskij, L. S. (1981). *Mind in Society: The Development of Higher Psychological Processes.* Harvard Univ. Press.

Wenger, E., McDermott, R. A., & Snyder, W. (2002). *Cultivating communities of practice: a guide to managing knowledge.* Harvard Business School Press.

White, M. (2007). *Maps of narrative practice* (1st ed.). W.W. Norton & Co.

White, M., & Epston, D. (1990). *Narrative means to therapeutic ends* (1st ed.). Norton.

Wilkinson, R. G., & Pickett, K. (2018). *The inner level: how more equal societies reduce stress, restore sanity and improve everyone's well-being.* Allen Lane.

Winslade, J. (2017). Narrative Mediation of Family Conflict. In A. Georgakopoulos (Ed.), *The Mediation Handbook, Research, Theory, and Practice* (pp. 87–96). Routledge. doi:10.4324/9781315648330-10

Winslade, J., & Monk, G. (2008). *Practicing narrative mediation: loosening the grip of conflict* (1st ed.). Jossey-Bass.

ADDITIONAL READING

Georgakopoulos, A. (Ed.). (2017). *The mediation handbook: research, theory, and practice.* Routledge, Taylor & Francis Group. doi:10.4324/9781315648330

Holstein, J. A., & Gubrium, J. F. (Eds.). (2008). *Handbook of constructionist research.* Guilford Press.

McNamee, S., & Gergen, K. J. (Eds.). (1992). *Therapy as social construction. Inquiries in social construction.* Sage Publications.

McNamee, S., & Gergen, K. J. (1999). *Relational responsibility: resources for sustainable dialogue.* Sage. doi:10.4135/9781452243733

Miller, L. (2015). *The Spiritual Child: The New Science on Parenting for Health and Lifelong Thriving.* St. Martin's Press.

Miller, L. (2021). *The awakened brain: the new science of spirituality and our quest for an inspired life.* Random House.

Smith, E. E. (2017). *The power of meaning: crafting a life that matters* (1st ed.). Crown.

KEY TERMS AND DEFINITIONS

Autoethnography: An ethnographic method where the author uses a biographical approach.

Community-Based Participatory Research: A form of participatory research that integrates community members in a participatory research process.

Duoethnography: An ethnographic method where authors incorporate their reflexive writing process in a shared text.

Earthship: Living in a conscious relationship with Earth.

Glocal: A global and local approach that takes into account global issues in local contexts.

Glovircal: The global and local linked through virtual landscapes.

Gnothi Seuton: Concept from the Greek Wisdom Tradition, "know thyself."

Holy Grail Way: Is a legend and metaphor referring to the questing process.

Homing In: Refers to the ability to find one's way by activating an inner compass.

Life-o-Grams: Holographic representations of life history.

Mediatorship: The function or position of a mediator, and a vessel of connectivity that contains an integrated framework of mediation practices.

Narrative Concrescence: A process that moves from coherency, to congruency, to concrescence or an intricate coming together of narrative strands in a form of increasing wholeness.

Noosphere: Planetary mind.

Transformagrams: Transformational processes.

Viriditas: The greening, generative power in nature.

ENDNOTES

1. https://avdm.ch Accessed February 28, 2022
2. https://www.sagw.ch/fileadmin/redaktion_seg-sse/Jahrestagungen/2021/SSEMeeting2021_full-program.pdf Accessed March 5, 2022. "Glovircal" is a term that was coined to illustrate how the global and local are connected through virtual landscapes, offering new forms of relating and connectivity.
3. https://susieriva.wixsite.com/mypage Senior Living Lab film Accessed March 8, 2022.
4. https://boasblogs.org/autor/susan-mossman-riva/?blog=curarecoronadiaries Curare Corona Diaries Project Accessed March 8, 2022.
5. http://www.uep.corep.it/esrea2018/papers/Riva.pdf Accessed October 29, 2021.
6. https://www.journeyoftheuniverse.org/film?gclid=Cj0KCQjwt-6LBhDlARIsAIPRQcIiQ2A-KUOvmRbbZn5aa5WeNipkkAA5CKlvnFALJ4biUabKrWixqdFwaAm6aEALw_wcB Accessed October 29, 2021.
7. https://fore.yale.edu Accessed October 29, 2021.
8. https://humanenergy.io/projects/noosphere-film-series/ Accessed October 29, 2021.
9. https://humanenergy.io/the-three-stories-of-the-universe/ Accessed October 29, 2021.
10. https://www.creighton.edu/about/what-jesuit-education Accessed November 3, 2021.
11. http://www.susanmossmanrivawrites.com Accessed November 12, 2021.
12. https://www.sagw.ch/fileadmin/redaktion_seg-sse/Jahrestagungen/2021/SSEMeeting2021_full-program.pdf Accessed February 28, 2022.

13 https://boris.unibe.ch/126517/2/elif_tibet_learning_to_be_freed.pdf Accessed November 11, 2021.

14 https://www.youtube.com/watch?v=n04Vbhg7PJY Abup talks, Sheila McNamee and « radical presence » Accessed March 8, 2022.

Chapter 17
Abr+a:
The Arts of Making Sense - The Discourse of Dragons

Deborah Green
Whitecliffe, New Zealand

ABSTRACT

Creative arts therapy, like dragon-riding, is poly-sensory and paradoxical. This variegated practice frequently falls prey to reductive research processes. Yearning for less dissonance between the what and how of research and greater congruence between the skill sets practiced in research and therapy, the author began exploring arts-based research and autoethnography. These methodologies now entangle under the investigational umbrella-term abr+a (arts-based research through autoethnography). In this chapter, the abr+a-dragon's tail is grasped for an escapade that: explores abr+a as performed by several researchers; revisits workshops facilitated at Whitecliffe (Aotearoa, 2017-2021), the BAAT/AATA Conference (London, 2019), and the ANZACATA Symposium (Brisbane, 2019); and theory-builds by tracing presence, poiesis, process, partnerships, pixellation, playfulness and psyche within abr+a. The intention is to express abr+a's emergent poietic-praxis and contribute to international intersectional conversations about creative research practices appropriate to therapy within a post-truth era.

INTRODUCTION AND BACKGROUND: THE RIDE BEGINS

A fellow-researcher and I are attempting to trace words around the numinous, embodied, perilous and poietic practice of abr+a – arts-based research through autoethnography. We're both animated: we peer puzzled into the air above us while clutching with both hands at something...something shaped like a rope, a cord...a tail?!

The metaphor arrives, unfolding leathery wings with a triumphant crack.

DOI: 10.4018/978-1-7998-9251-9.ch017

Practicing abr+a is, for me, like clasping the tail-tip of a winged dragon in flight – its shape-shifting magical body frequently obscured by rushing cloud, the ever-changing ground below flickering in and out of view, our destination largely a mystery.

Figure 1. Deborah Green 2019 "Taking flight". Digital collage.

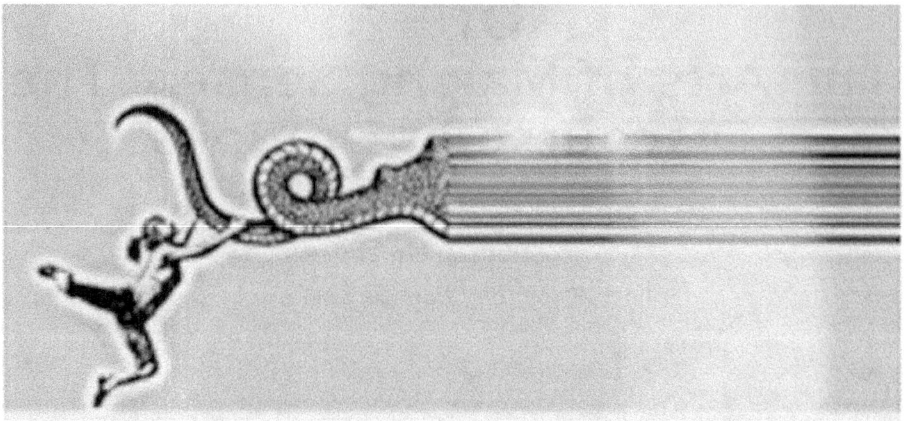

My[1] predominant experience of creative arts therapy (CAT) resembles dragon-riding – prismatic, parabolic, poly-sensory, and paradoxical. This variegated practice can fall prey, however, to rigid and reductive research processes. My yearning for less dissonance between *what* and *how* I was researching plus more congruent reciprocity between the skill-sets I was cultivating via both research and therapy, sent me questing. I stumbled across McNiff's (1998) words: "the process of research should correspond as closely as possible to the experience of therapy" (p.170). Riding the back of this exhortation, I discovered arts-based research (ABR) and autoethnography (Holman Jones, Adams & Ellis, 2016; Leavy, 2018; McNiff, 1998, 2013). Simultaneously a practice, process and product, ABR is an 'aesthetic way of knowing' (Greenwood, 2012): the researcher investigates a research question through artistic creating during data gathering/generation and/or analysis/translation and/or presentation. Autoethnography studies 'the culture of self' (Ricci, 2003), or others through self, encouraging "researchers to start with their own lived experiences as a way of uncovering new ways of knowing and understanding wider cultural beliefs" (Gray, 2011, p.67). The unpredictable adventures that arise when these methodologies are blended and used in conjunction with CAT awakens excited trepidation within me. I wish to infuse some of this frisky frisson into the journey we shall embark upon in this chapter and so I externalise this hope by arts-making in which I juxtapose unexpected media: apple, glitter and plasticine (figure 2).

Figure 2. Deborah Green 2019 "The paradox of a juicy journey..." Sugar paper, plasticine, apple, glitter, thread, digital alterations.

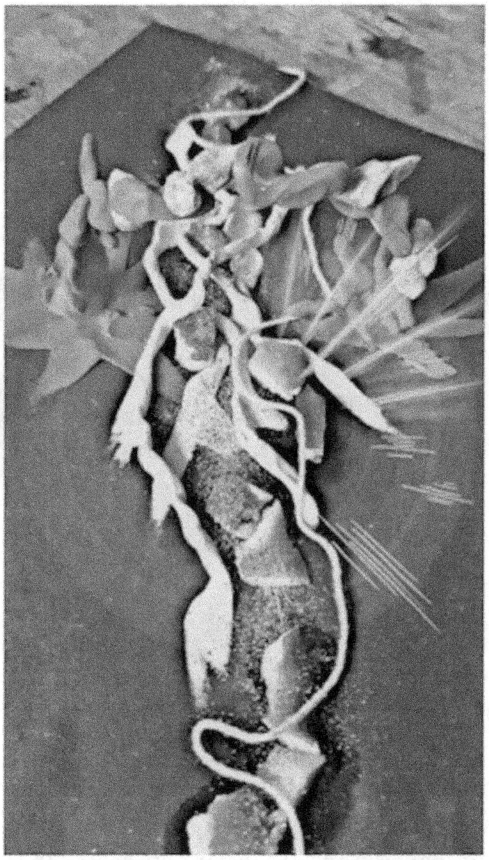

Experimenting with unexpected juxtapositions of ABR and autoethnography – including repurposing an increasing range of CAT processes as research – opens two juicy avenues for curiosity. Firstly, I wonder how we creative arts therapists (CATs) breathe our unique practice of arts-as-therapy into the arts within ABR and our unique knowledge of psychotherapy into the psyche-of-self within autoethnography. And secondly, I wonder how engaging with these research approaches may enhance our clinical practice of CAT. I thus entangle the poietic-praxis (Green, 2018) of these performative methodologies (Haseman, 2006) under the investigational umbrella-term *abr+a* (arts-based research through autoethnography).

Figure 3. Deborah Green 2020 "the essence of abr+a". Digital collage.

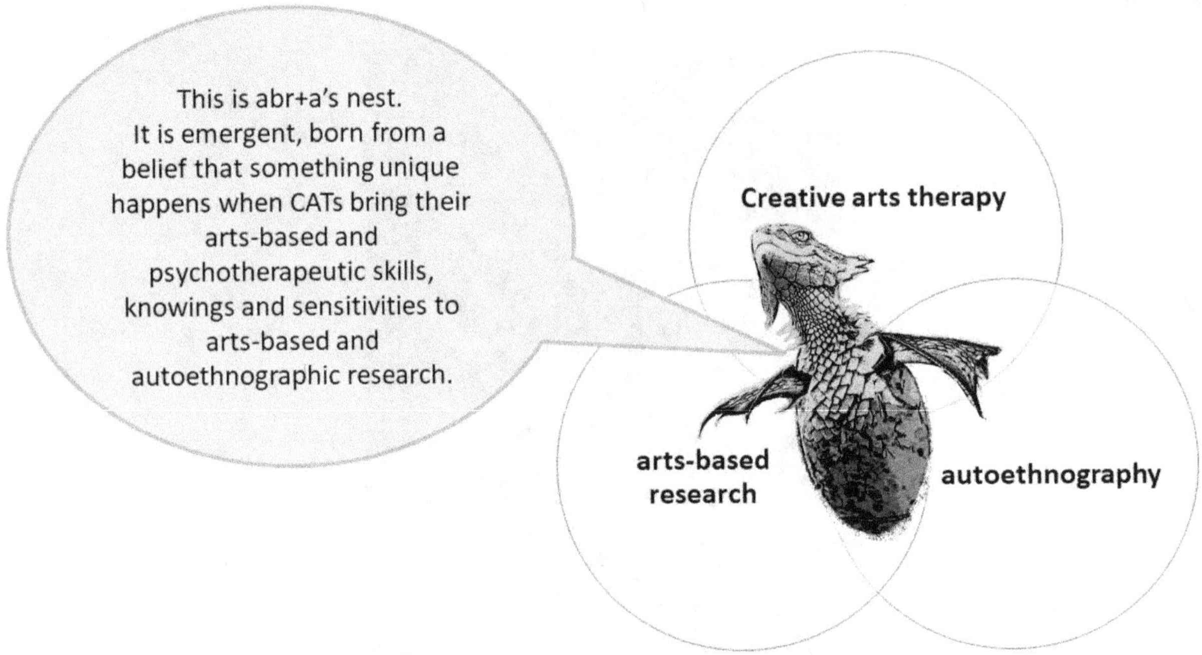

Drafting Our Flight Plan

The abr+a-dragon and I have been on many flights, both before and after it claimed the name abr+a in 2017. These sorties are various and, alongside several research escapades, we've flashed our scales and demonstrated our wingspan to five generations of Master's students[2], the majority of whom have conjured their own abr+a-dragons to complete dissertations. My dragon and I have also incited collaborative magic at the *Inaugural BAAT/AATA Conference* (London, 2019)[3] and the *ANZACATA Symposium* (Brisbane, 2019)[4]. At these events, I facilitated workshops to open transnational conversations regarding how abr+a may contribute to training art/s therapists, the art/s therapy profession[5], and how CAT-as-research may be useful for other disciplines. These various experiences lead me to believe that this abr+a-dragon is a frolicsome but robust creature worthy of sharing. With this chapter, I therefore hope to further these conversations. The arts-based nature of this dragon, however, brawled against chapter-esque ordering. "Boof! It's all there at once!" a student in one abr+a workshop cried in response to my question about what happens to research and therapy when the arts lead. Fashioning any abr+a is bedevilled by too-much-ness. Bullying words/paragraphs/images into coherent sequences feels like combing a dragon's mane while flying through a tornado.

A braying whinny roils back through the mist to where I'm clinging perilously white-knuckled to the fog-slick tail of my current dragon. I seldom get to see the whole beast – it seems to relish its mystery. And my companion critter in crafting this chapter is a particularly frisky and wayward creature. I'm asking it to assist me in making itself and its kin known, to reflect and reflex – but it's finding the notion comic. It's a 'don't fence me in' and 'you can't cage a thing with wings' diffractive kinda dragon. So here am I, holding on for dear life as it loop-the-loops and spiral dives and plunges in parabolas, casting prismatic and rhizomatic rainbows and shadows of confusion and misdirection through the whiteout whistling past.

As I straddle this all-at-once-ness, the tension between two dimensions becomes figural – a paradoxical push-and-pull between creativity's often-chaotic clarion call and the orderliness required to articulate in accessible ways. I yearn to honour, model and enact abr+a within this chapter – and this entails allowing the arts to lead while also wrangling with intelligibility and sequential structuring. Again, I turn to my creative practice for assistance: I free-write without pause for five minutes and then shape this into a mind-map, tracing words around the many tangled abr+a-esque elements and practices infusing this writing (figure 4).

Figure 4. Deborah Green 2021 "Elements of abr+a infusing this writing". Digital collage.

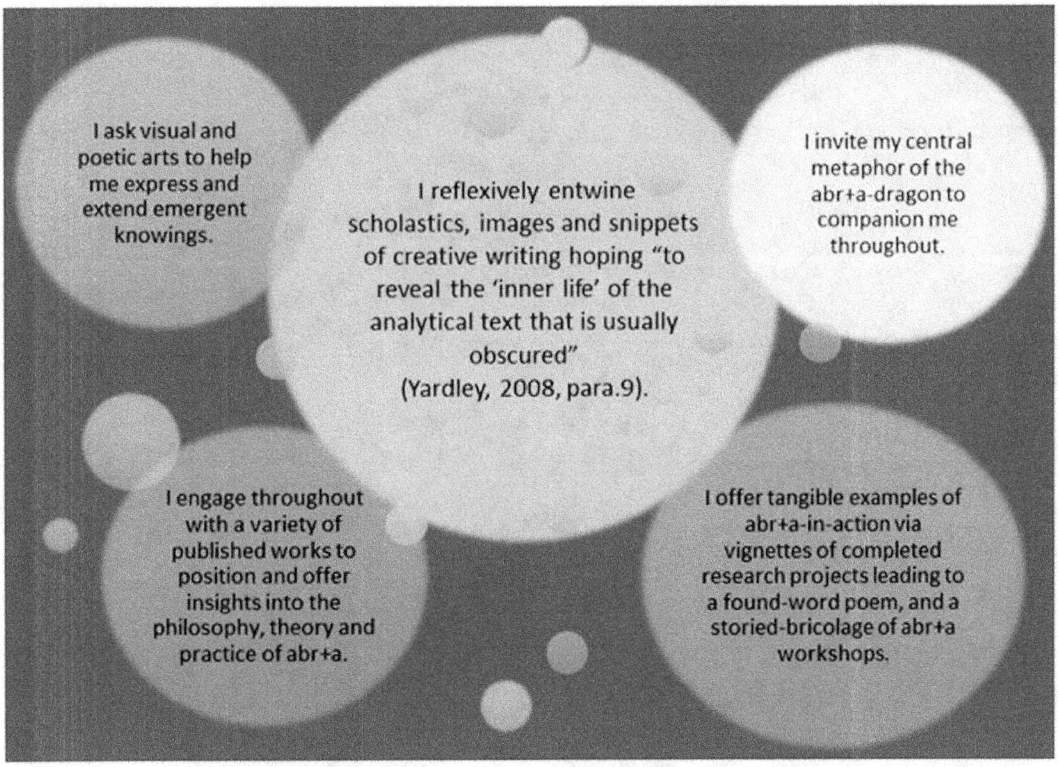

MAIN FOCUS OF THE CHAPTER

I then turn to digital collage endeavouring to visually express the sequential structuring of this work (figure 5). From these two creative capers, I deduce that the main focus of this chapter has conceded to take the following form:

- Firstly, in a section entitled **The Etiology of Dragon**, I outline abr+a's contextual, paradigmatic, and onto-epistemological foundations.

- In **Dragon's Gold**, I take a more applied turn and provide a dragon's-eye view of projects undertaken by my students and me before reflexively compiling a combined narration of the aforementioned workshops' interactive components.
- In **The Anatomy of Dragon**, I attempt to interweave theory and practice in emergent exploratory theory-building to begin making cognitive+affective+embodied+soulful+contextual-sense of abr+a.

I finally conclude by attempting a summary of salient arrivals and offer encouragement to "**Ride Your Own Dragon**."

Figure 5. Deborah Green 2019 "Rebellious contents." Digital collage.

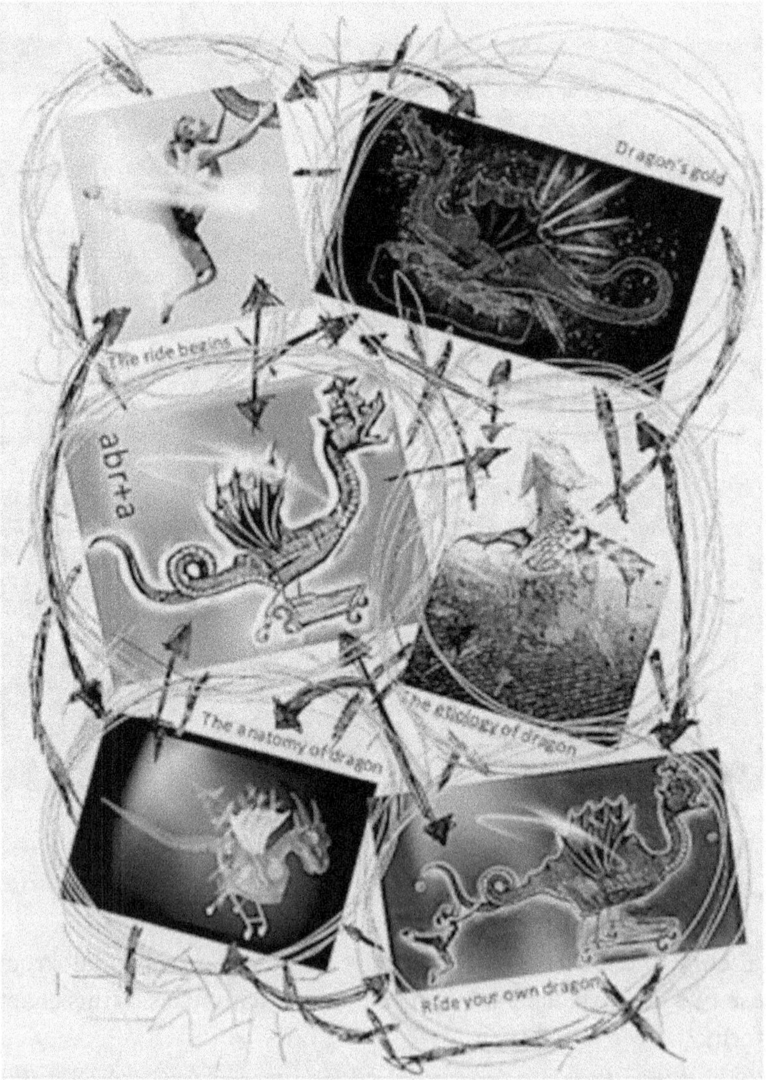

THE ETIOLOGY OF DRAGON

Grasping the lively-tail of abr+a requires orientating to our dragon's contextual, paradigmatic and onto-epistemological turns (Barad, 2007; Gerber, Biffi, Biondo, Gemignani, Hannes & Siegesmund, 2020).

Contextual Considerations

Before we locate abr+a in relation to established research practices, let's pan back a little to consider our dragon's positioning within the international arts therapy landscape. Our abr+a-dragon is infused with our particular practice of CAT, which occupies a complexified space. CAT's growth is ever-evolving within Aotearoa where Whitecliffe faculty and students, along with professional practitioners, are all actively engaging in pioneering work to develop a plethora of bespoke approaches suited to our local demographics. This postmodern/metamodern emergent eclecticism (Vermeulen & van den Akker, 2010) is mirrored throughout this chapter where I reference the works of numerous international arts therapy practitioners and researchers who espouse a variety of approaches. Our approach to CAT is not, however, a free-for-all. I tentatively name a few seminal psychotherapeutic antecedents as Jung's symbolism, Hillman's archetypal psychology, and Gendlin's philosophy of the implicit. Moving into the realm of arts therapy, our nascent approaches are influenced by the phenomenological leanings of Expressive Arts Therapists such as Knill, S. and E. Levine, McNiff and Rogers. Beyond these taproots, we are mycelial and will draw upon many sources, and thus, often featured are: Rappaport's approach to focusing; Kapitan's inter-cultural ecotonal explorations; Halprin's life/art processes; Fish's response art; Hinz's expressive therapies continuum; Whitehouse's authentic movement; Moon's existential art therapy; Chilton's positive art therapy; and Allen's Open Studio Project – to name but a few. Closer to home, there is a flourishing body of scholarship emerging from and informing our programmes that is exploring fruitful interactions between indigenous Māori health models and CAT – see for example O'Connor and Vlasić Manaia. We also draw inspiration from outside arts therapy literature and currently feminist-anthropologist-philosopher Haraway's thinking is informing CAT-reconfigurations. This is evident in rhizomatic explorations of how reflexivity *and* diffraction[6] may be entangled within our therapeutic and research processes. An expanded sense of this and the core elements of our CAT approach are mapped in our Emergent CAT Net (figure 14) and in **The Anatomy of Dragon** in which I use these features to begin abr+a theory-construction while also offering further insight to our positioning relative to international trends within arts therapy.

Now we drop-in to considerations of abr+a in context. Akin to many international arts therapy training institutions, Whitecliffe (Aotearoa New Zealand) is simultaneously tasked with producing well-equipped clinicians while providing evidence of the efficacy of our emergent profession. This suggests two competing research obligations. The first, 'deep journeying' research, appears to meet our obligation to train clinicians. The second, 'outcome/efficacy/evidence-based' research, aims to professionalise the field of CAT by providing legitimising evidence for CAT's disciplinary and applied status (personal communication, D. Fleming, 2019).

Swooping close-in to the deep journey, I spy support for abr+a. I've mentioned the desire for research that "correspond[s]…to the experience of therapy" (McNiff, 1998, p.170) to elicit less dissonance and breed more reciprocity between skill-sets cultivated through research and therapy. Our students state, by engaging with a plethora of CAT-informed/congruent research approaches, they simultaneously gain new content knowledge while developing aptitudes that markedly enhance their clinical practice. Both abr+a and CAT draw upon poietic creativity. Both involve the considered use of visual, performing and/or literary artistic practices to generate, analyse and communicate knowledge (Manders & Chilton, 2013; McNiff, 1998, 2013). Both stimulate 'flow state'[7] (Csikszentmihalyi, 1990), an optimal engagement that activates explicit and implicit/tacit information systems to process and integrate stimuli. Both CAT and autoethnography invite intimate self-examination allowing clients and clinicians to know themselves in more meaningful ways (Gray, 2011). Engaging abr+a thus forms part of the practitioner's learning triangle, combining personal experience and academic research to inform future practice and enhance the development of therapist identity (Skovholt, 2012). In addition, abr+a encourages the repurposing of CAT processes into research methods (McNiff, 2013) potentially gifting new creative research approaches to the broader research world. Plus, to "overlook the beauty of the soul's speech by turning exclusively to empirical analysis…is to expel the soul from art therapy" (McConeghey, 2017, p.19).

The second legitimising responsibility of our research requires that abr+a researchers ascend from the purely personal and harvest insights useful to our profession. While these forms of research still jostle for appreciation, there is growing support championing "the idea that knowledge of the world cannot and should not be reduced to words and numbers alone" (O'Connor & Anderson, 2015, p.23). Recognition is mounting for research that works from insider knowledge while disrupting and making taken-for-granted constructs visible. Such research forms are being increasingly valued as they foster engagement and create intersubjective response, offer expression to silenced voices and topics, and render academic knowledge more accessible to non-academics by turning social science inquiry into a non-alienating practice (Bochner, 2015; Gerber, Biffi, Biondo, Gemignani, Hannes & Siegesmund, 2020; Holman Jones, Adams & Ellis, 2016; Kara & Khoo, 2022).

Paradigmatic Performativity

Abr+a hatches from what Haseman (2006) calls the 'third methodological distinction', Lincoln and Denzin (2003) name the 'performative turn' and Adams St. Pierre (2014) refers to as the 'ontological turn' within research. Haseman (2006) believes the binary of the 'approved' quantitative and qualitative paradigms fails "to meet the needs of an increasing number of practice-led researchers, especially in the arts" (p.1). Challenging what has "become monolithic and stifling" (Adams St. Pierre, 2014, p.3) within these accepted approaches, abr+a uses creative means to reflexively and diffractively explore self/other/world through postmodern/metamodern lenses (Vermeulen & van den Akker, 2010) that view truth and reality as local, shifting/oscillating and co-constructed.

Figure 6. Deborah Green 2019 "Origins." Natural materials, paper, wire, string, digital collage.

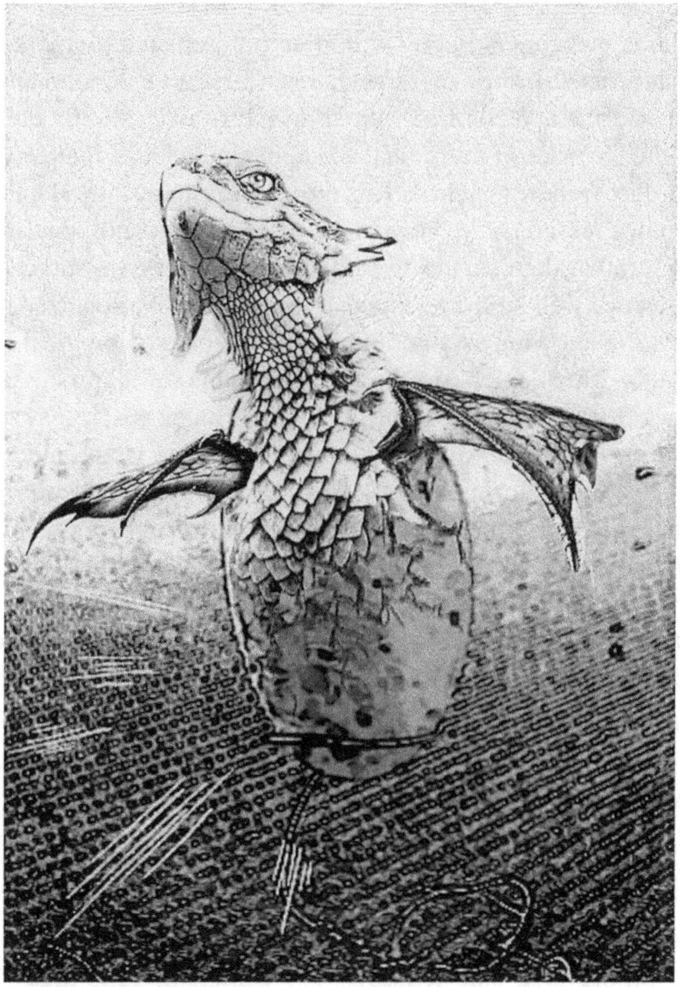

Abr+a thus alights within the 'performative paradigm' (Haseman, 2006). Performative researchers create new artistic forms to carry out intrinsically experiential practice-led research, ultimately understood "in terms of the performative force of art, that is, its capacity to effect 'movement' in thought, word and deed in the individual and social sensorium" (Bolt, 2016, p.130). Performative research recognises research acts are generative – they don't simply dis/un/cover what is already there, they create and/or transform both the researcher and researched (Adams St. Pierre, 2014; Green, 2018; Haseman, 2006). This aspect is alive as I create this inquiry into abr+a. What began as a playful digital collage escapade into dragon-creation becomes almost obsessive – a proliferative deep diving wrangle with multiple collaging apps, digital filters, Creative Commons dragon images combined with my own artworks, rich communing with the wisdoms both inherent in and evoked by the magical possibilities of my dragon metaphor. In this process, the dragon and I map new realities and l/edges of knowing (for examples see figures 1, 6, 15, 16 &17).

Onto-Epistemological Enactment

As this paradigm positions our abr+a-dragon within an onto-epistemology[8] somewhat foreign to the first and second research turns, therapist-researchers must first grapple with and expand how *knowing* may be construed and performed. When I permitted myself to live into my creative knowing, I began shedding what felt like the shackles of traditional academic knowledge that privileges positivist cognition and separates researcher from researched. This creative epistemological turn opened new ontological vistas for what becomes researchable, how I may research this and what intentions and outcomes I evoke. Placing *knowing* rather than *knowledge* at the heart of abr+a embraces knowing as an active, dynamic and ongoing practice well-suited to encounters with the 'ever-open edge' of the human psyche (Gendlin, 1997). Construing knowing as a gerund borrows from sociological imagination (Hegeman, 2015) and grounded theory which emphasise how verbal nouns reveal processes that otherwise might remain invisible (Charmaz, 2012). Focus on knowing disrupts modernist research epistemologies hinged upon the notion that *truth* is out there to be found and knowledge is an outcome, a commodity to be mastered. While knowledge in this form plays a role, CAT in practice calls for being hospitable to not-knowing rather than imposing facts upon clients. Knowing within abr+a thus privileges ambiguity and multiplicity, challenging conceptions that humans contain a single self by inviting communion with a chorus of selves (Levine, 2009). This isn't however a simple rejection of knowledge. Abr+a holds an open constructivist gaze while also being curious about truths that seem absolute and essential. Attentive to uniquely individualised knowing as well as normative knowledge, it oscillates between obscurity/messiness/entanglement and clarity/crispness/certainty. While "embodying pluralistic ontologies and eclectic epistemologies", by drawing on its ABR roots, abr+a "simultaneously resists rigid classifications and methodologies" (Gerber, Biffi, Biondo, Gemignani, Hannes & Siegesmund, 2020, para.13). Each researcher is thus encouraged to purposefully dialogue with their own ever-emergent epistemology again and again as they plan/propose, implement/enact and distil/interpret/curate their research projects.

The air is thin up here. My abr+a-dragon is riding cirrus cloud uplift and the earth's gritty tangible textures and tantalising multilayered experiences lurk indistinct and generalised far, far, far below...It's tempting to stay here, where crispness and clarity feel possible...but I'm becoming dizzy. I feel my hold slacken as, in my ears, my blood pounds and I hear my own voice intoning to students and workshop participants: 'Don't let theorising carry you away from your own unique body/heart/soul/story, stay close-in, experience-near, in the arts...too much heady abstraction can make us lose our vital grip on the magic of making...' My dragon takes pity and, with a whump! of its leathery wings, we begin our descent. Down, down, down towards the seafoam, the glittering windows of buildings, the swirl of cream on a good coffee, grass blades, the sob of a heart broken, salt of tears, smudge of paint, squish of clay, the dancer's achingly sweet gesture, that line of poetry that does and undoes in a few words, this riff that quickens the soul... and so we hover and come to rest in some lived examples.

DRAGON'S GOLD

Abr+a is practice-led, and so we are lured from the heady realms of paradigmatic-onto-epistemological loop-the-loops back to earth by some concrete examples. Each abr+a-dragon's practice generates unique bounty, so let's riffle through a treasure-trove as, in this section, I draw upon two sources. We begin with examples of research projects mounted by various student-researchers and then we harvest several workshops I've facilitated with diverse participants.

Alighting in Examples[9]

Quake Destruction / Arts Creation: Arts Therapy and the Canterbury Earthquakes

Deborah Green (2015)

For my PhD, I combine a/r/tography[10], fiction-based research[11], focusing-orientated arts therapy (FOAT)[12], and dialoguing with the images as angels/messengers[13] to investigate my experiences as quake-arts therapist during the Canterbury earthquakes. I use dance/movement, enactment, visual arts, nature-connected work[14] and creative/poetic writing[15] to revisit ways the quakes reopened older family wounds of murder, paralysis, cancer and suicide. I befriend myself as wounded-healer embracing how intimate knowledge of both wounding and healing helps me connect more deeply with wounding and healing in my clients as together we experience the enduing liminality of the quakes – and learn to fly kites from within the rubble.

Figure 7. Deborah Green 2014 "Kite-in-the-rubble." Digital collage, digital drawing, pastel on paper.

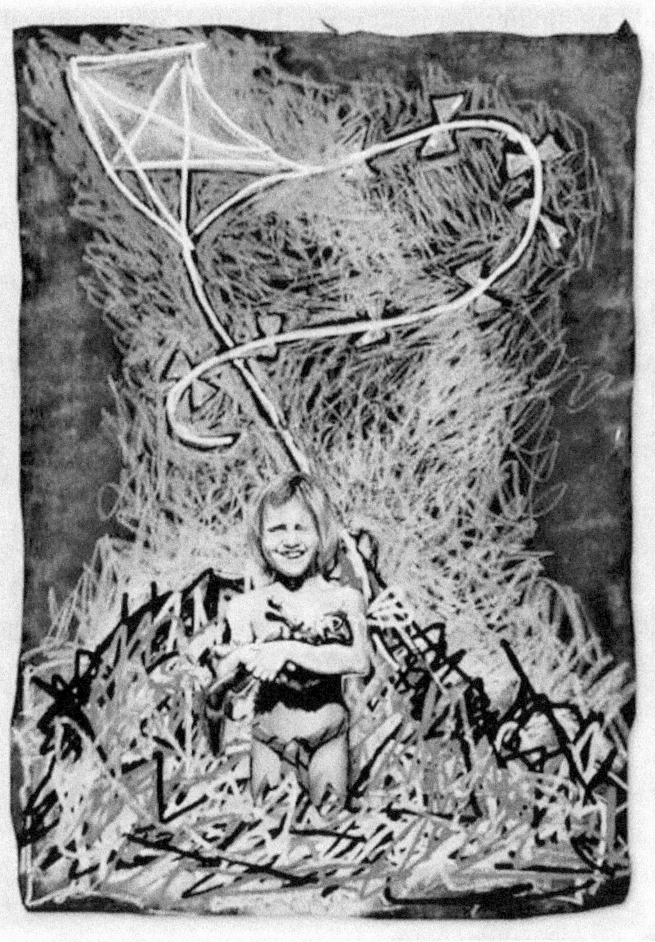

Liminal Space: Reverie and Matter - Using Arts-based Research to Explore the Liminal Spaces Within Arts Therapy

Ingrid (Ying) Wang (2017)

In New Zealand's Westernised culture, Ingrid's Chinese tongue struggles with English and silences her. In her sessions with clients, she lingers in the liminal spaces carved from these silences. Using abr+a, she pays attention to how this feels in her body. Chinese aesthetics, arts-materials, calligraphy, philosophy and spirituality begin arriving in her work – and are welcomed and embraced. Despite initially feeling afraid to immerse in ambiguous moments within arts-based exploration, by knowing and honouring her own thoughts, emotions, sensations and culture, Ingrid learns to appreciate the power of ambivalence. The process helps her reconcile her Chinese-self with her English-self.

Playing 'Hide-and-Seek' With Nana - An Autoethnographic, Arts-based Journeying Through Historical Grief

Kathrin Marks (2017)

Kathrin seeks to (re)establish a (lost) continuing-bonds connection with her deceased Nana. Her abr+a is held by an a/r/tographic framework, employing visual as well as performance art, movement, nature-hiking and creative writing. Crafting a fairytale, Kathrin writes in her final work: "I set out on this re/search to find nana. And I am finding her right where I started: Within myself. Nana is me as much as I am nana. Our souls have been dancing together for all my life. Sometimes, all it takes is opening my eyes to what is already there. To really look. And see. With all my heart and soul. I love you, nana. And I love myself."

Figure 8. Stefan Marks 2017 "Fairy wo/anderings 16: Meeting of souls". Photograph of performance.

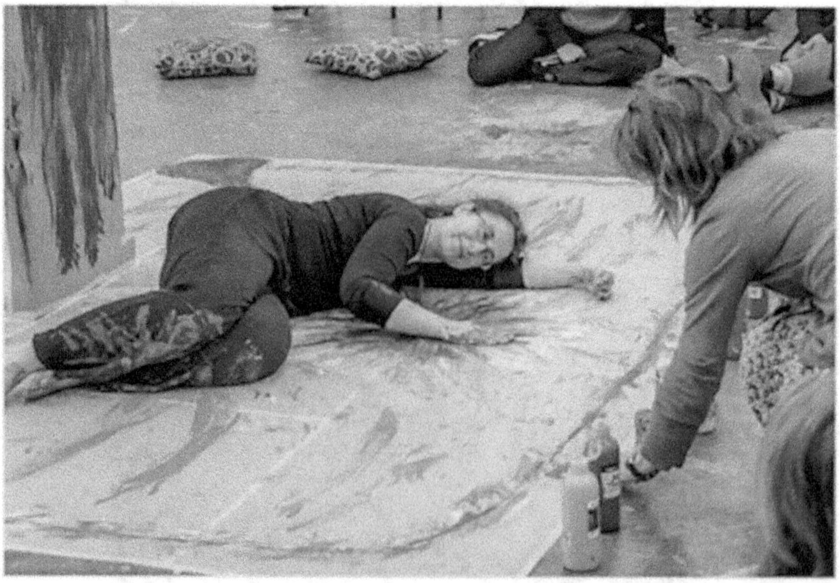

Using Creative Art Responses to Illuminate Intersubjective Processes With Violent Clients

Istvan Csata (2018)

Istvan performs abr+a using dramatic enactment, visual arts, dance/movement and creative fiction-based research. He explores his own counter-transferential responses to the violent outbursts from his clients on the spectrum and with profound multiple learning difficulties. He takes himself and his readers on a detailed and often wrenching journey through his oppressive and brutal Hungarian childhood, he stories several agonising encounters with clients, and learns how his body acts as a primary receptor of countertransference. By applying body/mind awareness and artistic creativity, Istvan learns how to transform potentially harmful emotions into creative energy.

Campfire: The Lived Experience of a Transnational Social Action Arts Therapist-in-Training - (*or* the Failings of the Western Hero Archetype)

Carrie Leigh Weston (2018)

Carrie transports her abr+a in a participatory action[16] form to South Africa, her birthplace. Here she revisits a rural village for orphaned and vulnerable children. She makes herself available – paying deep attention and coming creatively present to the felt-needs she encounters. Back in Aotearoa, she crafts an interactive installation sharing her writing, collages, assemblages and conversations. Her dissertation is a collection of interchangeable booklets storying the different selves (artist, therapist-in-training, researcher, expat) she encountered as she experienced and interrogated troubling Western concepts of humanitarian intervention such as arrogance and imposition.

Figure 9. Carrie Leigh Weston 2018 "Carrie in-stallation". Installation.

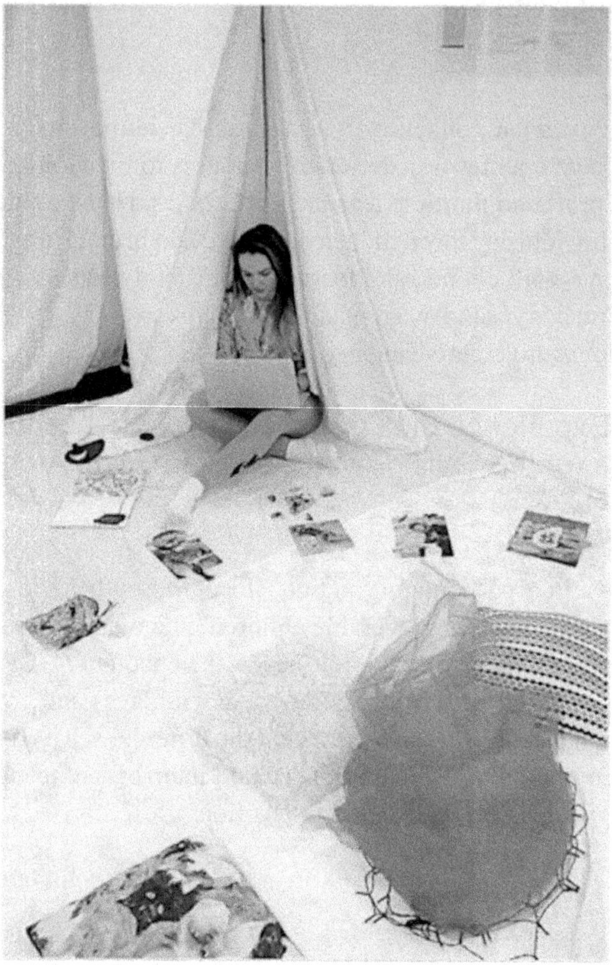

'Borderlines': Transforming Deviance Into Liminal-belonging - A Critical-autoethnographic Exploration of 'Madness' and Mysticism

Mary Teresa Weir (2018)

Mary explores their diagnosis of Borderline Personality Disorder (BPD) and several psychiatric admissions. After years of experimenting with the edges and boundaries of body as a circus performer, Mary now uses abr+a to reclaim back their soul from the weight of diagnostic labels – disentangling socio-cultural narratives of personality disorder from personal experiences of emptiness and spiritual growth through disintegration. Immersing in theologies, mysticism, feminist theory and radical acceptance as well as archetypes that speak in creatively complex and more compassionate ways of what is often labelled 'disorder'; they dance, draw, paint, and craft poetry. Each piece inviting us to shift, from viewing an absence of 'core-self' as scarred emptiness, to a fertile liminal space full of possibilities.

The Art of Curatus

Allie Manners (2018)

Allie uses abr+a to explore her history of self-harm. What she describes as her 'ramshackle' research process embraces resistance and reactance, creative non-fiction and poetic writing, visual arts, assemblage and work in nature. She anxiously circles the experience of her own childhood sexual violation. Finally, the story catches her in a heart-breaking poetic telling, entitled: *An open letter to a crocodile.* Her final dissertation is rich with imagery and takes us on an often-agonising journey through body-loathing into her process of anointing her self-harm scars with 24 carat gold-leaf and then enacting this powerful ritual blessing-of-the-wounds with willing participants in her women's group.

Self-Exposed: An Autoethnographic Exploration of World(s) and the Decentering Process as an Emergent Arts Therapist

Renée Barker (2019)

To twin utility with creativity, Renée decides to explore her sense of self-exposure as a non-native of the digital world working with clients for whom technology is seemingly innate. She struggles to find traction, however, and embraces heuristic research[17] and decentering[18]. This calls her inwards and backwards and she drops-into storytelling, collage, creative collaborations and construction to narrate her descent, several years previously, into soul-deadening depression and suicidal ideation. Themes of exposure, vulnerability and connection are harvested and carried over to the original topic of self-exposure, but the true power of her work emerges in her use and interrogation of decentering as a part of abr+a.

Endo-ME-Trio-Sis: An Arts-based Research, Autoethnographic Cello-portation

Kim Walker (2019)

Many years of undiagnosed agony call Kim to explore endometriosis. Her broken cello, Gertrude, soon begs entry into her research. Together they unexpectedly time-travel into Kim's childhood survival of abuse via artworks that blur boundaries between the endo-induced harm and that inflicted by her abuser. In alchemical hermeneutic spirals[19], Kim and Gertrude listen to cello music while creating poetic writings; collages using old x-rays; installations and sculptures using construction off-casts, hot wax, broken glass and rusted bolts; and huge paintings that arrive when Kim and Gertrude dance with a paintbrush strapped to Gertrude's endpin. Kim feels transformed in herself and her work as therapist as a result of bringing music and light to the dark stories lying in the trenches of her soul.

Figure 10. Kim Walker 2019 "Ritual amalgamation." Mixed media installation.

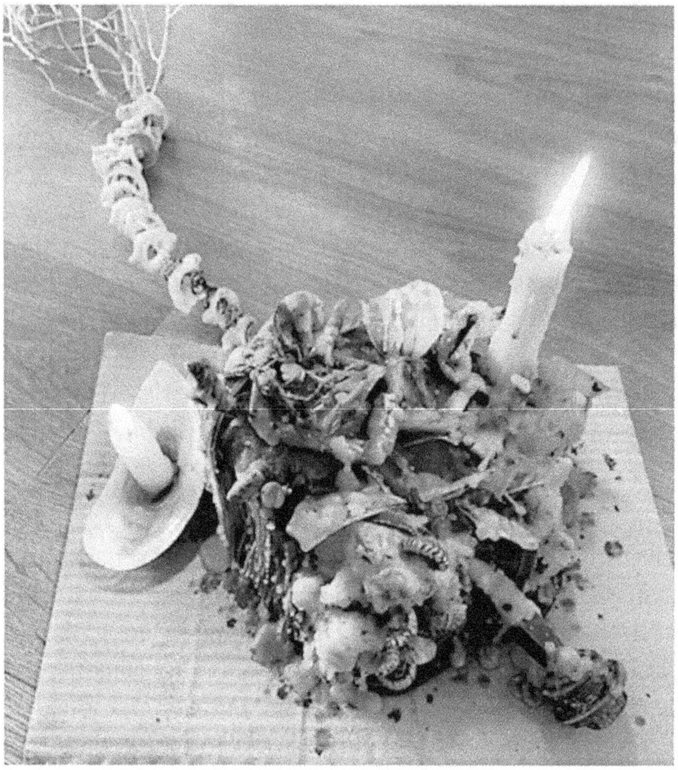

I revisit these vignettes with a gentle dancing gaze, inviting my eyes to alight upon words and phrases imbued with the felt-sense[20] of each piece. I highlight and extract and then arrange and rearrange these, reading and singing them aloud until I can hear the quiet but luscious tinkle of gold in their curation. This finally becomes a found-word poem (van Rooyen & d'Abdon, 2020).

Poeming Gold

Deborah Ingrid Kathrin Istvan Carrie Mary Allie Kim Renée
cartwheel through abr+a in
alchemical hermeneutic spirals, heuristic hullabaloos and 'ramshackle' research processes
using combinations of a/r/tography, fiction-based research, participatory action research, poetic inquiry
performed through FOAT, dialoguing with images as angels, decentering, dance/movement, enactment, visual arts and collage, nature-connected work, creative writing, interactive installations, assemblages and constructions, storytelling, performance art, and creative collaborations and conversations
which draw-upon/use/revisit/welcome/embrace/challenge/disrupt
multiple theologies, transference/countertransference,
Chinese aesthetics, calligraphy, philosophy and spirituality,
mysticism, feminist theory, archetypes and
radical acceptance
to explore

old family wounds,
liminal spaces, silences, and the power of ambivalence,
earthquake-arts therapy and wounded-healing,
grief, loss and broken bonds,
responses to violent outbursts from clients,
a brutal Hungarian childhood,
a South African rural village for orphaned and vulnerable children,
Western arrogance and imposition,
a diagnosis of BPD,
weighty diagnostic labels and psychiatric admissions,
body-loathing, self-harm, resistance and reactance,
childhood sexual violation,
a sense of self-exposure, and
soul-deadening depression and suicidal ideation.
These often-wrenching journeys pry open/explore/generate/interrogate
heart-breaking stories, laden with agonising imagery,
enduring liminality,
fear of immersion in ambiguous moments,
painful encounters of the body as primary receptor,
felt-needs and body boundaries,
emptiness and disintegration,
absence of a core-self,
struggles to find traction, and
blurred boundaries
which transform into the treasure of
intimate knowing and spiritual growth,
kites flying from within the rubble,
a Chinese mother-tongue befriended,
thoughts, emotions, and feelings honoured,
different selves storied,
body and soul reclaimed,
self-harm scars anointed with 24-carat gold,
and stories lying in soul-trenches finding light…
…all sprinkled with a mad-dash of glitter,
time-travel,
circus performance,
and dances with a broken cello named Gertrude.

WORKSHOP WO/ANDERINGS

Now that we've peered at the variegated gold clustered beneath the rumps of several nesting dragons, let's take a step or two back. In this section focussed on the practical implementation of this hybrid methodology, we will tinker with alchemy, exploring ways the raw materials may be gathered/generated, analysed/translated, and distilled/crafted into abr+a-dragon-gold. I demonstrate this by compounding inter-mingled accounts of the *dropping-in-to-knowing* activity I've facilitated in London (2019), Brisbane (2019) and New Zealand (2017-21)[21]. The unfolding process at the heart of these workshops provides a tangible example of abr+a-in-action. This activity emanates from my sense that abr+a is birthed when we commit to making-strange and thereby enliven our construction of *knowing* within research. The workshops engage a process I call *poietic-praxis* – shorthand for how the repeated cycles of Sullivan's (2006) 'create and critique' merge the doing-and-thinking of praxis within the creative aesthetic of Levine's (2009) poiesis[22].

To story these workshops, I employ creative non-fiction and a process of synthesis that mirrors heuristic phenomenology (Coles, 2014) to interlace factual and fictional narration (Leavy, 2013). With this amalgamated factional story, I hope to traverse from personal to communal by rendering visible tacit assumptions and happenings embedded in the lived experience (Denzin, 2013) of these workshops – while simultaneously protecting participants who travelled into unexpected places. I frame this storying in grey boxes to distinguish it from my other creative contemplations.

Each workshop begins with a welcome, an outline of intention/process, information about abr+a, and some research vignettes (see above). Then we get creative, opening our participatory process with a simple ritual to limber-up for entry into liminal creative spaces (Turner, 1969).

We stand in a circle, grounding through slow breaths. I introduce a creative community code to encourage containment. Respect for the land we're on, those who've gone before, our hosts, each other, ourselves and our artworks. Witnessing balanced with Experiencing to allow ourselves and others to titrate direct engagement as required to regulate and open different perspectives. And Risk balanced with Safety to edge-walk the creative playability where known and unknown meet.

Returning to our breath, I guide us inward to visit our current feeling-states. A delightful array of vocalisations and gestures arrive as we embody our here-and-now felt-sense – arms fly out, are hugged to bodies, hands flutter or clap; heads bob, droop or snap to-and-fro; torsos hunch or stretch. We're welcoming our whole selves, ready for creative action.

We then tackle the session's core intent: to explore the slippery concept of knowing that is vital to an a/effective researcher and therapist. Coming-to-know-your-own-knowing/not-knowing blends several CAT-derived approaches with ideas from ABR and autoethnography. To summarise: In *phase one,* we begin by dropping-in and a foundational image is created; this is surrounded/amplified and re/interpreted through various modalities/media in *phase two*, following which the artwork/s are engaged in dialogue and free-writing to capture insights, provocations and further curiosities to begin sense-making/interpretation/analysis; in *phase three,* composite-artworks are curated and shared in a process of sympoietic[23]/ collaborative sense-making, and the session is then creatively closed.

Phase one involves a CAT-informed process I call 'dropping-in-to-find-what-your-soul-is-doing' (Green, 2015a). This process interweaves Rappaport's (2008) FOAT, Hillman's (1983) attention to soul, Jung's (Jung & Chodorow, 1997) amplification using active imagination, McNiff's (2015) dialoguing with images as messengers/angels, and Fish's (2012) response art. Initial present-tense grounding in the physical senses is followed by inward focus to locate where the theme in question – in this case, knowing – is alive within. The felt-sense of this living location within is accepted and befriended with curiosity, invited to unfold and propose how it may be creatively expressed. Once a resonant symbolic representation arrives, this is externalised through arts-making. To deepen the experience while creating, the artist-researcher converses with the messenger-artwork using active imagination-based dialogue.

Participants emerge from the guided dropping-in – some blinking, others stretching and yawning. They cluster around the arts materials as soft music lilts. Some choose paper and pastels, others gather construction materials – wool, pipecleaners, plasticine, feathers. The natural materials I collected this morning prove popular: heady sprigs of lavender and rosemary, twigs, petals and leaves, stones of various shapes and colours. The room settles into the deep flow of creative-intent. After several minutes, I softly remind the artists to drop-in again and track their unfolding sense of knowing: How is it resonating with what's emerging in the artwork? Is anything shifting as the work progresses?

We slip into *Phase two* through ABR-informed iterative cycles of multi-modal creation. Participants are invited to do at least two of the following to further amplify/surround/explore their initial artwork:

- Craft a piece of creative writing;
- Dance/move the artwork;
- Dialogue with their artwork and write its answers using their non-preferred hand;
- Fossick online to find something about knowing;
- Borrow an idea from another participant;
- Notice something random;
- Come up with their own process of creative inquiry…

Using multi-modes/media embraces Sullivan's (2006) idea of "surrounding a problem" (p.19), Manders and Chilton's (2013) emphasis on evoking "multiple, emergent meanings" (p.2), and Springgay, Irwin and Wilson Kind's (2010) endorsement of excess and reverberation. Autoethnographic practices also infuse this process. Richardson's writing for discovery (as cited in Elizabeth, 2008) holds hands with Elizabeth's (2008) shifting of language from simply recording to a method of inquiry. Also present are Deleuze's (1994) rhizomatic thinking, and Davies' (2000) viewing of self from "multiple vantage points" (p.167) to generate what Rambo Ronai (1995) calls 'layered accounts' of self. This process of surrounding welcomes 'strong reflexivity' (Anderson & Glass-Coffin, 2016) and 'vulnerability with purpose' (Holman Jones, Adams & Ellis, 2016).

Movement fills the room as further materials are gathered, or artworks become engaged in dramatic enactment and dance. Some participants write, crafting poems. Some dialogue with their creations. Some wander the room, finding inspiration in the abundant creative-knowing that is manifest. Artworks transform and participant-researchers journey with them. One begins as a meandering trail of stones and string, evoking the transitional-nature of knowing. The artist dances this, discovering her knowing sometimes staggers, intuition's fluidity severed by critical thought. To this trail she adds scissors, some open to reveal sharp edges. Another participant experiences her head-knowing as warring with that in her bones and belly. Wanting to 'get it right', she privileges cognition, denying her being's ancestral wisdom. Her creation goes awry – it resembles a scaffold, so she creates a hanged figure. Weeping, she pens poetry to her Indigenous wisdom sacrificed to Western education. Quietly intent, another therapist-researcher lays a circle of bright rose-petals around her cross-legged form. She sits, feeling into her whole-bodied-knowing. She steps from her circle, fetches water, re-enters and gently places a drop into each petal's velvet-cup, honouring and nourishing intuitive and sensory knowing.

Phase three is a process of 'gatherings' (Gerber, Biffi, Biondo, Gemignani, Hannes & Siegesmund, 2020) and "collective attunement" (Stewart, 2010, p.340). Participants widen attention from their personal process to seek connections by collaboratively entangling and curating their emergent-knowing with that of others. This is led by the artworks letting us know where they need to be placed within a gestalt of knowing (figures 11 and 12).

Participants begin weaving intricately whimsical interconnections. Few words join us, expression and interaction happen through gesture and sound – this spirit of communitas[24]*, sparkling with playfulness, incites disruptions to previously sedimented ways of self-storying. One participant play-bows to her artwork. Another straps her creation to the arm of a willing playmate. Yet another, high on a chair, perches her sculpture aloft on the light-fitting. Drawings, sculptures and assemblages flit about the room, alighting here, taking off to journey further over there, as someone cheekily laces us together with string. Lilting music tinkles to silence. I invite stillness and we again drop-in to commune with our embodied sense of knowing. What's it up to now? Has it shifted and changed? What do we know about our knowing that we didn't when we began?*

Figure 11. Deborah Green 2019 "Workshop shenanigans". Digitally altered photographs.

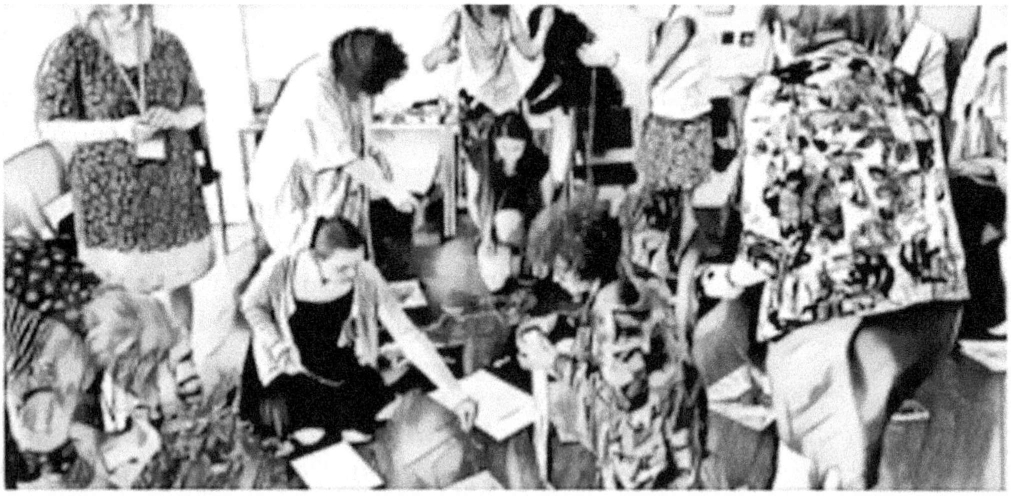

Figure 12. Deborah Green 2019 "Workshop shenanigans". Digitally altered photographs.

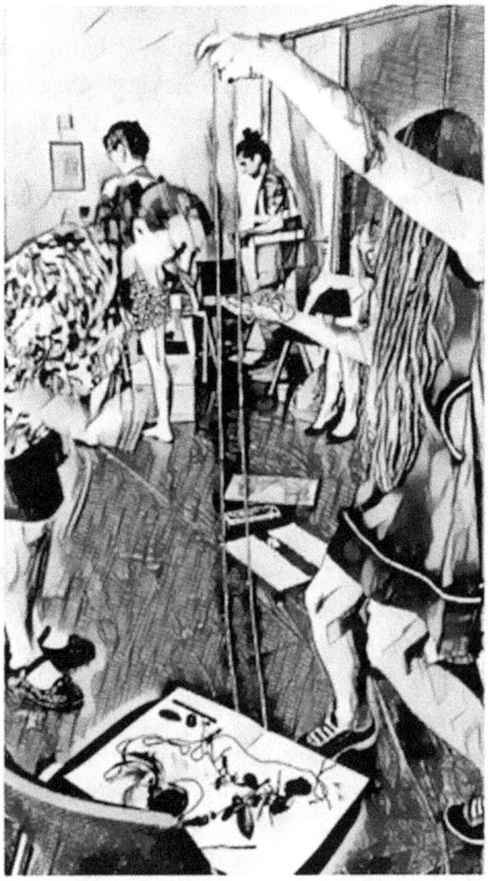

Through curating our creations using this "both show and tell" approach (Vaughan, 2009, p.15), we 'surround' the problem rather than 'solve' it (Sullivan, 2006). Instead of yielding definite single answers, this generates collections of ideas and images that enhance, challenge and diffract each other's meanings (Barad, 2007; Undurraga, 2021; Yardley, 2008) and suggest possibilities for further engagement.

I ask: What has arrived? In longer workshops we reflect deeply, in London and Brisbane[25] *each participant shares a sound, gesture and sentence to express their knowing as it is alive now. The room again fills with innovative noises, movements and words expressing intuition, embodiment, sensation, imagination, multiplicity, the ancestors, the collective soul, truths beyond language, trust and fear, formlessness, chaos, passion, hope, and lightness of touch.*

It seems we share the felt-sense that our explorations sing of "a new paradigm, one which doubles back on its self and wanders in spaces that have not yet been named" (Denzin, 2013, p.354). To close our session, we mirror our opening ritual – acknowledging and exiting the liminal space we entered to research together (Turner, 1969).

THE ANATOMY OF DRAGON

Now that we have some tangible examples under our wings, I shall attempt to bring thinking and doing together in exploratory theory-building and thus begin making sense of *abr+a* in interwoven cognitive +affective+embodied+soulful+contextual ways…

…and immediately my abr+a-dragon, so viscerally present throughout this process thus far, vanishes in a flurry of scales and smoke. Without its companionship, I'm swamped in doubt and too-much-ness. I breathe. I'll trust readers can visit the ever-expanding body of ABR and autoethnographic literature for what is already established, and I'll privilege what may be unique about abr+a, paying specific attention to how abr+a and CAT are mutually enhancing. My collywobbles ebb slightly, but the task still looms capaciously, causing cacophonous clamouring from my mind-monkeys.

You see, the abr+a-dragon shares my imaginal worlding with an ever-expanding array of critters – including a monkey-carousel in my head. When I sleep, the carousel-lights blink out one by one as the carousel slows into darkness and the monkeys pause. They're not sleeping, just waiting…a rolled eyeball glints, warm breath sighs. At around 2am, the calm is sullied as some silly bugger twitches. A snicker shivers through the hoard, a hairy finger creeps towards the light-switch and Pop! a bulb is illuminated. Furry bodies stretch delightedly, more lights pierce the gloom and soon the whole bloody carnivalesque-carousel is ablaze, spinning and wheezing tinny fairground-music as the monkey-mob shrieks and flings pooh...

On one such raucous night, following a day of trying to crowbar cantankerous abr+a-concepts into this bookish container, the monkeys offered help by deluging me with abr+a-describing words beginning with P.

Figure 13. Deborah Green 2019 "A plethora of P-pushing primates." Digital collage.

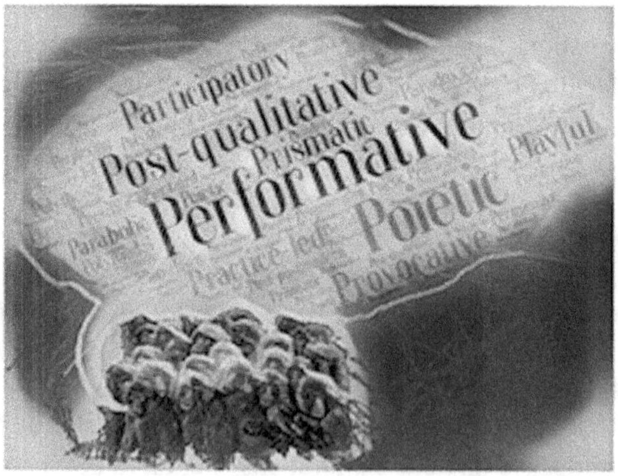

Dawn pinked the sky amidst a proliferation of perspicacious P-words…and (in a pernicious form of prevarication and procrastination or possibly a necessary preparation though peregrinatory decenter-

ing) for several days I trailed a comet-tail of newly arriving words as if a portal had opened into the P-dimension where words beginning with P propagate and promulgate.

Containing the torrent in an artwork (figure 13), I turn to our CAT Net (figure 14) to pare down the P's. This Net articulates the core practices guiding our Master's programme. These are:

- Presence,
- poiesis,
- process,
- partnerships,
- pixellation,
- playfulness
- and, of course, psyche.

Figure 14. Wendy Lawson on behalf of the School of CAT 2019 "Whitecliffe Emergent CAT Net". Digital image.

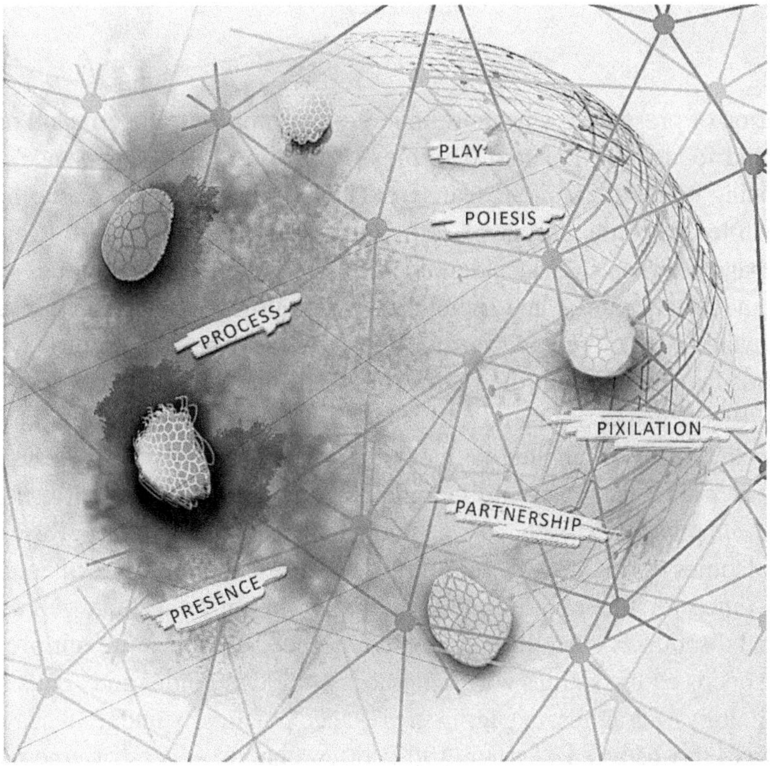

Psyche

Attention to psyche is the chi/qi[26] / mauri[27] enlivening and powering our abr+a-dragon. Psyche began life in Greek mythology, becoming synonymous with *soul* before succumbing to the early positivist leanings of psychology to become *mind*. Within abr+a, she returns to her original form, honouring suggestions that our core purpose as therapists is soul-building (Hillman, 1983; McNiff, 2004; Levine, 2009). Before the term *abr+a* *(CATdabra)* pestered me into adopting it, I called this emergence 'soul-based research' (Green, 2015a). Abr+a embraces the belief that creative expression is how the soul both communicates and heals itself (Jung & Chodorow, 1997) as "within a therapeutic context, artistic creativity can itself be understood as a form of soul-making which aims to restore sense to the world" (Levine, 2009, p.45). This is particularly important for therapists/researchers practicing in inter-cultural environs such as Aotearoa where health services may "lack recognition of taha wairua (the spiritual dimension). In a traditional Māori approach, the inclusion of the wairua [...is] as important as the physical manifestations of illness" (Vlasić Manaia, 2017, p.38). Poietic processes develop soul-language which communicates from different/deeper places than can be reached through cognitive processes alone (Hillman, 1983; Levine, 2009; McNiff, 2004). Care "of the soul is not solving the puzzle of life; quite the opposite, it is an appreciation of the paradoxical mysteries that blend light and darkness into the grandeur of what human life and culture can be" (Moore, 1992, p.xiv). Abr+a doesn't hinge upon a singular reductive definition of soul. Within our programme, training as a creative arts therapist/researcher involves repeatedly coming present to the multiplicit manifestations of one's own soul to cultivate robust intimacy with its unique quirks so one may hold space for clients to do the same.

Presence

Continuous cultivation of presence forms the spine of our approach to therapy and research. Borrowing from mindfulness and focusing-orientated therapies (Rappaport, 2014), presence is holistic and welcomes the whole being of the therapist-researcher. This wholeness is prismatic, holding postmodern and post-postmodern lenses to the gestalt-of-self, welcoming presence with/to/from multiple self/s in multiple roles. Slippage between Cartesian demarcations occurs in research processes: cognition blends with the physical, emotional, soulful, and social thereby heralding recognition of multi-layered 'worlding'[28] (Levine & Levine, 2017). Presence further opens research beyond empirical reasoning by being hospitable to artworks as presences in their own right (Hillman, 1983). Artworks may be engaged in dialogue (McNiff, 2015), further animated and 'surrounded' using other modalities/media (Levine & Levine, 2017; Sullivan, 2006) and invited to interact intersubjectively with their human creator/reader-viewer. Furthermore, 'presence' typed into Google leads to ghosts and hauntings, stirring generative reverie about the unseen presences that hover and haunt in research and therapy. Research engaging with/in liminal spaces welcomes the invisible (intuition/felt-sense and the sentience of nature and place), those not corporally here (ancestors/the deceased/those we carry in our bones), as well as cultural/religious/social-constructs and discourses corralling us (including theories informing our profession).

Abr+a therefore opens conversations with a plethora of hidden guides and goads and, in kinship with the mysterious mythology of dragons, engaging in presence poietically nudges research off well-trodden pathways into betwixt-and-between (Turner, 1969) often chaotic spaces of emergence (Bush, 2018). Abr+a invites communion with what is known and unknown, what is knowable but hidden, and what may remain unknowable. Simultaneously being present and making-strange conjures a state akin to what the expressive arts therapists call 'decentering' – shifting attention away from the immediate problem towards the "surprising-unpredictable-unexpected" worlds of imagination (Knill, 2011, p.55). This therapeutic decentering shares some resonances with research processes of phenomenological epoché/bracketing (Kapitan, 2018) and heuristic incubation (Moustakas, 1990). In abr+a, decentering becomes a parabolic iterative dance between centre and periphery. The therapist-researcher repeatedly retreats from the research question by entertaining the power of imagination, coming present to an alternative/liminal experience of worlding (Levine & Levine, 2017) and, upon return to the research problem, harvests this poietic escapade for innovative knowings.

Poiesis

Poiesis forms our abr+a-dragon's heartbeat, enlivening this decentered process of making-strange-to-rearrange. Within therapy and research, poiesis welcomes uncertainty and formlessness, facilitating coming-into-form of the chaos of meaning (Levine, 2009). Infusing research with poiesis opens transitional spaces (Winnicott, 1977) that inspire meaning-making "in the same way as we engage in creative work: by letting the new form emerge without controlling it" (Levine, 2009, p.139). This mirrors Heidegger's (1935/1975) use of poiesis. Rather than a wilful intellectual act, poiesis invites surrender to a process which requires relinquishing control, a paradoxical will-to-not-will as the therapist-researcher abandons critical intention and becomes receptive. It is an ecstatic threshold-occasion where familiar structures are void and new ones have yet to appear, inciting confusion and powerlessness. As Tapper (2021) describes: "When that unexpected visitor came scratching …, much like an unanticipated experience in art-making, I was called out of my comfort and known structures, into the unknown, and into the possibility of something new" (p.69).

Suddenly my dragon is back and, caught unprepared, I'm flailing! Fearing I'm losing my grip, my fingernails dig into wee notches between scales as the wind howls past, wrenching my hair and clothes. The dragon, feeling the intensity of my grasp and interpreting it rightly as my desire to control the process and outcome of its flight, is speeding up, whipping in twisty spirals, seeking out patches of damp face-scouring fog…

Figure 15. Deborah Green 2019 "Perilous practices." Digital collage.

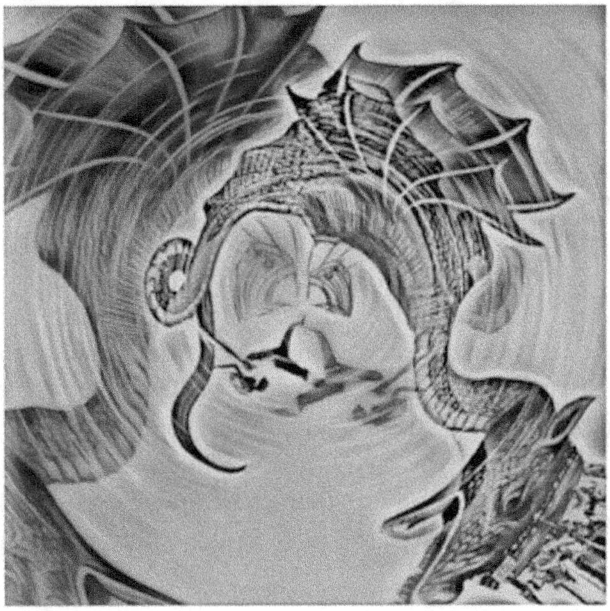

Poietic abr+a can be a perilous practice. It involves 'staying with the trouble' (Haraway, 2016) by clinging onto the dragon's-tail rather than sitting in the saddle with whips to bridle its exploratory yearnings. Viewed through our local indigenous lens, the abr+a-dragon evokes the felt-sense of Māori taniwha, supernatural creatures similar to serpents and dragons in other cultures. Taniwha are sometimes protective and sometimes terrifying manifestations of the mauri/life-force in physical form (Keane, 2007). Greer and Blair (2018) explore the 'discourse of danger' and reveal researchers construe creative research as either heroic pioneering of new territory or incursions into hazardous terrain. Mirroring Romanyshyn (2013) quoting Keats, poiesis invites us to dwell in the place of liminality as a "negative capability" created by a willingness to linger in "uncertainties, mysteries, doubts, without any irritable reaching after fact and reason" (p.77). Abr+a-researchers thus perch precariously between validity and vilification, evoking the previous deep journeying/legitimacy-building discussion.

In yet another incursion from my wayward imaginal worlding, I'm being haunted by shopping trollies. These conjure Pratchett's Reaper Man (1998): Death has abdicated leaving the life-force of dead humans to accumulate. This disruption exposes Ankh-Morpork to invasion by a parasitic lifeform that feeds on cities. It hatches from snowglobe-eggs, transforms into wobbly-wheeled shopping trollies, which coagulate into the third, city-devouring form, the shopping mall. I puzzle over why contemplating poiesis as a potentially perilous practice invites this mental invasion of trollies. I ruminate upon the dialectic between wayward trolley-wheels that frustrate linear progress – tugging the wire structure into digressive rhizomatic dances – and shopping malls containing soul-flattening, mass-produced, franchised-rows of one-size-fits-all-ness...

Process

Poiesis encourages tangents by bucking more formulaic shopping-mall-esque research approaches. This privileges process-orientated creativity which takes flight on wings that are proliferative and precipitative. This unpredictability means work-in-the-making can't be predicted – only afterwards may it make sense (Levine, 2009) – which requires deep trust in the creative process. Trusting the poietic process invites therapist-researchers to engage abr+a as an unfolding practice in which possibilities arise for still points of completion/certainty among ongoing transition/uncertainty (McNiff, 2015). As in therapy, this process of appreciative curiosity – ever asking: what more? what else? what if? – is a tangle of simultaneity. This proliferative concurrency, mirroring the worlding brought into therapy by most clients, isn't pared back as in traditional more reductionist research. Rather, it's invited into art where its paradoxical and diffractive all-there-at-once-ness may find temporary resting-points. It can then be pixellated and decentered from different angles and distances and through various mediums/modalities. This peregrinatory near-far-near-again helps cultivate reflexivity, criticality and capacity to be with too-much-ness in titrated and pendulated[29] ways (P. Levine, 2010) beneficial to both therapy and research.

Of further benefit to therapy and research is an embrace of meaning/sense-making as more than rational-cognitive. Abr+a disrupts and multiplies the process of making-sens/e. The five physical senses are plumbed for embodied knowing. The tacit, implicit sixth soul-sense/felt-sense is courted. Attention goes to the sensual expressive qualities of various arts modalities/mediums/processes/products. And the French word 'sens' – meaning direction – invites therapy and research to create life-forward orientation (Levine, 2009; Rappaport, 2014). The abr+a research process thus encourages us to engage all these sens/es to generate, translate/interpret, challenge/contradict, and articulate nascent knowing (Green, 2015; Green et al., 2022).

This prismatic sens/e-making forges additional bonds between therapy and research through reimagining CAT practices as research processes. (I'm currently experimenting by weaving CAT into the magician's traditional declaration of abra*cadabra*, rendering this now as abr+a^{CATabra}.*)* My use of CAT-as-research to generate and analyse/interpret research material has included poiesis and playfulness (Levine, 2009), focusing/FOAT (Gendlin, 1997; Rappaport, 2013, 2014), active imagination (Jung & Chodorow, 1997), the life/art process[30] (Halprin, 2003), dialoguing with images (McNiff, 2015), open studio[31] (Allen, 1995), response art (Fish, 2012), inter-modality/multiple-mediums (Levine & Levine, 2017; Rogers, 1999) and decentering (Levine & Levine, 2017) (see Green, 2019, 2018, 2018a, 2018b, 2017, 2017a, 2015, 2015a; Green et al., 2018; Green & Evans, 2018; Wang & Green, 2017). Whitecliffe faculty and students have employed nature-connected arts therapy (Evans, 2018), puppetry, the expressive therapies continuum[32] (Hinz, 2009), collage (Chilton & Scotti, 2014), authentic movement[33] (Whitehouse, 1963), body-casting, drama-therapeutic enactment, storytelling…the list is ever-expanding.

Repurposing therapeutic processes as research may ameliorate some of the risk involved when self-as-subject research entails expeditions into painful and precarious places. Holman Jones, Adams and Ellis (2016) name 'vulnerability with purpose' as a core autoethnographic process – yet traversing places of pain willy-nilly can cause harm. CAT-as-research may be especially useful to other non-therapeutic disciplines that may be less-equipped to navigate these spaces, opening possibilities for trans- and poly-disciplinary partnerships.

Figure 16. Deborah Green 2019 "Descent into shadows." Digital collage.

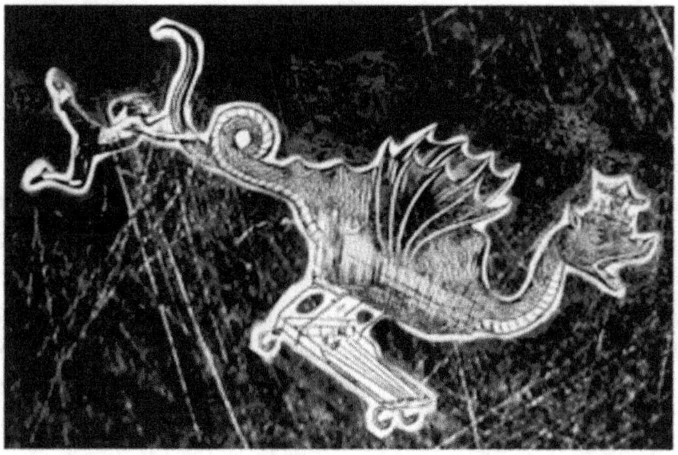

Partnerships

Practicing various sympoietic partnerships breathes life into the flexible ribcage of our abr+a-dragon. Foremost is the intrapsychic partnership instigating participation of the whole gestalt of therapist-researcher – mind/soul/body/affect/context and the imagical-dragon, the wonky-shopping trollies, the entire carousel plus monkeys... Research may use self-as-subject and/or include others, but the self/s-of-the-researcher is always present. Rigour arises from reflexivity rather than attempted objectivity (Adams St. Pierre, 2014) and purposeful vulnerability is pivotal (Holman Jones, Adams & Ellis, 2016). Connections radiate from this into the inter/extra-psychic partnerships researchers forge with other beings (alive, dead, imagined), constructs/discourses, and creative processes/modalities/mediums/artworks.

These abr+a partnerships privilege parabolic reciprocity, recognising all involved may be altered (Moon, 2016). This influences informed consent for participation. Student-researchers are encouraged to design and sign informed consent to participate in their own research. Feedback suggests this helps them deeply consider personal risk alongside the necessary trajectory of research which may publicly expose their intimate utterances. They also lean into holistic Māori and indigenous ontological cosmologies which emphasise spiritual connections between the living and non-living (O'Connor, 2018) and develop consent processes for others, living and/or dead and/or non-human, who may be implicated. While engaging the living is common practice, requesting consent from the deceased and the non-human is unusual. Feedback again suggests this enhances ethicality, responsibility, cultural sensitivity and compassion.

Abr+a's polytheistic and polyamorous nature may ignite perplexing and fricative dialectical partnerships. This often manifests in a tussle between established knowledge and emergent knowing. Student-researchers frequently rail against academic requirements to situate their work through referencing established theorists, believing their newly-hatched and tentative voices may be bullied from the nest by the more assured tones in published texts. In these instances, abr+a nurtures dinner-table-partnerships that nestle into reciprocity. This encourages emergent-researchers to respectfully de-reify recognised thinkers by imagining a meal, a few wines and a yarn being shared – creating partnerships that dwell at the ever-opening-edge of something new.

Pixellation

These paradoxical partnerships share characteristics with pixellation, a technological term indicating images crafted through constellations of small parts. In abr+a, pixellation indicates two key features.

Firstly, it embraces purposeful cyclical shifting of perspective between intimate individuated pixels and the larger patterned gestalt. This may be spied in the glittering dragon-eye of metamodern-esque oscillation (Vermeulen & van den Akker, 2010), theme-near/theme-far decentering (Knill, 2010), and titration and pendulation (P. Levine, 2010). As poietic engagement often results in a deluge of data, such reflexive processes may assist therapist-researchers to metabolise into meaning this proliferation of 'artifactual' material (Gerber, Biffi, Biondo, Gemignani, Hannes & Siegesmund, 2020, para.14).

This excess is often birthed through abr+a's embrace of living inquiry (Springgay, Irwin, Leggo & Gouzouasis, 2008). Such inquiries often originate in the researcher's everyday experience, and, in teaching abr+a, I use Whyte's (2006) poem *Start Close In* to encourage student-researchers to heed their present-lived experience for alluring urges, mysteries and stories. This prompts them to pixellate-in and "commence practising to see what emerges" (Haseman, 2006, p.6). While these emergences are idiosyncratically individualistic – hence attracting the critique of 'solipsistic narcissism' (Coffey, 1999) – this may be wrangled through pixellation. Abr+a doesn't "work without larger agendas or emancipatory aspirations, but...eschew[s] the constraints of narrow problem setting and rigid methodological requirements at the outset" (Haseman, 2006, p.4). Abr+a inter-braids evocative with analytic and critical autoethnographic approaches (Pace, 2012; Tilley-Lubbs, 2016). Researchers must raise their gaze from their navels and seek ways their personal ruminations may alight meaningfully in the public sphere, ensuring deep journeys birth new knowledge that contributes to our profession. This introduces the second element of pixellation: diffraction (Barad, 2007; Haraway, 2016). The multiple byways of sense-making within both CAT and abr+a appear to entangle reflexivity *and* diffraction – two approaches that are often held in contention (Undurraga, 2021). Reflexivity is alive in our autoethnographic, recursive loops into communing-with-self. And diffraction raises and prisms the researcher's gaze by "thinking through or with the stories and artworks as a material encounter" (Thomson 2019, p.86). This diffractivity infuses the process with divergent perspectives of difference opened by communing with/through: multiple arts modalities/processes/mediums/products; an eclectic selection of literature/theorists; and others – be they participants, fellow-researchers, and/or the range of unseen-yet-felt presences that may be evoked during our inquiries.

Playfulness

The repetitive diffractive reflexivity of pixellation may be better endured through playfulness. This spirit of playfulness, ignited by the mythical whimsy of the abr+a-dragon, grants permission for numerous qualities useful to therapy and research. The pragmatic imagination of play (Sarder, 2010) – including characteristics of risk, experiment, imagination, extension, innovation, and dissension (Finneran, 2013) – becomes a fruitful way to endure and even frolic within the poietic chaos of abr+a. It invites abr+a-researchers to grasp the map lightly, adventuring into the void like the Fool abreast a shopping-trolley with wonky-wheels that frequently veers from the pre-planned linear path into unpredictable rhizomatic twists and tangents (Deleuze, 1994). Playfulness can help researchers navigate these potentially perilous, perturbing, pandemonium-laden spaces by balancing gravity's pull with the lightness of levity. Self-focused research sometimes assumes weighty mythical-hero's-journey undertones (Campbell, 1995) becoming Persephone's descent into Hades, the unending agony of Prometheus on his crag, or form-shifting like Proteus. As playfulness, imagination and creativity belong to health (Poynton, 2012; Winnicott, 1977), bringing these to such pugnacious themes can ventilate their shadows by changing "passive experiences into active ones" (Ablon, 1996, p.545). This tugs us into the present moment and transforms us from those who are done-to into the doers (Levine, 2009).

I sigh and nod a thanks to my perceptive P-eeking monkeys – this emergent process of attempting to articulate abr+a feels well-held within the string-figuring CATs-cradle of presence, poiesis, process, partnerships, pixellation, playfulness and psyche. My dragon seems to agree and our hurtling jaunt through obscuring-mist slows, and the steady beat of wings calls us to clamber along the dragon's muscular sun-warmed back and perch between its powerful wings. We mustn't get too comfortable – this calm is temporary. But for now, the fog clears momentarily, and a virgin-world comes crisply into view as we float over lush landscape…

CONCLUSION: RIDE YOUR OWN DRAGON

And thus, it's time to pause and reflect upon our dragon-ride. This journey to know abr+a has characterised CAT as poly-sensory, parabolic and paradoxical thus requiring research practices that match. We've contemplated ways abr+a strives for less dissonance between the *what* and *how* of research, facilitating greater congruence between the skill-sets practiced in research and therapy. Layered multi-imaged storyings accompanied our scholarly explorations as we pondered the innovative reciprocity that may happen when CATs bring their unique poietic and psychotherapeutic skills, knowings and practices to arts-based and autoethnographic research. And my best hope is I've planted seeds for further conversations about ways abr+a may contribute to training creative therapists, the CAT profession, and how CAT-as-research (CATabra) may take flight in the research worlding of others.

Metaphors racket about my mind, bumping sharp edges into soft flesh. A dragon, a monkey-carousel, a wonky-wheeled trolley – so much for avoiding mixed metaphors…but woah, this is abr+a where imagination dons provocatively disparate demeanour, taunting me to be curious about the haphazardly-haywire alongside the neatly-tucked-in.

I hop on my bicycle to decentre these seemingly unrelated poietic metaphors. I grunt uphill – the ocean on my right and cliffs on my left, passing turgid stinky lumps of kamikaze-possum – and I free my soul to play with dragons and trolleys and monkeys and carousels. Whooping precariously home down a gravelled descent, these notions become words…

A Perambulative and Partially-Packaged Postscript

Here be dragons…
And today we met one.
We grasped its tail and took flight,
precariously clinging
on a juicy journey of too-much-ness.
A roller-coaster-ride that feels
perilous, precocious, prescient…
…and familiar…
A sibling to therapy when the arts lead.
But wait, there's more…
We quest for ways of knowing that 'correspond as closely as possible' to this poiesis.
Our ears prick to the clarion call of arts-based research and autoethnography.
We swoop and become entangled+enlivened by abr+a.
Might this offer deep journeying and legitimacy?
We encounter performative ways of knowing:
knowing that renews with each wingbeat;
knowing that unleashes many mess-and-merriment-making monkeys;
knowing that doesn't prescribe but responds creatively to this chaos;
living, sensory, expansive and wayward knowing…
Psyche inhales and soul-chi simmers through this knowing;
Presence stretches a limber spine, re/flexing appreciative curiosity towards seen and unseen, the gestalt-of-self, the arts, stories and concepts that shape;
Poiesis responds from the heart, surrenders, becomes receptive, creating with what is given;
Process spreads iridescent wings, trusting the unfolding through prismatic sens/e-making, riding the updrafts of CAT-as-research;
Partnerships breathe knowing into the flexible ribcage of our dragon, purposefully vulnerable communion with whole-self/others/arts/theories;

Pixellation shifts perspective through multifaceted eyes, gazing inward and outward asking 'where will this knowing alight? how might it make a difference?'; and

Playfulness whoops a loop-the-loop, the whimsy of our magical-dragon, permissive, opening imagination and decentering into alternative worldings.

All while we cling to a scaly tail, mist streaming by, startling sudden birds,
landing gear crafted from a wibbly-wheeled shopping-trolley
offering scant assurance
that the work will land safely in a world
where the sedimented sharp edges of tradition
still loom like teeth...

Figure 17. Deborah Green 2020 "Your abr+a-dragon?" Digital collage.

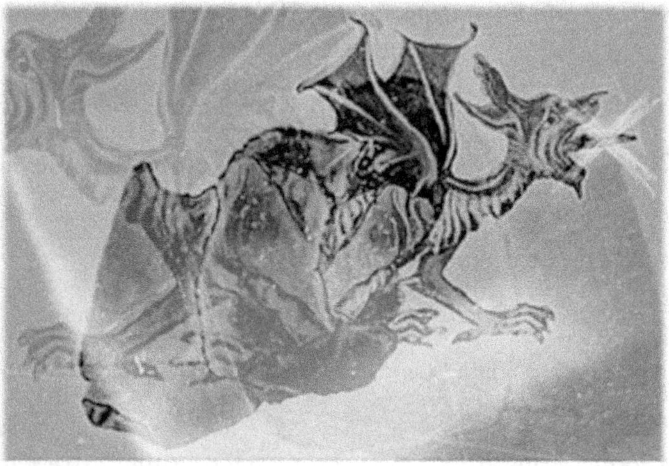

REFERENCES

Ablon, S. L. (1996). The therapeutic action of play. *Journal of the American Academy of Child and Adolescent Psychiatry*, *35*(4), 545–547. doi:10.1097/00004583-199604000-00022 PMID:8919718

Adams St. Pierre, E. (2014). A brief and personal history of post qualitative research: Toward "post inquiry". *Journal of Curriculum Theorizing*, *30*(2), 2–19.

Allen, P. B. (1995). *Art is a way of knowing*. Shambhala.

Anderson, L., & Glass-Coffin, B. (2016). I learn by going. In S. Holman Jones, T. E. Adams, & C. Ellis, (Eds.), Handbook of autoethnography (pp. 57-83). Routledge.

Barad, K. (2007). *Meeting the universe halfway: Quantum physics and the entanglement of matter and meaning*. Duke University Press. doi:10.2307/j.ctv12101zq

Bochner, A. P. (2016). Autoethnography's existential calling. In S. Holman Jones, T. E. Adams, & C. Ellis (Eds.), Handbook of autoethnography. (pp. 50-56). Routledge.

Bolt, B. (2016). Artistic research: A performative paradigm. *Parse Journal*, *3*, 129–142.

Bush, S. (2018). Emergence, resonant felt sensing and the arts: With/in relational spaces of us. *ANZJAT Australia and Journal of Arts Therapy*, *13*(1 & 2), 125–129.

Campbell, J. (1995). *Reflections on the art of living: A Joseph Campbell companion*. Harpercollins.

Charmaz, K. (2012). The power and potential of grounded theory. *Medical Sociology Online, 6*(3).

Chilton, G., & Scotti, V. (2014). Snipping, gluing, writing: The properties of collage as an arts-based research practice in art therapy. *Art Therapy: Journal of the American Art Therapy Association*, *31*(4), 163–171. doi:10.1080/07421656.2015.963484

Coffey, A. (1999). The ethnographic self. *Sage (Atlanta, Ga.)*.

Coles, A. (2014). 'Being time': An exploration of personal experiences of time and implications for art psychotherapy practice. *International Journal of Art Therapy*, *19*(2), 71–81. doi:10.1080/17454832.2013.844184

Csikszentmihalyi, M. (1990). *Flow: The psychology of optimal experience*. Harper and Row.

Csikszentmihalyi, M. (2004). *Mihaly Csikszentmihalyi on flow*. https://www.ted.com/talks/mihaly_csikszentmihalyi_on_flow

Davies, B. (2000). *(In)scribing body/landscape relations*. Altamira Press.

Deleuze, G. (1994). *Difference and repetition* (P. Patton, Trans.). Athlone.

Denzin, N. K. (2013). The death of data? *Cultural Studies « Critical Methodologies, 13*(4), 353-356. doi:10.1177/1532708613487882

Elizabeth, V. (2008). Another string to our bow: Participant writing as research method. *FQS, 9*(1). https://www.qualitative-research.net/index.php/fqs/article/view/331

Evans, B. (2018). Earthbound teaching nature connected arts therapy. *Creative Arts Education and Therapy*, *4*(2), 164–173. doi:10.15212/CAET/2018/4/26

Finneran, M. (2013, October). Keynote presentation. In *Critical journeys in applied theatre*. University of Auckland.

Fish, B. J. (2012). Response art: The art of the art therapist. *Journal of the American Art Therapy Association*, *29*(3), 138–143. doi:10.1080/07421656.2012.701594

Geerts, E., & van der Tuin, I. (2016). *Diffraction & Reading Diffractively.* https://newmaterialism.eu/almanac/d/diffraction.html

Gendlin, E. T. (1997). *Experiencing and the creation of meaning*. Northwestern University Press.

Gerber, N., Biffi, E., Biondo, J., Gemignani, M., Hannes, K., & Siegesmund, R. (2020). Arts-based research in the social and health sciences: Pushing for change with an Interdisciplinary Global Arts-Based Research Initiative. *FQS*, *21*(2). Advance online publication. doi:10.17169/fqs-21.2.3496

Gray, B. (2011). Autoethnography and arts therapy: The arts meet healing. *Australia and New Zealand Journal of Arts Therapy*, *6*(1), 67–80.

Green, D. (2015). Exploring and sharing arts therapy experiences through fiction-based research. *Australia and New Zealand Journal of Arts Therapy*, *10*(1), 33–42.

Green, D. (2015a). *Quake destruction/arts creation: arts therapy and the Canterbury earthquakes* (Unpublished doctoral thesis). University of Auckland, New Zealand.

Green, D. (2017). Imagical play: arts therapy and trauma. In P. O'Connor & C. R. Gómez (Eds.), *Playing with possibilities* (pp. 200–222). Cambridge Scholars.

Green, D. (2017a). Quake destruction/arts creation: Arts therapy and the Canterbury earthquakes. *Australia and New Zealand Journal of Arts Therapy*, *12*(1), 40–45.

Green, D. (2018). Arts therapy, imagical play, and trauma: Exploring arts therapy during the canterbury earthquakes. *The International Journal of the Arts in Society: Annual Review, 13*(1). doi:10.18848/1833-1866/CGP

Green, D. & Evans, Bettina. (2018). Kites and shaking hearts in the rubble. *Australia and New Zealand Journal of Arts Therapy*, *13*(1&2), 35–46.

Green, D. (2018a). Making-sense of poietic presense in arts therapy and education. *Creative Arts in Education and Therapy*, *4*(2), 139–148. doi:10.15212/CAET/2018/4/21

Green, D. (2018b). Reclaiming messy-mudpies & magic through poiesis, education & arts therapy. *The International Journal of Arts in Education,* 31-57.

Green, D. (2019). Communitas and soul-healing: arts therapy within the loss-upon-loss of natural disaster. In M. J. M. Wood, B. Jacobson, & H. Cridford (Eds.), *The international handbook of art therapy in palliative and bereavement care* (pp. 340–356). Routledge. doi:10.4324/9781315110530-35

Green, D., Levey, A., Evans, B., Lawson, W., & Marks, K. (2022). The arts of making-sense in uncertain times: arts-based research and autoethnography. In H. Kara & S. Khoo (Eds.), *Qualitative and digital research in times of crisis: methods, reflexivity, and ethics* (pp. 59–77). Policy Press.

Green, D., Pears-Scown, N., Weir, M., Csata, I., Heney, R., McGeever, M., Lambert, R., Marks, K., & Wang, I. (2018). The arts of making sens/e. *Australia and New Zealand Journal of Arts Therapy*, *12*(1), 112–130.

Greenwood, J. (2012). Arts-based research: Weaving magic and meaning. *International Journal of Education & the Arts*, *13*(1). http://www.ijea.org/v13i1/

Greer, G.-H., & Blair, L. (2018). Arts-based research and the discourse of danger. *Studies in Art Education*, *59*(3), 243–255. doi:10.1080/00393541.2018.1479824

Halprin, D. (2003). *The expressive body in life, art and therapy. Working with movement, metaphor and meaning*. Jessica Kingsley.

Haraway, D. (2016). *Staying with the trouble: Making kin in the Chthulucene*. Duke University Press.

Haseman, B. (2006). A manifesto for performative research. *Media International Australia Incorporating Culture and Policy, Theme Issue Practice-led Research*, (118), 98–106.

Hedges, F. (2010). *Reflexivity in Therapeutic Practice*. Bloomsbury. doi:10.1007/978-1-137-12293-3

Hegeman, S. (2015). A sociological imagination. *Studia Neophilologica, 87*(sup1), 97–103. doi:10.1080/00393274.2014.981960

Heidegger, M. (1935/1975). *Poetry, language, thought* (A. Hofstadter, Trans.). Harper & Row, Perennial Library.

Hillman, J. (1983). *InterViews: Conversations with Laura Pozzo on psychology, biography, love, soul, the gods, animals, dreams, imagination, work, cities, and the state of the culture*. Spring Publications.

Hinz, L. D. (2009). *Expressive therapies continuum: A framework for using art in therapy*. Routledge. doi:10.4324/9780203893883

Holman Jones, S., Adams, T. E., & Ellis, C. (2016). *Handbook of autoethnography*. Left Coast Press Inc.

Jung, C. G., & Chodorow, J. (1997). *Jung on active imagination*. Princeton University Press. doi:10.1515/9781400866854

Kapitan, L. (2013). Editorial. Reexamining the map: Extending and disrupting art therapy assumptions of representation. *Art Therapy: Journal of the American Art Therapy Association, 30*(3), 96–97. doi:10.1080/07421656.2013.819548

Kapitan, L. (2014). *Introduction to art therapy research*. Routledge.

Kapitan, L. (2018). *Introduction to art therapy research* (2nd ed.). Routledge.

Kapitan, L., Litell, M., & Torres, A. (2011). Creative Art Therapy in a Community's Participatory Research and Social Transformation. *Art Therapy: Journal of the American Art Therapy Association, 28*(2), 64–73. doi:10.1080/07421656.2011.578238

Kara, H., & Khoo, S. (Eds.), *Qualitative and digital research in times of crisis: methods, reflexivity, and ethics*. Policy Press. doi:10.2307/j.ctv2321kdr

Keane, B. (2007). Taniwha. *Te Ara - the Encyclopedia of New Zealand*. http://www.TeAra.govt.nz/en/taniwha

Knill, P. (2011). Communal art-making and conflict transformation. In E. Levine & S. K. Levine (Eds.), *Art in Action* (pp. 53–77). Jessica Kingsley.

Knill, P. J., Levine, E. G., & Levine, S. K. (2005). *Principles and practice of expressive arts therapy, toward a therapeutic aesthetics*. Jessica Kingsley.

Kotler, S. (2015). *The Neurochemistry of flow states*. Think Big. https://www.youtube.com/watch?v=aHp2hkue8RQ

Leavy, P. (2013). *Fiction as research practice: Short stories, novellas, and novels (Developing qualitative inquiry)*. Left Coast Press.

Leavy, P. (2018). *Handbook of arts-based research.* The Guildford Press.

Levine, E. G., & Levine, S. K. (2017). *New developments in expressive arts therapy: The play of poiesis.* Jessica Kingsley.

Levine, P. A. (2010). *In an unspoken voice: How the body releases trauma and restores goodness.* North Atlantic Books.

Levine, S. K. (2009). *Trauma, tragedy, therapy: The arts and human suffering.* Jessica Kingsley.

Lincoln, Y. S., & Denzin, N. K. (2003). *Turning points in qualitative research: tying knots in a handkerchief.* Altamira Press.

Manders, E., & Chilton, G. (2013). Translating the essence of dance: Rendering meaning in artistic inquiry of the creative arts therapies. *International Journal of Education & the Arts, 14*(16). http://www.ijea.org/v14n16/

McConeghey, H. (2017). Art and soul (2nd ed.). Spring.

McNiff, S. (1998). *Art based research.* Shambhala.

McNiff, S. (2004). *Art heals: How creativity cures the soul.* Shambhala.

McNiff, S. (2013). Art as research: Opportunities and challenges. *Intellect.*

McNiff, S. (2015). *Imagination in action: secrets for unleashing creative expression.* Shambhala.

Moon, B. (2016). *Art-based group therapy: Theory and practice.* Charles C Thomas Ltd.

Moore, T. (1992). Introduction. In *Archetypal Imagination (Introduction).* Lindisfarne Press.

Moustakas, C. (1990). Heuristic Research: Design, methodology and applications. *Sage (Atlanta, Ga.).*

O'Connor, N. (2018). Visual whakapapa: An arts therapy experiential. *Australia and New Zealand Journal of Arts Therapy, 13*(1&2), 63–66.

O'Connor, P., & Anderson, M. (2015). *Applied theatre: research: radical departures.* Bloomsbury. doi:10.5040/9781472513489

Pace, S. (2012). *Writing the self into research: Using grounded theory analytic strategies in autoethnography. Creativity: Cognitive.* Social and Cultural Perspectives.

Palmer, H., & Hunter, V. (2018). *Worlding.* https://newmaterialism.eu/almanac/w/worlding.html

Poynton, M. (2012). "We should be playing, not talking": Play, self-agency and moving towards depressive moments. *Journal of Child Psychotherapy, 38*(2), 185–198. doi:10.1080/0075417X.2012.684488

Pratchett, T. (1998). *Reaper man.* Transworld, Ltd.

Rambo Ronai, C. (1995). Multiple reflections of child sex abuse: An argument for a layered account. *Journal of contemporary ethnography, 23*, 395-426.

Rappaport, L. (2008). *Focusing-oriented art therapy: Accessing the body's wisdom and creative intelligence.* Jessica Kingsley.

Rappaport, L. (2013). Trusting the felt sense in art-based research. In S. McNiff (Ed.), *Art as research: Opportunities and challenges* (pp. 201–208). Intellect. doi:10.1386/9781783200016_24

Rappaport, L. (2014). Focusing-orientated arts therapy: Cultivating mindfulness and compassion, and accessing inner wisdom. In L. Rappaport (Ed.), *Mindfulness and the arts therapies: Theory and practice* (pp. 193–207). Jessica Kingsley.

Ricci, R. J. (2003). Autoethnographic verse: Nicky's boy: A life in two worlds. *Qualitative Report*, *8*(4), 591–596. http://www.nova.edu/sss/QR/QR8-4/ricci.pdf

Rogers, N. (1999). The creative connection: A holistic expressive arts process. In S. K. Levine & E. G. Levine (Eds.), *Foundations of expressive arts therapy theoretical and clinical perspectives* (pp. 113–131). Jessica Kingsley.

Romanyshyn, R. D. (2013). *The wounded researcher: research with soul in mind*. Spring Journal, Inc.

Sarder, Z. (2010). *Welcome to postnormal times*. https://ziauddinsardar.com/2011/03/welcome-to-postnormal-times/

Shankar, S. (2020). *Emotions as the new ethical turn in social research*. https://items.ssrc.org/covid-19-and-the-social-sciences/social-research-and-insecurity/emotions-as-the-new-ethical-turn-in-social-research/

Skovholt, T. M. (2012). *Becoming a therapist: On the road to mastery*. John Wiley & Sons, Inc.

Springgay, S., Irwin, R. L., Leggo, C., & Gouzouasis, P. (Eds.). (2008). *Being with a/r/tography*. Sense. doi:10.1163/9789087903268

Springgay, S., Irwin, R. L., & Wilson Kind, S. (2005). A/r/tography as living inquiry through art and text. *Qualitative Inquiry*, *11*(6), 897–912. doi:10.1177/1077800405280696

Stewart, K. (2010). Worlding refrains. In M. Gregg & G. J. Siegworth (Eds.), *The affect theory reader* (pp. 339–353). Duke University Press. doi:10.1215/9780822393047-015

Sullivan, G. (2006). Research acts in art practice. *Studies in Art Education*, *48*(1), 19–35. doi:10.1080/00393541.2006.11650497

Tapper, H. (2021). Uninvited guests, soul-filled skies and universes beneath my toes: Exploring poiesis at the confluence of the arts and self for arts therapy research. *Journal of Creative Arts Therapies*, *16*(2), 52–67.

Thomson, J. (2019). Working with death through art and story: A collective biography. *ANZJAT*, *14*(1), 77–90.

Tilley-Lubbs, G. A. (2016). Critical autoethnography and the vulnerable self as researcher. In G. A. Tilley-Lubbs & S. Bénard Calva (Eds.), *Re-telling our stories: Critical autoethnographic narratives* (pp. 3–5). doi:10.1007/978-94-6300-567-8_1

Turner, V. W. (1969). *The ritual process: Structure and antistructure*. Aldine.

Undurraga, J. K. A. S. (2021). What if reflexivity and diffraction intra-act? *International Journal of Qualitative Studies in Education*, 1–14. Advance online publication. doi:10.1080/09518398.2021.1900622

Van Rooyen, H., & d'Ablon, R. (2020). Transforming Data into Poems: Poetic Inquiry Practices for Social and Human Sciences. *Education as Change, 24*(8103). https://upjournals.co.za/index.php/EAC

Vaughan, K. (2009). A home in the arts: From research/creation to practice or The story of a dissertation in the making, in action – so far! *International Journal of Education & the Arts, 10*(13). http://www.ijea.org/v10n13/

Vermeulen, T., & van den Akker, R. (2010). Notes on metamodernism. *Journal of Aesthetics & Culture, 2*. http://aestheticsandculture.net/index.php/jac/article/viewArticle/5677

Vincent, A. (2018) is there a definition? Ruminating on poetic inquiry, strawberries, and the continued growth of the field. *Art/Research International: A Transdisciplinary Journal, 3*(2), 48-76. doi:10.18432/ari29356

Vlasić Manaia, A. (2017). Kaupapa Māori arts therapy. *Australia and New Zealand Journal of Arts Therapy, 12*(1), 27–39.

Waller, D., & Sibbett, C. H. (Eds.). (2008). Art therapy and cancer care. KakJiSa/OUP.

Walsh, A. (2022). Beyond extraction: co-creating a decolonial and feminist research practice in post-conflict Guatemala. In H. Kara & S. Khoo (Eds.), *Qualitative and digital research in times of crisis: methods, reflexivity, and ethics* (pp. 235–246). Policy Press.

Wang, I., & Green, D. (2017). Stitching East and West. *Creative Arts in Education and Therapy – Eastern and Western Perspectives, 3*(1). https://caet.quotus.org/article/2017/1/4

Whitehouse, M. (1963). The Tao of the body. In P. Pallaro (Ed.), Moving the body, moving the self, being moved: A collection of essays (2nd ed., pp.51-57). Jessica Kingsley.

Whyte, D. (2006). *River flow: new and selected poems*. Many Rivers Press.

Winnicott, D. W. (1977). *Playing and reality*. Tavistock.

Yardley, A. (2008). Piecing together—A methodological bricolage. *FQS, 9*(2). https://www.qualitative-research.net/index.php/fqs/article/view/416/902

KEY TERMS AND DEFINITIONS

Creative Arts Therapist (CAT): A term adopted by ANZACATA to recognise the range of modalities used by uni-modal and multi-modal arts therapists within the regions of Australia, New Zealand and Asia. Terminology used in other countries and regions may vary and may include art therapy, arts therapy, expressive arts therapy and creative therapy.

Decentering: The use of creative making to move from stuckness into the alterative logic of the imagination.

Diffraction: A term used metaphorically and methodologically within feminist and new materialist research to indicate a critical and difference-attentive approach in which emergent ideas overlap, interfere with, and co-establish one another and divergences are encouraged.

Poiesis: A Greek word that means roughly the same as 'art' in English, both signifying a medium and a making. This term is used to make-strange, expose hidden assumptions and arouse fresh insights. When applied to both therapy and creative research, poiesis implies the human capacity to respond to and change the world through the act of shaping what is given.

Reflexivity: Critical examination of the impact of the researcher's/therapist's worlding (taken-for-granted values, assumptions, and behavioural patterns and practices) upon research/therapeutic processes. Reflexivity may also include feedback loops that explore the reciprocal influence of these processes upon researcher/therapist's worlding.

Sympoiesis: A concept that embraces intersubjectivity combined with creative arts-making. Sympoiesis means 'making with' and infers 'becoming with'.

Worlding: An embedded and enacted process, a way of being in the world, an individual's whole-person act of 'staying with the trouble' and attending to the world that removes the boundaries between subject and environment.

ENDNOTES

1 Throughout this chapter I use first person rather than attempting objective third person. Emphasising objectivity is deemed essential in traditional scholarship for both ethics and rigour, based on assumptions that emotion/subjectivity impedes knowledge-creation (Walsh, 2022). Creative auto-ethnographic research, however, views emotions as productive for human understanding (Shankar, 2020), inviting the purposefully vulnerable presence of the multiplicit-researcher/author-self (Holman Jones et al., 2015). Rigour arises from reflexivity rather than attempted objectivity (Adams St. Pierre, 2014).

2 At the School of Creative Arts Therapy, Whitecliffe, Aotearoa New Zealand.

3 The British Association of Art Therapy (BAAT) and the American Art Therapy Association (AATA).

4 The Australian, New Zealand and Asian Creative Arts Therapy Association (ANZACATA) session included the creative participation of eight Master's students: Elizabeth Love, Shanti Brown, Elske-Reyneke-Barnard, Rachel Baker, Heleina Dalton, Lyndy Broughton, Kumi Nakamura and Hilary Tapper.

5 ANZACATA has adopted the term 'creative arts therapy' (CAT) to recognise the range of modalities used by uni-modal and multi-modal arts therapists within this region. Terminology used in other countries and regions may vary and may include art therapy, arts therapy, expressive arts therapy and creative therapy.

6 *Reflexivity* involves critically examining the impact of the researcher's/therapist's worlding (taken-for-granted values, assumptions, and behavioural patterns and practices) upon research/therapeutic processes. Reflexivity may also include feedback loops that explore the reciprocal influence of these processes upon researcher/therapist's worlding (Hedges, 2010). *Diffraction* is used metaphorically and methodologically within feminist and new materialist research to indicate a critical and difference-attentive approach in which emergent ideas overlap, interfere with, and co-establish one another and divergences are encouraged (Geerts & van der Tuin, 2016). There is some contention between reflexivity and diffraction, which are often seen as opposing.

7 Csikszentmihalyi (1990, 2004) began researching the *flow* phenomenon when he realised how absorbed artists can become in creative processes. He identified various characteristics exhibited by flow. Action and awareness become merged through a task that is challenging, yet achievable. The activity provides an autotelic experience – it is worth doing for its own sake. Self-consciousness is lost, paradoxically resulting in a stronger sense-of-self. Attention is centred and focused, and kinaesthetic awareness is heightened resulting in a loss of ego. The experience of time is transformed, and the activity engenders a feeling of empowerment by providing the possibility rather than the actuality of control (Waller & Sibbett, 2008). Flow state can be richly charged with pleasure, releasing an array of helpful neurotransmitters including norepinephrine, dopamine, anandamide, serotonin and endorphins (Kotler, 2015).

8 *Onto-epistemology* references new materialist relational thinking in which ontology is no longer categorised as separate from epistemology (Barad, 2007). Rather, they become entangled together within the inherent pluralistic and eclectic onto-epistemic of ABR (Gerber, Biffi, Biondo, Gemignani, Hannes & Siegesmund, 2020, para.2). In other words, as the researcher is of the world, there exists no privileged position from which knowledges may be produced.

9 These collaboratively generated vignettes are presented on a grey background to distinguish them from other creative writing segments in this chapter. Consents have been gained from all researchers for inclusion of their work. All these finished theses and dissertations can be obtained on request from the Whitecliffe Library: https://www.whitecliffe.ac.nz/whitecliffe-library

10 *A/r/tography* (Springgay, Irwin, Leggo & Gouzouasis, 2008) is a form of practice-based research in which the researcher engages their interacting roles of artist/researcher/teacher to render intertwined writing and art making (in any artform).

11 *Fiction-based research* (Leavy, 2013) is an adaptation of arts-based research in which researchers write creative fiction to generate data, perform analysis/translation, and/or present research outcomes in ways that invite empathetic engagement (Green, 2015).

12 *FOAT* (Rappaport, 2008, 2013, 2014) is a mindfulness-informed therapy that uses creative making to express and inquire into the felt-sense of an experience or idea.

13 McNiff (2004) encourages us to view artworks as messengers, entities in their own right with whom we may dialogue and from whom we may learn.

14 *Nature-connected arts therapy* (Evans, 2018) invites nature into creative collaboration by recognising the sentience of nature through use of natural materials and creating in natural spaces.

15 *Poetic inquiry* (Vincent, 2018) is an artistic practice that, while implemented within a research framework, does not diminish the critical/aesthetic qualities of poems as poetry.

16 *Participatory action research* (Kapitan, 2018) forms part of an anti-oppressive movement in research that believes research and action must be done 'with' people and not 'on', 'to' or 'for' people. Subjects are co-researchers in diverse research stages and processes where they become the masters of explorations into underlying features and causes of the happenings in their worlds (Kapitan, Litell, & Torres, 2011).

17 *Heuristic research* (Moustakas, 1990) is an approach to phenomenological research that focuses on the meanings given to significant human experiences by the humans themselves.

18 *Decentering* (Levine & Levine, 2017) uses creative making to move from stuckness into the alterative logic of the imagination.

19 *Alchemical hermeneutics* (Romanyshyn, 2013) refers to a form of phenomenological research in which artworks become 'texts' in a process of interpretation that makes a particular place for the unconscious.

20 *Felt-sense* is the term used by phenomenological psychologist, philosopher, and creator of Focusing, Gendlin (1997), to describe an 'all there at once', internal knowing which is directly experienced but not yet in words.

21 Inaugural BAAT/AATA Conference; ANZACATA Symposium; and Whitecliffe seminars with creative arts therapy Master's students and trainee supervisors.

22 The Greek word *poiesis* means roughly the same as 'art' in English, both signifying a medium and a making. I borrow Levine's (2009) use of poiesis to make-strange, expose hidden assumptions and arouse fresh insights. When applied to both therapy and creative research, I follow Levine (2009) believing that "ultimately the ground of our work is not psychology, the theoretical understanding of the mind, but poiesis, the human capacity to respond to and change the world through the act of shaping what is given to us" (p.25). Originally developed by Aristotle, further elaborated by Heidegger (1935/1975), and then by Knill, Levine, and Levine (2005), poiesis involves a creative caper with chaos as it entails meaning- and soul-making by shaping "ourselves in the same way as we engage in creative work: by letting the new form emerge without controlling it" (Levine, 2009, p.139).

23 *Sympoiesis*, borrowed from Haraway (2016), embraces intersubjectivity combined with creative arts-making. Sympoiesis, at its heart, means 'making with' and infers 'becoming with'; it is "a word proper to complex, dynamic, responsive, situated, historical systems. It is a word for worlding-with, in company" (Haraway, 2016, p.58).

24 *Communitas* is used by Turner (1969) to describe the unique quality of full, unmediated communion that can arise between liminal neophytes during rituals.

25 Ninety minutes in total, including the introduction and information section at the beginning.

26 *Chi/qi* refers to a real and empirical creative force moving through all of life. According to expressive arts therapist McNiff (2015), chi aligns with the process of artistic expression and is therefore a core focus of arts therapy.

27 *Mauri* in te reo Māori refers to life force / ethos (Vlasić Manaia, 2017).

28 *Worlding* can be defined as an embedded and enacted process, a way of being in the world, an individual's whole-person act of 'staying with the trouble' (Haraway, 2016) and attending to the world. New materialists, Palmer and Hunter (2018) write that "worlding, is the setting up of the world. Worlding is a particular blending of the material and the semiotic that removes the boundaries between subject and environment…Worlding affords the opportunity for the cessation of habitual temporalities and modes of being" (para.8).

29 *Titration* and *pendulation* are terms used to describe specific approaches within Somatic Experiencing, a form of trauma therapy. Titration refers to graduated exposure by working with only small parts of difficult experiences at a time. Pendulation indicates shifting of body sensations or emotions between expansion and contraction (P. Levine, 2010).

30 The *life/art process* developed by Halprin (2003) is movement-based arts therapy that integrates movement/dance, visual arts, performance techniques, creative writing and therapeutic practices.

31 The *Open Studio Process* developed by Allen (1995) is a group therapy approach grounded in equality, self-determination and freedom that flattens client-therapist hierarchy, and is directive-free but held by a framework involving witness-writing, creation, further witness-writing and sharing.

[32] The *expressive therapies continuum* (ETC)(Hinz, 2009) offers theory and practical guidelines that detail how clients process information during their interactions with art materials.

[33] *Authentic movement* developed by Whitehouse (1963) encourages participants to focus attention on inner feeling-states and express the flow of these through improvised dance movements with their eyes closed to reduce distractions.

Chapter 18
Rewriting a Lost Story:
The Truth in the Narratives of Balkan Immigrants

Bozkurt Koç
https://orcid.org/0000-0002-6295-8009
Ondokuz Mayıs University, Turkey

Doğan Güneş Temli
https://orcid.org/0000-0002-9786-0052
Ondokuz Mayıs University, Turkey

Aysu Gül Şanli
Ondokuz Mayıs University, Turkey

Eren Trabzon
Ondokuz Mayıs University, Turkey

ABSTRACT

The phenomenon of migration appears as an incontrovertible reality of social life today as it was in the past. While social, cultural, political, economic, etc. factors constitute the causes of migration, they are seen as the psycho-social dynamics most affected by migration. In this study, the narratives regarding the migration process of the Balkan immigrants living in Samsun were evaluated from a social psychological perspective in the context of the post-migration adaptation process. The narratives of the Balkan immigrants were examined in depth using thematic analysis method. As a result of the analysis, the narratives were evaluated within the framework of the themes of "basic needs," "cultural characteristics," and "acculturation." It has been determined that with the effect of features such as cultural similarities, sense of belonging, empathy, and cooperation, Balkan immigrants mostly do not experience problems in the adaptation process relatively different from other migration processes.

DOI: 10.4018/978-1-7998-9251-9.ch018

INTRODUCTION

Almost every country in the world has been affected by immigration. The issue of migration is on the agenda not only in the countries receiving immigration, but also in all geographies where globalization is felt or intensely experienced. Especially in the second half of the 20th century, mass population movements took place and the immigrant population has increased rapidly in the last half century (R.o.Tr. General Directorate of Migration Management, 2017). According to the data of The UN Refugee Agency for 2021, 82.4 million people around the world had to migrate forcibly (The UN Refugee Agency, 2021).

Like many countries in the world, Turkey has been affected by migration movements throughout history and has hosted many immigrants. According to the 2016 Turkey Migration Report, Anatolian geography opened its doors to a large number of immigrants between 1492 and 1922. Arrival of approximately 1 million 185 thousand people from Greece, the Balkans and Germany during the republic period, between 1922-1945; and also approximately 900 thousand people from Iraq, Bulgaria, Bosnia and Kosovo to Turkey between 1988 and 2000 is among the most concrete examples of Turkey's migration history (R.o.Tr. General Directorate of Migration Management, 2017). According to United Nations Refugee Agency 2021 data, in 2020 Turkey hosted more than 3.6 million people, mostly Syrians (The UN Refugee Agency, 2021; McAuliffe, & Triandafyllidou, 2021). According to the international migration statistics for 2019 published by the Turkish Statistical Institute (TURKSTAT) on July 17, 2020, of the foreign nationals who came to Turkey in 2019 are 14.5% Iraqi, 13.8% Turkmenistan, 8.2% Afghanistan, 7.5% Syria and 7.3% Iranian citizens (Turkish Statistical Institute, 2019).

As it can be understood from the data on international migration, some of the immigrants hosted by Turkey are Balkan immigrants. Since the end of the nineteenth century, there has been an intense migration movement from the Balkans to Anatolia and this migration movement continued in the republic period. Between 1923 and 1938, there was a migration to Turkey from Balkan countries such as Bulgaria, Romania and Yugoslavia (Duman, 2009). These migration movements have turned into mass migration as a result of the Turks' desire to return to their homeland due to the pressure, persecution and assimilation they have been subjected to in Balkan countries such as Greece, Bulgaria, Yugoslavia and Romania where Turks live intensely. Therewithal, it is seen that the resettlement policies of the Turkish state and the policy of increasing the population by bringing Turks living in the Balkans to Turkey are effective in this regard (Aksoy, 2016). It is seen that 1.204.205 people who immigrated from the Balkans to Turkey between 1923 and 1960 were composed of immigrants, refugees and exchanged people. During the said period 407.788 people of which 384.000 "Exchanged" were from Greece; 374.478 people from Bulgaria; 269.101 people from Yugoslavia-Macedonia and 121.351 people from Romania immigrated to Turkey (Geray, 1962). These immigrants were settled in the low-density regions of Thrace and Anatolia for reasons such as security, population policy, opening the idle lands to production and contributing to the economy within the scope of the settlement policy. All the problems of immigrants, especially sheltering, were tried to be solved by the state and necessary measures were taken to help them become producers (Duman, 2009).

All migrations, including migrations from the Balkans to Turkey, are at the center of international debates today, as in the historical process (Mbaye, 2017). The phenomenon of migration, which has a multidimensional feature (Bauloz, Vathi, & Acosta, 2019) and expresses a complex process that covers large time (Landau, 2017) is a dynamic process that has short- and long-term effects on both immigrant individuals and groups and the receiving societies (Dovidio, & Esses, 2001). In other words, all countries are affected by immigration in a positive or negative way. Among the positive effects of migration, the improvement of the economic conditions of the immigrants and the economic development of the receiving countries can be shown. Among the negative effects of migration are the loss of qualified citizens due to brain drain for the sending countries; for the countries that receive immigration, there are conflicts due to reasons such as ethnic origin and religious belief differences (Sam, & Berry, 2006).

At the same timeas one of the factors that determine the cultural characteristics of a society and their impact on the person (Kağıtçıbaşı, & Cemalcılar, 2014), migration is also effective in the formation of today's multicultural society structure (Berry, 2009; 2020) and cultural diversity. Depending on the migration, social, cultural, ethnic, religious etc. differences emerge and social heterogeneity increases (Appave, & David, 2017). This multicultural and heterogeneous structure that emerged after migration inevitably brings along acculturation and social adaptation processes. Acculturation encompasses the contact between individuals and groups with different cultural backgrounds, in other words, all the changes that occur after migration (Sam, 2006). Individuals and groups who encounter new and different cultural situations after migration experience some psychological and social changes in the acculturation process (Cabassa, 2003; Gemicibasi, & Yilmaz, 2021). The acculturation process produces different results at the individual and group level. While the effects of acculturation at the group level emerge in the form of changes in collective activities and social institutions; individual-level effects include changes in individuals' behaviors, attitudes, values, identities, or affects (Sam, & Berry, 2010).

Social adaptation which is of vital importance especially for immigrants and host societies (Appave, & David, 2017), can occur within the acculturation process (Berry, Phinney, Sam, & Vedder, 2006). Ensuring social adaptation is an important requirement for a healthy migration process (Goodman, 2010). Settling in a new community, temporarily or permanently, requires immigrants to adapt to a new culture, traditions, social values and language. The social adaptation of immigrants with the host society also depends on the the attitudes of the host society towards phenomenon of immigration and immigrants (Bauloz, Vathi, & Acosta, 2019). In addition to economic and political adaptation, social adaptation also includes adaptation facilitating factors such as belonging to the country of immigration, recognizing the country's culture and social values, and language proficiency (Goodman, 2010).

Therefore, when examining the phenomenon of migration, historical, cultural, political, social and economic differences of immigrant and host communities, the impact of the relationships shaped by these differences and of host culture's making sense of the migration process should be taken into account. The phenomenon of migration, which includes individual, interpersonal and intergroup processes, is basically psychological (Dovidio, & Esses, 2001). However, although handled by different disciplines such as anthropology, sociology, economy, politics, history and geography, it is noteworthy that the phenomenon of migration has not been adequately examined in terms of psychology (Berry, 2001 It is asserted that psychology as a discipline can make important contributions to the study of the phenomenon of migration, which includes social psychological factors (Ward, & Masgoret, 2008).

The Aims of the Present Study

In this study, the phenomenon of migration and the post-migration adaptation process are evaluated from a social psychological perspective, specific to Balkan immigrants. In this context, the study was carried out to determine the post-migration adaptation processes of the Balkan immigrants living in Samsun, based on their narratives about the problems brought by migration and the post-migration adaptation process (basic needs, cultural characteristics and acculturation).

METHOD

Participants

The sample of the study consists of Balkan immigrants (Greece, Bulgaria, Yugoslavia and Romania) living in Samsun. Data were collected from 62 participants within the sample. The ages of the participants ranged from 23 to 98 years ($M = 51.17$; $SD = 18.35$). Thirty-three (53.2%) of the participants were women and 29 (46.8%) were men.

The data of the study were obtained through semi-structured interviews that held with each participant individually and face to face. In the interview, a standard interview form consisting of 2 demographic information questions, 30 open-ended questions and 6 multiple-choice questions prepared by the researchers for the purpose of the study was applied to each participant. The interviews lasted an average of 60 minutes. The answers of the participants were noted one-on-one by the researchers using paper and pencil during the interview. The interviews were held in the participants' own homes and in local associations established by Balkan immigrants. Before the interview, each participant was informed about the purpose of the study, and it was informed that their personal information would not be collected and the information obtained would not be used outside of the study. Responses of Balkan immigrants to these themes were included in the analyses. These responses included both the immigrants' own experiences of the migration process and the narratives conveyed to them by their family elders.

Data Analysis

Thematic analysis method, which is one of the qualitative methods, was used in the analysis of the participants' narratives. The multi-stage standardized thematic analysis method proposed by Braun and Clarke (2006) was used in the coding and analysis of the data obtained from the participants as a result of the interviews.

Written notes about the participants' narratives were checked by the researchers for spelling mistakes etc. and than transferred to an electronic text document. The content related to the migration and adaptation process, which is the main problem of the research, has been extracted and compiled in a single document. In the first step after this, the content related to migration has been defined to include narratives about the problems brought by migration and the post-migration adaptation process. Obtained themes were evaluated in the context of topics such as basic needs, cultural characteristics and acculturation. In the second stage of the analysis, the researchers have read the content repeatedly to become familiar with the content on the migration process. In the third stage, the first codes related to the content were determined. These codes, determined by inductive reasoning, were then grouped according to their similarities and similar codes were combined to form overarching themes. Finally, the preliminary themes were examined by the researchers in terms of both internal homogeneity and external heterogeneity (Patton, 2014), and the extent to which the themes were related to the data set as a whole was evaluated. After consensus was reached, the final themes were named and defined.

RESULTS AND DISCUSSION

The adaptation process of the Balkan immigrants, which is the main problem of the study, was evaluated under three main themes based on the answers of the participants. These themes were discussed under the headings of (1) basic needs, (2) cultural characteristics, and (3) acculturation (Figure 1). The basic needs theme includes narratives about economic, sheltering, security and health topics; cultural features theme includes narratives on language, appearance and values topics; the acculturation theme includes narratives on prejudice and integration topics. For each theme, sub-themes were evaluated by making sample quotations under separate headings and supported by the findings of different studies.

Figure 1. Themes about the adaptation process of Balkan immigrants

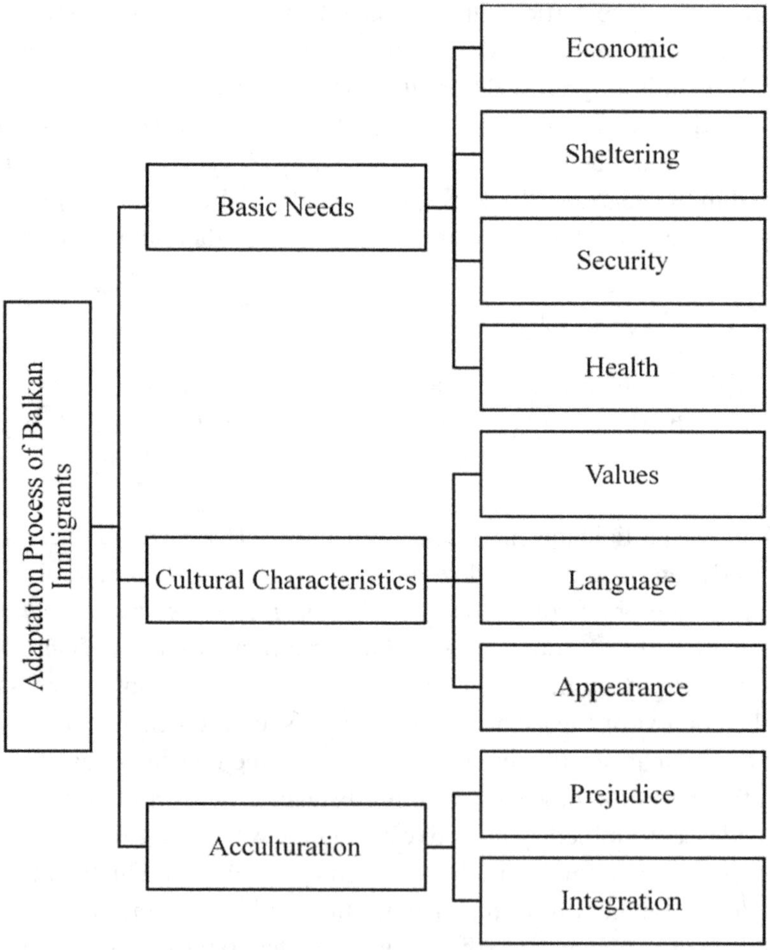

Theme 1: Basic Needs

Theme 1.1: Economic

It is seen that Balkan immigrants mostly evaluate economic needs topic in terms of finding a job, assets and livelihoods. In the narratives of the participants, it is seen that although the vast majority of the immigrants did not experience problems with economic needs after their arrival in Turkey, some of them had problems in this regard.

In the narratives of the participants, who stated that they did not have any problems with the economy, it is noteworthy that they did not have problems in finding a job in Turkey, they were successful in the fields in which they made a living, and if the necessary training was received, job opportunities have emerged where they can work:

Even though they have problems economically, they are generally satisfied (Male, 27 years old).

They had no problems finding a job. They even had set an example because they were more successful in agriculture than the natives. He/she was able to work in any job with the necessary education (Female, 48 years old).

However, in their narratives, some participants state that they experienced economic difficulties due to establishing a new business order, having to leave their assets in the country they came from or having to undersell them:

They had difficulty in finding a job, they had tried to establish their own businesses, and they had lived in poverty from time to time (Male, 50 years old).

When they were a wealthy family in the Balkans, they had left everything behind when they came to Samsun. They had problems because they were engaged in agriculture and the place where they settled was not suitable for this. They had to relocate (Female, age 21).

They had experienced economic difficulties because they left their assets and gave their goods at the expense of nothing in Greece (Male, 39 years old).

When the narratives of the economic needs sub-theme are evaluated as a whole, it is seen that although Balkan immigrants generally did not have problems in finding a job in Turkey, they also sometimes experienced problems due to the facts that they had to leave their assets in the country they come from and tried to establish a new business order. At the same time, to the multiple-choice question asked whether they had a problem in finding a job in Turkey because they are Balkan immigrants, some participants stated that they had problems, but the majority (90.3%) stated that they did not have any problems in finding a job, which supports these narratives. As a matter of fact, a participant's narrative on the topic of economic needs shows that the economic problems experienced stemmed from the difficult conditions the country was in at that time:

What prominent is Turkey's difficult conditions at that time and difficulties that experienced (Male, 62 years old).

When the literature on the topic is examined, besides the monetary aid collected, so that the Balkan immigrants who came to Turkey could cope with the problems related to their economic needs; clothing, blankets, beds, supplies, medical tools, medicines, vehicles for their transportation, tents, shelters, hospitals and soup kitchens were provided and distributed to the immigrants in need (İpek, 2000). Agricultural lands have been allocated to the Balkan immigrants, especially who were engaged in agriculture, so that they could practice agriculture (İpek, 2012). Seeking to make migrants producers, the government has provided seed wheat aid to immigrants by implementing legal regulations regarding seed aid since the first days of mass migration. In addition, farm and harness animals were given by the government, as well as necessary agricultural tools and equipment for the farmer immigrants to work the land. At the same time, capital aid was given to immigrants dealing with trade and art so that they could establish businesses. Aid campaigns were launched throughout the country in this period in order to ensure the contribution of the public as well as the aid from the state budget (Duman, 2009).

Theme 1.2: Sheltering

Sheltering topic is generally discussed by Balkan immigrants in terms of sheltering conditions, health conditions related to sheltering conditions and state aids. Considering the narratives about the sheltering topic, it is seen that there were problems with sheltering right after the migration, but the sheltering problem was resolved by making the necessary regulations and taking the necessary precautions by the state; and sheltering opportunities such as houses were offered to immigrants:

Not my parents, but their parents had suffered a lot. They had stayed in tents until their house was built. Tents had drawn water from the bottom. Many had died. (Female, 81 years old).

Thanks to Atatürk, they had no problems. They came to ready-made houses. (Female, 83 years old).

The state had built new houses. (Female, age 69).

In the literature, it is seen that guesthouses were established by the Hilal-i Ahmar Society (Turkish Red Crescent Society) in order to prevent the Balkan immigrants from experiencing sheltering problems until they were transported to their places of permanent residence and efforts were made to meet the sheltering needs of the immigrants (Arı, 1991). Within the scope of the resettlement policy, the sheltering problems of the immigrants who were placed in regions with low density were tried to be solved by the government. Some of the immigrants were temporarily placed with the local people as guests so that they would not experience sheltering problems (Duman, 2009). In addition, the Ministry of Exchange, Development and Housing provided assistance to immigrants in the repair and construction of residences where they would settle permanently, and despite the difficulties and deficiencies experienced, these aids were largely successful in solving the sheltering problems of immigrants (Erdal, 2006).

Theme 1.3: Security

When the narratives of the Balkan immigrants are examined, it is seen that they did not have problems with security. It is stated that the policies and practices of the president of the time, Gazi Mustafa Kemal Atatürk, regarding immigrants; at the same time, the migration of different nations residing in Turkey to their own countries within the scope of exchange agreements were effective in not experiencing security-related problems:

No one does anything because we are fellow townsmans of Atatür. (Male, 50 years old).

The sending of the Greeks in the settled region to their countries had prevented the problems. Thanks to Atatür. (Female, 83 years old).

It is noteworthy that the security of Balkan immigrants is taken into account to a great extent (Duman, 2009). The "Composite Exchange Commission", which was formed to accompany the migration process and to realize the liquidation of the movable and immovable properties of immigrants, carried out activities to prevent problems related to human rights, life and property safety and to take necessary measures (İpek, 2000). In addition, efforts were made by the Ministry of Exchange, Development and Housing for the protection and security of Balkan immigrants, among other purposes (İpek, 2012).

Theme 1.4: Health

When the narratives of the Balkan immigrants are examined, it is seen that the immigrants include narratives about the various health problems related to sheltering in the process immediately after the migration:

They had stayed in the tent for a while, got sick. The property had remained there. (Female, 69 years old).

Malaria and tuberculosis due to swamp. (Male, age 79).

Health problems of Balkan immigrants in Turkey were also closely dealt with (Duman, 2009). Balkan immigrants were vaccinated against diseases such as dysentery, smallpox and plague by undergoing a health check upon their entry to Turkey. For example, a dispensary was established in Samsun and served to immigrants, doctors were appointed and sent to villages to deal with the treatment of immigrant patients. The Ministry of Settlement has carried out works to send the migrants living in the swamps to more sheltered areas and to drain the swamps (İpek, 2012). Tents were distributed and Turkish bath was allocated for those who were been homeless (İpek, 2000).

It is seen that the narratives of Balkan immigrants about basic needs in the post-migration period are concentrated under the headings of economic, sheltering, security and health needs. Based on these narratives, it can be said that the problems they had experience regarding basic needs were mainly in the fields of economy and sheltering. Balkan immigrants state that their economic situation was very good before they migrated, and that they experienced economic difficulties (poverty) and problems due to economic difficulties after migration. They had to leave their real estates such as housing, workplace and land, large and small cattle, agricultural implements and household goods in the country they migrated from. Considering the narratives about the sheltering topic, it is seen that there were problems with sheltering right after the migration, however, when planning the settlement of the immigrants, both with the Settlement Law enacted by the state and the necessary regulations and measures taken by the state depending on the process, the sheltering problem was resolved and the sheltering facilities such as house etc. were provided to immigrants. As seen in the narratives of the immigrants, although they did not encounter many economic and accommodation difficulties in general, they had faced problems specific to immigration such as having to rearrange their lives and losing their existing livelihoods. The state has provided the necessary assistance in order to ensure that the immigrants were permanently resettled and became producers as soon as possible. Immigrants were settled by considering the climate and living conditions of the places they came from and their previous occupations. While the Balkan immigrants were settled, various aids were given to them and they became producers in a short time (Sarınay, 2011). Until the immigrants were transferred to the regions where they would be settled permanently, they were placed in guesthouses consisting of tents and their basic needs such as sheltering, health and nutrition were tried to be met to a large extent (Arı, 1991).

Theme 2: Cultural Characteristics

Theme 2.1: Language

When the narratives of immigrants about language were examined, it is seen that they focused on their unique speaking styles and the differences in the Turkish used. For instance, one participant stated that he had problems in the first period after immigration due to their unique way of speaking, while another participant stated that she had problems due to the fact that the Turkish she used was Ottoman Turkish:

I had problems in my youth because of the idiosyncratic way of speaking of the exchanged people. (Male, 43 years old).

I did not know the language. My existing Turkish was the old Ottoman Turkish… (Female, 46 years old).

When the literature is examined, although there were dialect differences, Balkan immigrants did not have significant language differences and generally did not experience language problems, since the language they used were Turkish or languages related to Turkish; moreover, it is seen that they used their unique speech styles in their speech and this speech style is perceived by the local people as a sympathetic situation rather than a problem (Sağır, & Aktaş, 2019; Ünal, 2008).

Theme 2.2: Appearance

When the narratives of immigrants about appearance are examined, it is seen that immigrants focus on their clothing styles, skin and eye color. For example, some participants state that they were alienated because of the differences in their dressing styles:

My grandmother had excluded because of her dressing style. (Female, 54 years old).

That they had problems with clothing, that Turkey was conservative when it comes to open dressing… (Female, 22 years old).

Some participants, on the other hand, state that they did not experience any problems due to differences in clothing, or that the problems they experienced due to differences in clothing styles were temporary, and adaptation with the society occurs in the next process:

Initially they were despised for their clothing. But they got used to it later... (Female, 74 years old).

I have not heard that they had many problems in terms of clothing, speech, attitude and behavior... (Male, 62 years old).

One participant states that the problems about appearance stem from issues such as skin color and eye color, and therefore she was stigmatized:

Ha! It's obvious, you're an immigrant, sometimes they say. They say that you are not one of me, even if it is rare and few. Sometimes they consider different from themselves because of the differences in skin and eye color. (Female, 48 years old).

Although it is seen in their narratives that Balkan immigrants occasionally encounter problems arising from differences in appearance, these differences had not always been met with prejudice by the local people. With the accruing of mutual social adaptation in the process, it is seen that these differences did not continue to be a problem. Similarly, it is stated in the literature that although the local people perceived the Balkan immigrants' clothing style and physical characteristics differently, such differences in appearance were not seen as a problem, on the contrary, Balkan immigrants were sympathetically welcomed in the society (Sağır, & Aktaş, 2019).

Theme 2.3: Values

It is seen that the narratives related to the sub-theme of values are handled through value differences and similarities. In the narratives of the participants, it is seen that there were no difference in terms of cultural values; on the contrary, the similarities in cultural values reflected positively on their social relations:

We played together in the neighborhood, we went to the teacher to read the Qur'an together. We used to visit each other easily day and night. There was no distinction as Muhajir or others. (Female, 74 years old).

We are socially integrated, we are no different. (Female, 54 years old).

One participant stated that although there are cultural similarities, there are also differences between their own cultural values and the cultural values of the Turkish society:

Although the cultures are similar, they are not exactly the same. Some of the things that are inherited to us by our grandfathers are not considered important in Turkey. (Female, 21 years old).

It was observed that some participants emphasized values such as modernity, open-mindedness, hard work and reliability as the prominent features of Balkan immigrants:

No. Immigrant women consider themselves to be more modern and more open-minded. That's how the locals look at them too. (Female, age 48).

It is difficult to find people as hardworking and reliable as Balkan Turks. (Male, 41 years old).

The narratives of the Balkan immigrants about cultural characteristics focused on the issues of appearance, language and values. It is noteworthy that Balkan immigrants occasionally encountered various differences and problems arising from these differences with the local people in terms of appearance, language and values in the post-migration process, but in general, they mostly emphasized the similarities in cultural characteristics as well as these differences. The fact that Balkan immigrants had common cultural roots, norms and values with the Turkish society has prevented many problems that may be experienced in the adaptation process (Ünal, 2008).

Theme 3: Acculturation

Theme 3.1: Prejudice

It is seen that Balkan immigrants mostly discussed the topic of prejudice within the framework of narratives such as in-group/out-group, stigmatization, social pressure, discrimination, and isolation. In the narratives of the participants, it is seen that although the vast majority of immigrants did not experience problems with prejudice after their arrival in Turkey, some of them had problems in this regard.

In the narratives of the participants, who stated that they did not have a problem with prejudice, it is seen that they were not exposed to discrimination thanks to the shared values and positive social interactions with the Turkish society; although they experienced exclusion at the beginning of the process after immigration, adaptation with Turkish society was achieved and the initial prejudices disappeared:

We played together in the neighborhood, we went to the teacher to read the Qur'an together. We used to visit each other easily day and night. There was no distinction as Muhajir or others. (Female, 74 years old).

They had not experience any problems because they came in collectively. (Female, 98 years).

First they had been excluded, then they had been relieved. (Female, 47 years).

The people around them had excluded them, they had not accept them. However, the process of adaptation has gradually started. (Female, 48 years old).

Some participants, who stated that there were mutual problems between Balkan immigrants and Turkish society on topics such as in-group/out-group, stigmatization, social pressure, discrimination and isolation, stated the following in their narratives:

My mother and grandmother had been excluded, they had saw them as strangers. Immigrants also call other people 'native' and separate them. (Female, age 54).

People in Samsun had said 'lousy immigrants', sometimes. (Female, 98 years old).

Because I am an immigrant, I am happy that my son has wived an immigrant bride. I would prefer my bride to be an immigrant. (Female, 74 years old).

I had went to welcome a neighbor. I felt that an old woman who was there was a Muhajir and I asked her if she was a Muhajir. When I got the answer yes, I felt closer to her, I made friends with her more quickly and talked to her more often in the following processes. (Female, 74 years old).

I am sometimes exposed to prejudiced sentences such as no girls can be taken from exchanges, they talk a lot. (Female, 21 years old).*

That people in Turkey see the newcomers as a separate society. (Male, 51 years old).

We were defined as giaours. They did not accept that we are Turkish. (Female, age 46).

We are addressed as Bulgarians. (Male, 27 years old).

They had felt alone. They only had communicated with Balkan immigrants. (Female, 48 years old).

It is difficult to find people as hardworking and reliable as Balkan Turks. (Male, 41 years old).

When the narratives on the theme of prejudice are evaluated as a whole, it is seen that Balkan immigrants did not always have problems about the topics associated with the theme of prejudice (such as in-group/out-group, stigmatization, social pressure, discrimination, isolation), but some participants sometimes had problems about these topics. At the same time, to the multiple-choice question asked whether they were exposed to discriminatory behavior in Turkey because they were Balkan immigrants, some participants stated that they had problems, but the majority (87.1%) stated that they were not exposed to discriminatory behaviors. Another multiple-choice question asked to the participants, who stated that they were not exposed to discrimination and prejudiced behaviors, to determine their evaluations about the reasons for this; having the same religion (77.4%), speaking the same language (72.6%), cultural similarities (66.1%), having the same nationality (62.9%), similarity in customs and traditions (50.0%), similarity in clothing (46.8%) answers are given. Based on all these, although it is seen that Balkan immigrants were exposed to prejudice and discrimination from time to time, it can be said that these similarities were an important factor in preventing prejudice and discrimination from being a general attitude towards them.

In the literature, international migrations are generally associated with prejudice (Çakırer Özservet, & Yurtsever, 2017). It is stated that these prejudices are generally caused by differences in religious beliefs, spoken language, traditions, cultural values, clothing and appearance observed between immigrants and the society they migrate to; depending on the prejudices, immigrants are seen as the cause of unemployment, crimes and diseases (Castles, & Miller, 2008). In different countries, it is seen that the host society exhibits negative attitudes towards immigrants and immigration (Facchini, & Mayda, 2008). However, regarding Balkan immigrants, it is seen that there was a positive perspective towards immigrants in the evaluations of Balkan immigrants in the national newspapers of the period in Turkey (Ulus Gazetesi, 1938). For example, the following statements made by Suphi Tanrıöver, the Turkish

Ambassador of Bucharest at the time, to the local press summarize the Turkish government's positive attitude towards Balkan immigrants:

...Tall, broad-shouldered and straight-headed, you sense the incomprehensible force of the great storm powers that come from the middle of Asia. Very welcoming, never lies. His/her skin is white, forehead is light and has mostly hazel eyes. Not frowning at all. When smiles, his/her white pearl teeth attract the heart. Is thrifty, but never stingy. Eats well, dresses well and lives well. Naturally passionate about music, reading and fine arts. In love with nature and homeland. Very attached to his/her home...(Eren, 1936).

Based on these evaluations reflected in the press, it can be said that positive attitudes and policies towards Balkan immigrants were also reflected in the public, and thus positive attitudes towards Balkan immigrants were developed and played a positive role in the integration process for immigrants.

Theme 3.2: Integration

It is seen that Balkan immigrants mostly deal with the integration topic through issues such as belonging, state policies, adaptation motivation of immigrants, social contact and cooperation. In the narratives of the participants about integration, it is seen that the vast majority of immigrants strove to adapt to the Turkish society, they had social contact with the Turkish society by mutual positive interactions, their sense of belonging to the Turkish homeland and society was high, and state policies facilitated the adaptation process.

It is seen that Balkan immigrants made an effort to adapt to Turkish society and culture in the post-migration process:

My grandmother, had dressed like them. They made themselves loved by keeping their neighborly relations closer. My grandmother and mother were described as being generous people. (Female, age 54).

They had made a change in clothing. By observing people living in Turkey, they had tried to be like them. (Male, 27 years old).

By paying attention to and observing their every behavior, by following whatever shameful thing is seen. (Female, 46 years old).

I preserved the language characteristics in the conversations between the exchanges, but I took care not to use such words in different communities. (Male, 43 years old).

They took off the abayas (veil) and started to dress like the locals. (Female, 74 years old).

They had changed their clothing, dressed like the people around them. Of course not right away. By sharing more what they eat and drink, by sharing the products they planted and produced, grains, local dishes, etc., they had tried to establish a close relationship. (Female, age 48).

These adaptation efforts have brought social interactions between Turkish society and Balkan immigrants, and this is also seen in the social contact narratives of the participants:

We played together in the neighborhood, we went to the teacher to read the Qur'an together. We used to visit each other easily day and night. There was no distinction as Muhajir or other. (Female, 74 years old).

In the beginning, they were despised because of their clothing (because they wore a black abaya). However, they got used to it later, and they had given and taken girls (intermarry). (Female, 74 years old).

It is noteworthy that in the narratives of the Balkan immigrants, they felt that they belonged to the Turkish homeland and society and that they saw themselves in their own homeland:

There is no problem in the homeland" (Male, 50 years old).

I was born into this society, I was like them. I did not feel any difference. (Female, 48 years).

I don't feel like an immigrant or an exchanger. I am a citizen of Turkish Republic, I am a Muslim-Turk. (Female, age 54).

In the process of social adaptation between Balkan immigrants and Turkish society, it is seen that another important factor in ensuring the positive interactions mentioned above was the state policies that support the provision of cohesion, and state policies that adopt the immigrants are expressed as follows in the narratives of the participants:

The state had built new houses. (Female, 69 years old).

No. Each family was given fields according to their number" (Male, 84 years old).

No, we didn't. We built our house ourselves. The state gave as much land in Turkey as they has in Greece. (Female, 98 years).

When the narratives of the Balkan immigrants are evaluated as a whole, it is seen that both the efforts made by them to ensure adaptation and the implementation of policies supporting the adaptation process by the state facilitate the integration of immigrants. In the integration process, it is also thought that social contact between immigrants and Turkish society and the immigrants' feeling of belonging to the Turkish society and homeland played an important role.

In addition, when the answers given by the participants to the multiple-choice question about whether they could adapt to social life in Turkey are examined, it is seen that the vast majority of Balkan immigrants (87.1%) did not have problems in adapting to social life in Turkey. To another multiple-choice question asked about the reasons why they did not have problems in adapting to social life in Turkey; participants had given answers of speaking the same language (80.6%), having the same religion (77.4%), having the same nationality (74.2%), cultural similarities (69.4%), similarity in clothing (56.5%) and similarity in customs and traditions (54.8%). Based on all these, it can be said that although Balkan immigrants sometimes experienced social adaptation problems, these similarities were an important factor in facilitating social adaptation.

At the same time, when the answers given to the multiple-choice question asked to the participants about how they define their social identities are examined, it is seen that the majority of Balkan immigrants (83.9%) identified themselves as a Turkish Republic citizen. Other social identity definitions are followed as exchanged (71.0%), Muslim-Turkish (40.3%), Balkan Turk (19.4%), muhajir (12.9%) and immigrant (6.5%), respectively. When evaluated in terms of social identity, it is noteworthy that Balkan immigrants did not have problems with social adaptation in terms of social identity definitions.

The following narrative of a participant summarizes the fact that Balkan immigrants did not face prejudice and discrimination in Turkey, as they show great similarities with Turkish society in terms of their culture and social identities, and that they did not have problems in social adaptation:

I married with a Balkan immigrant woman. I never thought about whether she was a Muhajir or not, I did not have a problem. The people around me did not criticize me about it. Culturally, we were very similar. Cultural differences did not bother me. Even their food cultures, invitation cultures, hospitalities, strong family ties, and etc. were among the factors that affected me a lot. In addition, these people were hardworking and self-sacrificing people. They were generally smiling, calm and cheerful people. Neighborhood relations were very good. My wife's relatives did not want her to marry me because I am not an immigrant. We did not have any cultural problems in marriage. I lived and live a happy life with my wife. We lived a happy life for 54 years… (Married to an immigrant woman, 76 years old male, university graduate, retired teacher).

Acculturation refers to a multidimensional process, including physical, psychological, social, economic, language and family adaptation (Mui, & Kang, 2006). It is stated that immigrants' adaptation to the culture of the society they migrate to without breaking away from their own culture and the integration strategy determined by the host country for immigrants has an important role in ensuring integration (Akıncı, Nergiz, & Gedik, 2015). On the other hand, facing different cultural norms can cause acculturation stress (Berry, 2006b; Oh, Koeske, & Sales, 2002).

According to Berry (2006a), acculturation strategies include attitudes and behaviors that emerge when individuals from different cultures come together. Acculturation strategies may include immigrants' contact with the dominant cultural group or their attitudes and behaviors to increase cultural similarity, as well as avoiding contact with the dominant cultural group or maintaining cultural differences. Therefore, these strategies consist of all positive or negative psychological reactions of immigrants towards the new dominant culture.

The acculturation process can be shaped in four different ways depending on different strategies for non-dominant ethnocultural groups. The first of these, assimilation, defines individuals' unwillingness to maintain their cultural identity and not seeking daily interaction with other cultures. In contrast, the separation strategy refers to individuals avoiding interaction with others, despite remaining loyal to their original culture. The integration strategy describes the desire of individuals both to maintain their own unique culture and to engage in daily interactions with other groups. Integration refers to individuals' trying to be an integral part of a larger social network as a member of an ethnocultural group, while maintaining a degree of cultural integrity. Finally, the marginalization strategy states that individuals are less likely to preserve their culture and are not interested in establishing relationships with others (Berry, 2006a; Van Oudenhoven, Ward, & Masgoret, 2006). These strategies vary depending on whether migration is forced or not, how the migration is experienced, and the time elapsed since migration (Yeh, 2003; Berry, Kim, Minde, & Mok, 1987).

The acculturation process can be shaped in four different ways for dominant cultures too, depending on different strategies. In the assimilation strategy, dominant groups may try to impose their own culture.

In a separation strategy, the dominant group may allow minority groups to preserve their culture, but may not want to interact with them. The marginalization strategy, on the other hand, may emerge as a form of exclusion imposed by the dominant group. Finally, integration represents the caring about of cultural diversity by the society and a strategy of mutual adaptation (Berry, 2006a).

Along with these social factors, many psychological variables can also be effective in the acculturation process. For example, before cultural contact, individuals' prior knowledge of a new language and culture, previous experiences of intercultural encounters, their motivation for cultural contact (voluntary or involuntary contact), attitudes towards acculturation (positive or negative), education and employment levels, values and self-esteem are important factors that determine how individuals under acculturation pressures will respond to the acculturation process (Williams, & Berry, 1991).

Studies show that immigrants may experience acculturation stress due to language problems, lack of employment opportunities, and difficulties with education, which negatively affects the integration process (Joyce, & Liamputtong, 2017). It is stated that communication skills, motivation to learn a new language and the capacity to acquire the social skills necessary to integrate with a new language are important in the integration process of immigrants (Hernandez, 2009). Language skills play an important role in for immigrants in establishing interpersonal relationships in the country they migrate to, as they affect the quality and quantity of intercultural interactions (Masgoret, & Ward, 2006).

Social psychological approaches to language communication assume a relationship between second language proficiency/use and social identity. It is seen that social contact and the ability of immigrants to use the language of the country they migrate to play an important role in both identity changes that occur in immigrants and the host society, and social adaptation (Clément, Noels, & Deneault, 2001).

Socio-cultural adaptation requires immigrants not only to be proficient in language, basic communication and social interaction skills, but also to adapt to the new environment, norms, values and worldviews (Masgoret, & Ward, 2006). Sociocultural adaptation is affected by the time spent in a new culture, cultural similarities and differences, host-immigrant relations and acculturation strategies. It is stated that this situation is compatible with research findings that evaluate the cross-cultural transition based on the culture learning approach and reveal the importance of cultural differences (Ward, & Kennedy, 1993). Cultural learning theory also focuses on social inadequacies rather than psychological inadequacies during cultural contact and change (Ward, 1997).

Social support that immigrants receive from their friends, family, ethnic groups, and wider regional communities helps them to cope with acculturation stress (Joyce, & Liamputtong, 2017). Therefore, social support systems are of vital importance in the acculturation process (Batista-Pinto Wiese, 2010).

One of the important factors affecting the social adaptation process of immigrants is the attitudes of the host society towards the phenomenon of migration and immigrants (Bauloz, Vathi, & Acosta, 2019). As adaptation of immigrant individuals to the basic characteristics of the host society, the fact that the host society accepts immigrants, contacts them and builds schools and hospitals for them, encourages the host society to contact immigrants by using education or similar channels, also positively affects the acculturation and adaptation processes of minority group members (Saygın, & Patient, 2018).

Successful integration of immigrants into the society they live in is closely related to how both immigrants and the host society position themselves within the social identity pattern. The full realization of socio-psychological integration depends on the immigrants creating an identity in which they can balance the requirements of adaptation to the society they migrated to (Türker, & Yıldız, 2015). Based on the social identity theory (Tajfel, & Turner, 1979), Hurtado and colleagues states that the post-migration adaptation process depends on the clarity of group boundaries between immigrants and members of the host society, social classifications, in-group and inter-group contact, communication, competition, cooperation, and social comparisons. Economic conditions, government policies and demographic distribution determine how these factors will affect the adaptation process (Hurtado, Gurin, & Peng, 1994).

When evaluated in general, it is seen that the post-migration adaptation processes of immigrants are evaluated as a three-dimensional process related to each other. Post-migration adaptation first refers to a legal process involving the granting of rights and entitlements to immigrants by the host state. This legal process includes the right of immigrants to seek employment, engage in other income-generating activities, receive education, ownership and disposal of property, enjoy freedom of movement and access such public services. Integration is also considered as an economic process. As migrants acquire legal rights and authorizations, they also develop their economic potential, such as creating sustainable livelihoods, achieving self-sufficiency, and becoming less and less dependent on government or humanitarian aid. Accordingly, the fact that there are barriers to participation in the local economy and that their living standards are permanently lower than that of the poorest members of the host society indicate that integration has not been achieved for immigrants. Finally, post-migration adaptation is a social process in which there is no systematic discrimination by the authorities or citizens of the host country, and where migrants can live in or next to the host population without fear of intimidation or exploitation. Therefore, this process includes both immigrants and the host society (Crisp, 2004).

When the adaptation process of Balkan immigrants in Turkey is evaluated by considering these criteria; with the Turkish state implementing the Settlement Law in order to ensure the adaptation process of Balkan migrants, it is seen that basic rights are provided to Balkan migrants without separating them from their own citizens by making legal arrangements on issues such as finding jobs, acquiring property and granting them educational freedoms. While the Turkish state offers opportunities such as finding a job, acquiring property, and getting education, it has made legal regulations regarding the adaptation process of Balkan immigrants both as a state and through aid organizations and has put these regulations into practice at the local and national level.

These practices, which can be considered as an indicator that the Turkish state does not separate Balkan immigrants from its own citizens, had played an important role in the realization of the adaptation process of Balkan immigrants with the host society. The economic aids made by the Turkish government to the Balkan immigrants also had facilitated the adaptation process. Within the framework of the said economic aid, the state had provided the immigrants with houses for their sheltering and agricultural land, animals and seeds to earn their livelihood. In the literature, it is stated that the success of immigrants in the fields of education and work in the country they migrated to is an indicator that they can adapt to the culture of the society they migrated to (Nguyen, & Benet-Martinez, 2013).

At the same time, the post-migration adaptation process can also be evaluated in terms of frustration-aggression theory. As is known, according to the frustration-aggression theory (Dollard, Doob, Miller, Mowrer, & Sears, 1939), aggressive behaviors emerge as a result of frustration. In their study, Wilson and Magam (2018) also determined that disappointments resulting from frustration can turn into hostility towards foreign nationals, based on the explanations of the frustration-aggression theory. As these explanations show, the fact that both the members of the host society and the immigrants encounter various obstacles can cause interpersonal conflicts and aggressive behaviors. However, it is seen that both the Balkan immigrants and the Turkish society were mostly not hindered due to immigration, and therefore, aggressive behaviors did not occur. Therefore, it is seen that the Balkan immigrants mostly did not experience frustrations in terms of basic needs such as economic, sheltering, health and security, as well as cultural similarities and acculturation, and thus, they did not experience problems with social adaptation. In this case, it can be stated that both social and economic aid and support provided by the Turkish state to Balkan immigrants were effective.

At the same time, the Turkish state used positive expressions towards Balkan immigrants in its oral and written statements in order to facilitate the post-migration adaptation process and contributed to the development of positive attitudes towards Balkan immigrants in the public. The Turkish society also adopted the positive statements of the state towards Balkan immigrants, had positive interpersonal relations with the Balkan immigrants who came to their country, and did not prejudice or discriminate against them.

On the other hand, when the relevant literature is examined, it is stated that obstacles may develop in ensuring social adaptation between immigrants and host societies due to reasons such as religious belief differences, and the host society may perceive immigrants as a threat (Kaufmann, 2017). Studies on this subject show that immigrants encounter identity threats while trying to adapt to a new culture and give different coping responses to these threats (Timotijevic, & Breakwell, 2000). However, it clearly shows that this is not the case for the Balkan immigrants who migrated to Turkey. The absence of religious belief differences between the Balkan immigrants and the Turkish society and the high cultural similarities had facilitated the adaptation process.

At the same time, factors such as not having communication problems because they speak the same language, having similar values, not seeing their own identity as different from the host identity, having a high sense of belonging, seeing themselves as an in-group, positive social contact, social assistance, absence of mutually stigmatizations, not encountering negative behaviors such as prejudice and discrimination also affected the adaptation of Balkan immigrants to Turkish society.

At the same time, it can be said that the absence of mutual prejudices and discriminatory behaviors is mostly effective in the realization of adaptation between Balkan immigrants and Turkish society. As it is known, differences between communities with different cultures in ethnicity, appearance, religious belief, culture, etc. can lead to prejudices against external groups and consequently discriminatory behaviors (Aronson, Wilson, & Akert, 2010; Hogg, & Vaughan, 2018; Kağıtçıbaşı, & Cemalcılar, 2014). However, social contact theories reveal that contact between groups with differences can be effective in reducing prejudice and discrimination (Küçükkömürler, & Sakallı-Uğurlu, 2017). However, social contact between these groups does not always lead to the complete elimination of prejudices and discriminatory behaviors. The basic conditions put forward by Allport (1954) for social contact to reduce prejudice include equality of status between groups, cooperation between groups towards a common goal, and state support for intergroup contact. When evaluated from this point of view, in the social contact between Balkan immigrants and Turkish society, it is seen that these basic conditions could be met to a great extent. As seen in the narratives of Balkan immigrants, the absence of social adaptation problems mostly between Balkan immigrants and Turkish society can be considered as an indicator of this.

CONCLUSION

As in every migration process, it is seen that the migration from the Balkans to Turkey has some unique features. These features, which distinguish different migrations from each other, highlight the spirit of the time when the migration took place. In other words, in order to fully understand a migration process in terms of social sciences and especially social psychology, it is clear that the circumstances such as historical, political, economic, social, etc. must be taken into account. In this context, it is seen that the spirit of the time (zeitgeist) of immigration is clearly included in the narratives of immigrants. Therefore, depending on the spirit of the time, it turns out that just as each migration process has its own unique narrative, as well as migrants who experience the same migration process can have different narratives. Every different narrative about migration has a unique value in revealing the truth about migration. From this point of view, beyond the "numbers" or "percentages" of immigrants moving from one country to another, it can be thought that they are the main heroes who directly experience the problems brought by migration or the adaptation process after it, and that they are beacons that shed light on the truth about the migration process with their sincere narratives about the process.

In this study, the narratives of Balkan immigrants are discussed within the framework of basic needs, cultural characteristics and acculturation themes. These themes were evaluated within the framework of topics such as economy, sheltering, health, spoken language, traditions-customs, religious belief, prejudice, discrimination, in-group/out-group, social cooperation, and social contact. All these evaluations were examined from a social psychological perspective, based on both the immigrants' own experiences of the migration process and the narratives conveyed to them by their family elders. As a result, it has been seen that there were mostly no problems in the adaptation processes of Balkan immigrants, relatively different from other migration processes, with the effect of features such as cultural similarities, sense of belonging, empathy and cooperation. At the same time, these results reveal that governments, public institutions and organizations, non-governmental organizations, the press and social media have important duties and responsibilities in the adaptation process of immigrants.

In this study, the adaptation processes of Balkan immigrants were evaluated within the framework of basic needs, cultural characteristics and acculturation. In other studies to be carried out on this issue, an interdisciplinary examination of Balkan immigrants within the framework of different themes will enrich the literature. Likewise, similar studies to be carried out in different cultures will contribute to the understanding of the post-migration adaptation process. In addition, by using qualitative methods in studies that will deal with migration and integration issues, the meaning of migration and integration processes for immigrants will be discovered in all their aspects.

REFERENCES

Akıncı, B., Nergiz, A., & Gedik, E. (2015). An assesment on process of adaptation: Migration and social acceptance [Uyum süreci üzerine bir değerlendirme: Göç ve toplumsal kabul]. *Göç Araştırmaları Dergisi, 1*(2), 58–83.

Aksoy, E. (2016). Turkey's population structure and policies after World War I (1919-1955) [1919-1955 yılları arasında Türkiye'nin nüfus yapısı ve uygulanan nüfus politikaları]. *Hacettepe Üniversitesi Türkiyat Araştırmaları Dergisi, 24*, 27–44.

Allport, G. W. (1954). *The nature of prejudice*. Addison-Wesley.

Appave, G., & David, I. (2017). Integration that values diversity - exploring a model for current migration dynamics. In M. McAuliffe & M. Klein Solomon (Eds.), *Migration research leaders' syndicate: Ideas to inform international cooperation on safe, orderly and regular migration* (pp. 151–158). International Organization for Migration.

Arı, K. (1991). The problem of transporting exchange immigrants to Turkey and the immigrants of Izmir (1923-1924) [Mübadele göçmenlerini Türkiye'ye taşıma sorunu ve İzmir göçmenleri (1923-1924)]. *Çağdaş Türkiye Tarihi Araştırmaları Dergisi, 1*(1), 13-46.

Aronson, E., Wilson, T. D., & Akert, R. M. (2010). *Social psychology* (7th ed.). Pearson Prentice Hall.

Batista-Pinto Wiese, E. (2010). Culture and migration: Psychological trauma in children and adolescents. *Traumatology, 16*(4), 142–152. doi:10.1177/1534765610388304

Bauloz, C., Vathi, Z., & Acosta, D. (2019). Migration, inclusion and social cohesion: Challenges, recent developments and opportunities. In M. McAuliffe & B. Khadria (Eds.), *World Migration Report 2020* (pp. 185–206). International Organization for Migration.

Berry, J. W. (2001). A psychology of immigration. *The Journal of Social Issues, 57*(3), 615–631. doi:10.1111/0022-4537.00231

Berry, J. W. (2006a). Contexts of acculturation. In D. L. Sam & J. W. Berry (Eds.), *The Cambridge handbook of acculturation psychology* (pp. 27–42). Cambridge University Press. doi:10.1017/CBO9780511489891.006

Berry, J. W. (2006b). Stress perspectives on acculturation. In D. L. Sam & J. W. Berry (Eds.), *The Cambridge handbook of acculturation psychology* (pp. 43–57). Cambridge University Press. doi:10.1017/CBO9780511489891.007

Berry, J. W. (2009). Living together in culturally-plural societies: Understanding and managing acculturation and multiculturalism. In S. Bekman & A. Aksu-Koç (Eds.), *Perspectives on human development, family, and culture* (pp. 227–240). Cambridge University Press. doi:10.1017/CBO9780511720437.017

Berry, J. W. (2020). How shall we all live together? In S. Safdar, C. Kwantes, & W. Friedlmeier (Eds.), *Wiser world with multiculturalism: Proceedings from the 24th Congress of the International Association for Cross-Cultural Psychology.* Retrieved from https://scholarworks.gvsu.edu/iaccp_papers/284

Berry, J. W., Kim, U., Minde, T., & Mok, D. (1987). Comparative studies of acculturative stress. *The International Migration Review, 21*(3), 491–511. doi:10.1177/019791838702100303

Berry, J. W., Phinney, J. S., Sam, D. L., & Vedder, P. (2006). Immigrant youth: Acculturation, identity, and adaptation. *Applied Psychology, 55*(3), 303–332. doi:10.1111/j.1464-0597.2006.00256.x

Braun, V., & Clarke, V. (2006). Using thematic analysis in psychology. *Qualitative Research in Psychology, 3*(2), 77–101. doi:10.1191/1478088706qp063oa

Cabassa, L. J. (2003). Measuring acculturation: Where we are and where we need to go. *Hispanic Journal of Behavioral Sciences, 25*(2), 127–146. doi:10.1177/0739986303025002001

Çakırer Özservet, Y., & Yurtsever, B. (2017). *Research on prejudice against immigrants.* (International Migration and Social Cohesion Research Series: 1) [*Göçmenlere yönelik önyargı araştırması.* (Uluslararası Göç ve Toplumsal Uyum Araştırmaları Serisi: 1)]. İstanbul: Marmara Üniversitesi Kent sorunları ve Yerel Yönetimler Uygulama ve Araştırma Merkezi. Retrieved from https://www.researchgate.net/publication/324834708_Gocmenlere_ Yonelik_Onyargi_Arastirmasi

Castles, S., & Miller, J. M. (2008). *The age of migrations, international migration movements in the modern world* [Göçler çağı, modern dünyada uluslararası göç hareketleri]. İstanbul Bilgi Üniversitesi.

Clément, R., Noels, K. A., & Deneault, B. (2001). Interethnic contact, identity, and psychological adjustment: The mediating and moderating roles of communication. *The Journal of Social Issues, 57*(3), 559–577. doi:10.1111/0022-4537.00229

Crisp, J. (2004). *The local integration and local settlement of refugees: A conceptual and historical analysis* (New Issues in Refugee Research Working Paper No. 102). United Nations High Commissioner for Refugees.

Dollard, J., Doob, L., Miller, N., Mowrer, O., & Sears, R. (1939). *Frustration and aggression.* Yale University Press. doi:10.1037/10022-000

Dovidio, J. F., & Esses, V. M. (2001). Immigrants and immigration: Advancing the psychological perspective. *The Journal of Social Issues, 57*(3), 375–387. doi:10.1111/0022-4537.00219

Duman, Ö. (2009). The settlement efforts of Balkan immigrants in Atatürk's era (1923-1938) [Atatürk döneminde Balkan göçmenlerinin iskân çalışmaları (1923-1938)]. *Ankara Üniversitesi Türk İnkılâp Tarihi Enstitüsü Atatürk Yolu Dergisi, 11*(43), 473–490. doi:10.1501/Tite_0000000299

Erdal, İ. (2006). Aid activities for Turk emigrant in Turkish-Greece exchange of population. [Türk Yunan nüfus değişiminde Türk mübadillere yapılan yardım faaliyetleri]. *Tarih Araştırmaları Dergisi, 25*(40), 203–214. doi:10.1501/Tarar_0000000255

Eren, A. A. (1936, October 14). What will immigration policy bring to the country? [Göç politikası memlekete neler kazandıracaktır?]. *Tan Gazetesi*, p. 5. Retrieved from https://www.gastearsivi.com/gazete/tan/1936-10-14/5

Facchini, G., & Mayda, A. M. (2008). From individual attitudes towards migrants to migration policy outcomes: Theory and evidence. *Economic Policy, 23*(56), 651–713. doi:10.1111/j.1468-0327.2008.00212.x

Gemicibasi, U., & Yilmaz, R. (2021). Meta-narrative of immigration: A study on migration and the presentation of immigration in Fatih Akin's films. In R. Yilmaz (Ed.), *Handbook of research on narrative interactions* (pp. 63–85). IGI Global. doi:10.4018/978-1-7998-4903-2.ch005

Geray, C. (1962). *Migration and resettlement of immigrants from and to Turkey (1923-1961), Turkish Economic Development Research Project* [Türkiye'den ve Türkiye'ye göçler ve göçmenlerin iskanı (1923-1961), Türk İktisadi Gelişmesi Araştırma Projesi]. Siyasal Bilimler Fakültesi Maliye Enstitüsü.

Goodman, S. (2010). Integration requirements for integration's sake: Identifying, categorising and comparing civic integration policies. *Journal of Ethnic and Migration Studies, 36*(5), 753–772. doi:10.1080/13691831003764300

Hernandez, M. Y. (2009). Psychological theories of immigration. *Journal of Human Behavior in the Social Environment, 19*(6), 713–729. doi:10.1080/10911350902910898

Hogg, M. A., & Vaughan, G. M. (2018). *Social psychology* (8th ed.). Pearson.

Hurtado, A., Gurin, P., & Peng, T. (1994). Social identities-A framework for studying the adaptations of immigrants and ethnics: The adaptations of Mexicans in the United States. *Social Problems*, *41*(1), 129–151. doi:10.2307/3096846

İçişleri Bakanlığı, Müdürlüğü, Politika, & Başkanlığı. (2017). *2016 Turkey migration report* [2016 Türkiye göç raporu] (Publication No. 40). Retrieved from https://www.goc.gov.tr/kurumlar/goc.gov.tr/YillikGocRaporlari/2016_yiik_goc_raporu_haziran.pdf

İpek, N. (2000). *Exchange and Samsun* [Mübadele ve Samsun]. Türk Tarih Kurumu.

İpek, N. (2012). *Exchanged people from Thessaloniki to Samsun* [Selanik'ten Samsun'a mübadiller] (2nd ed.). Samsun Büyükşehir Belediyesi, Kültür ve Sosyal İşler Daire Başkanlığı.

Joyce, L., & Liamputtong, P. (2017). Acculturation stress and social support for young refugees in regional areas. *Children and Youth Services Review*, *77*, 18–26. doi:10.1016/j.childyouth.2017.03.016

Kağıtçıbaşı, Ç., & Cemalcılar, Z. (2014). *Human and people from past to present: Introduction to social psychology* [Dünden bugüne insan ve insanlar: Sosyal psikolojiye giriş] (16th ed.). Evrim.

Kaufmann, E. (2017). Why values, not economics, hold the key to the populist right-and to crafting new migration narratives. In M. McAuliffe & M. Klein Solomon (Eds.), *Migration research leaders' syndicate: Ideas to inform international cooperation on safe, orderly and regular migration* (pp. 183–188). International Organization for Migration.

Küçükkömürler, S., & Sakallı-Uğurlu, N. (2017). Social contact theories to regulate intergroup relations: Intergroup, extended, imagined contact [Gruplar arası ilişkileri düzenlemede sosyal temas kuramları: Gruplar arası, yayılmacı ve hayali temas]. *Nesne Psikoloji Dergisi*, *9*(5), 1–31. doi:10.7816/nesne-05-09-01

Landau, L. B. (2017). Southern urbanism, legalization, and the limits of migration law. In M. McAuliffe & M. Klein Solomon (Eds.), *Migration research leaders' syndicate: Ideas to inform international cooperation on safe, orderly and regular migration* (pp. 33–36). International Organization for Migration. doi:10.1017/aju.2017.39

Masgoret, A. M., & Ward, C. (2006). Culture learning approach to acculturation. In D. L. Sam & J. W. Berry (Eds.), *The Cambridge handbook of acculturation psychology* (pp. 58–77). Cambridge University Press. doi:10.1017/CBO9780511489891.008

Mbaye, L. (2017). Supporting communities under migration pressure: the role of opportunities, information and resilience to shocks. In M. McAuliffe & M. Klein Solomon (Eds.), *Migration research leaders' syndicate: Ideas to inform international cooperation on safe, orderly and regular migration* (pp. 91–96). International Organization for Migration.

McAuliffe, M., & Triandafyllidou, A. (Eds.). (2021). *World migration report 2022*. International Organization for Migration.

Mui, A. C., & Kang, S. Y. (2006). Acculturation stress and depression among Asian immigrant elders. *Social Work*, *51*(3), 243–255. doi:10.1093w/51.3.243 PMID:17076122

Nguyen, A. M., & Benet-Martinez, V. (2013). Biculturalism and Adjustment: A Meta-analysis. *Journal of Cross-Cultural Psychology*, *44*(1), 122–159. doi:10.1177/0022022111435097

Oh, Y., Koeske, G. F., & Sales, E. (2002). Acculturation, stress, and depressive symptoms among Korean immigrants in the United States. *The Journal of Social Psychology, 142*(4), 511–526. doi:10.1080/00224540209603915 PMID:12153126

Patton, M. Q. (2014). *Qualitative research & evaluation methods: Integrating theory and practice* (4th ed.). Sage.

Sağır, A., & Aktaş, Z. (2019). The sociological analysis of the relationship between Turkish immigrants from Romania and the Turkish community: The period of 1934-1938 in the Turkish newspapers [Romanya'dan Türkiye'ye gelen göçmenlerle Türk toplumu arasındaki ilişkinin sosyolojik çözümlemesi: Türk yazılı basınında 1934-1938 dönemi]. *Atatürk Araştırma Merkezi Dergisi, 35*(1), 141–214.

Sam, D. L. (2006). Acculturation: Conceptual background and core components. In D. L. Sam & J. W. Berry (Eds.), *The Cambridge handbook of acculturation psychology* (pp. 11–26). Cambridge University Press. doi:10.1017/CBO9780511489891.005

Sam, D. L., & Berry, J. W. (2006). Introduction. In D. L. Sam & J. W. Berry (Eds.), *The Cambridge handbook of acculturation psychology* (pp. 1–7). Cambridge University Press. doi:10.1017/CBO9780511489891.003

Sam, D. L., & Berry, J. W. (2010). Acculturation: When individuals and groups of different cultural backgrounds meet. *Perspectives on Psychological Science, 5*(4), 472–481. doi:10.1177/1745691610373075 PMID:26162193

Sarınay, Y. (2011). Migrations from the Balkan countries to Ankara during the republican period (1923-1990) [Cumhuriyet döneminde Balkan ülkelerinden Ankara'ya yapılan göçler (1923-1990)]. *Atatürk Araştırma Merkezi Dergisi, 27*(80), 351–388.

Saygın, S., & Hasta, D. (2018). Migration, acculturation and adaptation [Göç, kültürleşme ve uyum]. *Psikiyatride Güncel Yaklasimlar, 10*(3), 312–333. doi:10.18863/pgy.364115

Tajfel, H., & Turner, J. C. (1979). An integrative theory of intergroup conflict. In W. Austin, & S. Worchel (Eds.), The social psychology of intergroup relations (pp. 33-48). Brooks/Cole.

The UN Refugee Agency. (2021). *Figures at a glance*. Retrieved February 18, 2022, from https://www.unhcr.org/en-us/figures-at-a-glance.html

Timotijevic, L., & Breakwell, G. M. (2000). Migration and threat to identity. *Journal of Community & Applied Social Psychology, 10*(5), 355–372. doi:10.1002/1099-1298(200009/10)10:5<355::AID-CASP594>3.0.CO;2-Y

Türker, D., & Yıldız, A. (2015). Socio-psychological integration analysis of immigrants [Göçmenlerde sosyo-psikolojik entegrasyon analizi]. In B. D. Şeker, İ. Sirkeci, & M. M. Yüceşahin (Eds.), *Göç ve uyum* (pp. 23–34). Transnational Press London.

Türkiye İstatistik Kurumu (TÜİK). (2019). *International Migration Statistics, 2018* [Uluslararası Göç İstatistikleri, 2018]. Retrieved February 17, 2022, from https://data.tuik.gov.tr/Bulten/Index?p=Uluslararasi-Goc-Istatistikleri-2018-30711

Ulus Gazetesi. (1938, January 19). *Muhajir* [Muhacir]. Retrieved from https://www.gastearsivi.com/gazete/ulus/1938-01-19/1

Ünal, S. (2008). *An evaluation on the Balkans migrants in Turkey in the context of social integration and identity (a sample from İzmir)* [Sosyal bütünleşme ve kimlik bağlamında Türkiye'deki Balkan göçmenleri üzerine bir değerlendirme (İzmir'den bir örneklem)] [Master's thesis]. Retrieved from Council of Higher Education Thesis Center. (Thesis No. 219894)

Van Oudenhoven, J. P., Ward, C., & Masgoret, A. M. (2006). Patterns of relations between immigrants and host societies. *International Journal of Intercultural Relations*, *30*(6), 637–651. doi:10.1016/j.ijintrel.2006.09.001

Ward, C. (1997). Culture learning, acculturative stress, and psychopathology: Three perspectives on acculturation. *Applied Psychology*, *46*(1), 58–62. doi:10.1111/j.1464-0597.1997.tb01094.x

Ward, C., & Kennedy, A. (1993). Where's the "culture" in cross-cultural transition? Comparative studies of sojourner adjustment. *Journal of Cross-Cultural Psychology*, *24*(2), 221–249. doi:10.1177/0022022193242006

Ward, C., & Masgoret, A. M. (2008). Attitudes toward immigrants, immigration, and multiculturalism in New Zealand: A social psychological analysis. *The International Migration Review*, *42*(1), 227–248. doi:10.1111/j.1747-7379.2007.00119.x

Williams, C. L., & Berry, J. W. (1991). Primary prevention of acculturative stress among refugees: Application of psychological theory and practice. *The American Psychologist*, *46*(6), 632–641. doi:10.1037/0003-066X.46.6.632 PMID:1952422

Wilson, R., & Magam, L. (2018). Frustration-aggression, afrophobia and the psycho-social consequences of corruption in South Africa. In A. O. Akinola (Ed.), *The Political Economy of Xenophobia in Africa* (pp. 93–107). Springer. doi:10.1007/978-3-319-64897-2_8

Yeh, C. J. (2003). Age, acculturation, cultural adjustment, and mental health symptoms of Chinese, Korean, and Japanese immigrant youths. *Cultural Diversity & Ethnic Minority Psychology*, *9*(1), 34–48. doi:10.1037/1099-9809.9.1.34 PMID:12647324

ADDITIONAL READING

Berry, J. W. (1997). Immigration, acculturation, and adaptation. *Applied Psychology*, *46*(1), 5–34. doi:10.1111/j.1464-0597.1997.tb01087.x

Berry, J. W., Kim, U., Power, S., Young, M., & Bujaki, M. (1989). Acculturation Attitudes in Plural Societies. *Applied Psychology*, *38*(2), 185–206. doi:10.1111/j.1464-0597.1989.tb01208.x

Hogg, M. A., & Abrams, D. (1998). *Social identifications: A social psychology of intergroup relations and group processes*. Routledge.

Mahalingam, R. (Ed.). (2006). *Cultural psychology of immigrants*. Lawrence Erlbaum Associates Inc.

Montreuil, A., & Bourhis, R. Y. (2001). Majority acculturation orientations toward "valued" and "devalued" immigrants. *Journal of Cross-Cultural Psychology*, *32*(6), 698–719. doi:10.1177/0022022101032006004

Pettigrew, T. F. (1997). Generalized intergroup contact effects on prejudice. *Personality and Social Psychology Bulletin, 23*(2), 173–185. doi:10.1177/0146167297232006

Verkuyten, M. (2018). The benefits of studying immigration for social psychology. *European Journal of Social Psychology, 48*(3), 225–239. doi:10.1002/ejsp.2354

Worchel, S., & Austin, W. G. (Eds.). (1986). *Psychology of intergroup relations* (2nd ed.). Nelson-Hall Publishers.

KEY TERMS AND DEFINITIONS

Acculturation: The processes by which individuals or groups adjust the social and cultural values, ideas, beliefs, and behavioral patterns of their culture of origin to those of a different culture.

Acculturative Stress: Stress caused among migrants by having to deal with a culture different than one's own.

Discrimination: Differential treatment of different racial, ethnic, age, sex, or other groups. Discrimination is the behavioral manifestation of prejudice. Involves negative and hostile treatment of the members of rejected groups.

In-Group: Any group to which one belongs, which contrasts with other groups toward whom one tends to feel superior or competitive.

Integration: Integration refers to a pattern of cultural change in which an individual engages with a new cultural group and adopts its characteristics while maintaining a strong connection to the original cultural group.

Out-Group: Any social group which an individual identifies as one to which he/she does not belong. Out-group is usually judged as inferior to the social group with which one identifies one's self.

Prejudice: A set of negative attitudes and beliefs toward another person or group which ignores within-group diversity and is resistant to contrary evidence.

Social Adaptation: The adjustment of individual and group behavior to conform with the prevailing system of norms and values in a given society, class, or social group. Also includes friendly or cooperative relations among people or groups.

ENDNOTE

1 It is used in the sense of "do not marry the women of the refugees".

Compilation of References

Corporation Research. (2001). *3M Corporation Research*. http://www.3m.com/meetingnrtwork/readingroom/meeting-guide_press.html

AA. (2022). *Russia-Ukraine crisis in 5 questions* [5 soruda Rusya-Ukrayna krizi]. Retrieved from https://www.aa.com.tr/tr/dunya/5-soruda-rusya-ukrayna-krizi/2203164

Abel, J. P., Buff, C. L., & Burr, S. A. (2016). Social media and the fear of missing out: Scale development and assessment. *Journal of Business & Economics Research*, *14*(1), 33–44. doi:10.19030/jber.v14i1.9554

Abels, P., & Abels, S. L. (2001). *Understanding narrative therapy: A guidebook for the social worker*. Springer Publishing Company.

Ablon, S. L. (1996). The therapeutic action of play. *Journal of the American Academy of Child and Adolescent Psychiatry*, *35*(4), 545–547. doi:10.1097/00004583-199604000-00022 PMID:8919718

Adams St. Pierre, E. (2014). A brief and personal history of post qualitative research: Toward "post inquiry". *Journal of Curriculum Theorizing*, *30*(2), 2–19.

Adams, T. E., Jones, S. H., & Ellis, C. (2015). *Autoethnography*. Oxford University Press.

Adanır, O. (2007). *Audio and Visual Meaning Production* [İşitsel ve Görsel Anlam Üretimi]. Turkey: +1Book Publications.

Adaval, R., & Wyer, R. Jr. (1998). The Role of Narratives in Consumer Information Processing. *Journal of Consumer Psychology*, *7*(3), 207–246. doi:10.120715327663jcp0703_01

Afiş. (n.d.). https://www.britannica.com/dictionary/poster

Afonskij, S. A. (2016). Naličie i harakter arhetipov v iskusstve russkogo plakata, sozdannogo v period Velikoj Otečestvennoj vojny 1941-1945 gg [The presence and nature of archetypes in the art of Russian posters created during the Great Patriotic War of 1941-1945]. *Vestnik Rossijskogo èkonomičeskogo universiteta im GV Plehanova*, *3*(87), 159–169.

Ağaoğlu, M. (2017). *A Keeper in a Nonsense World: Albert Camus [Saçma Dünyada Bir Kaleci: Albert Camus]*. Üvercinka Journal. August.

Aguilera, L., Reed, K., & Goulding, J. (2020). Experiences of engaging in therapeutic storytelling. *Mental Health Review (Brighton)*, *25*(1), 47–61. doi:10.1108/MHRJ-11-2018-0036

Akbulut, T. N. (2004). Women's Discourse on Turkish Television [Türk Televizyonunda Kadın Söylemi]. *Kadın Çalışmalarında Disiplinlerarası Buluşma, Vol*, *2*, 157–162.

Akıncı, B., Nergiz, A., & Gedik, E. (2015). An assesment on process of adaptation: Migration and social acceptance [Uyum süreci üzerine bir değerlendirme: Göç ve toplumsal kabul]. *Göç Araştırmaları Dergisi*, *1*(2), 58–83.

Akkuş, K., Kütük, B., & Samar, B. Ş. (2020). Narrative therapy: Philosophical and theoretical foundations, therapy techniques and efficacy [Öyküsel terapi: Felsefi ve kuramsal temelleri, terapi teknikleri ve etkinliği]. *Akdeniz İnsani Bilimler Dergisi, 10*, 27–37. doi:10.13114/MJH.2020.515

Akmeşe, E. (2021). An Archetypal Analysis on the Transformation of the Individual in Play with Fire [Ateşle Oyun Filminde Bireyin Dönüşümü Üzerine Arketipsel Bir Analiz]. *İNİF E-Dergi, 6*(2), 325-339.

Akmeşe, Z. (2020). *The Effect of Framing on the Production of Content and Meaning in Television [Televizyonda Çerçevelemenin İçerik ve Anlam Üretimine Etkisi]* (E. Sirer, Ed.). Literatürk Publication.

Akmeşe, Z. (2020a). The Effect of Framing in Television on Content and Meaning Production. In *Television 4.0 Society 5.0 New Curriculum New Audience*. Literatürk Publication.

Akmeşe, Z. (2020b). Framing in Television Main Newsletters: Türk Telekom Advertising Film Example [Televizyon Ana Haber Bültenlerinde Çerçeveleme: Türk Telekom Reklam Filmi Örneği]. *Middle Black Sea Journal of Communication Studies, 5*(1), 37–49.

Akşar, T. (2005). *Industrial Football [Endüstriyel Futbol]*. Literatür Publications.

Aksoy, E. (2016). Turkey's population structure and policies after World War I (1919-1955) [1919-1955 yılları arasında Türkiye'nin nüfus yapısı ve uygulanan nüfus politikaları]. *Hacettepe Üniversitesi Türkiyat Araştırmaları Dergisi, 24*, 27–44.

Alaniz, J. (2010). *Komiks: Comic Art in Russia*. University Press of Mississippi. doi:10.14325/mississippi/9781604733662.001.0001

Alekseeva, T. P., & Vinickaja, N. V. (2018). Fol'klornye tendencii sovetskogo ideologičeskogo plakata [Folklornye tendencies of the Soviet ideological poster]. *Vestnik Tomskogo gosudarstvennogo universiteta. Kul'turologija i iskusstvovedenie*, (29), 5-22.

Alexa. (2022). *Top Sites in Turkey*. Retrieved from https://www.alexa.com/topsites/countries/TR

Alicea-Planas, J. (2016). Listening to the Narratives of Our Patients as Part of Holistic Nursing Care. *Journal of Holistic Nursing, 34*(2), 162–166. doi:10.1177/0898010115591396 PMID:26088595

Allen, P. B. (1995). *Art is a way of knowing*. Shambhala.

Allianz Turkiye. (2019, Oct 8). *Allianz Life Cycle* [Video]. YouTube. https://www.youtube.com/watch?v=D9L6WkhZz3w

Allport, G. W. (1954). *The nature of prejudice*. Addison-Wesley.

Alpay, Y. (2017). *The Politics of Lies: Legitimating Lies, Trivializing Truth, and Fraudulent Reasoning Techniques* [Yalanın Siyaseti: Yalanın Meşrulaştırılması, Hakikatin Önemsizleştirilmesi ve Hileli Akıl Yürütme Teknikleri]. Destek Yayınları.

Alpay, Y. (2019). *The Politics of Lies [Yalanın Siyaseti]*. Destek Publication.

Alt, D. (2015). College students' academic motivation, media engagement and fear of missing out. *Computers in Human Behavior, 49*, 111–119. doi:10.1016/j.chb.2015.02.057

Althusser, L. (2016). İdeoloji ve Devletin İdeolojik Aygıtları [Ideology and State Ideological Devices]. İthaki Yayınları.

Altun, F. (2022, January). A Critical Approach to the Post-Truth Narrative in the Framework of Sociological Theory. *Research Article. Journal of Erciyes Communication., 9*(1), 249–267.

Alutaybi, A., Al-Thani, D., McAlaney, J., & Ali, R. (2020). Combating fear of missing out (FoMO) on social media: The FoMO-R method. *International Journal of Environmental Research and Public Health, 17*(17), 1–28. doi:10.3390/ijerph17176128 PMID:32842553

Amerikan Psikiyatri Birliği (APA) (2014). *Diagnostic and Census Manual of Mental Disorders 5* [Ruhsal Bozuklukların Tanısal ve Sayımsal Elkitabı 5]. Hekimler Yayın Birliği.

Andersen, T. (1992). Reflections on reflecting with families. In S. McNamee & K. J. Gergen (Eds.), *Therapy as Social Constructionism* (pp. 54–68). Sage.

Anderson, L., & Glass-Coffin, B. (2016). I learn by going. In S. Holman Jones, T. E. Adams, & C. Ellis, (Eds.), Handbook of autoethnography (pp. 57-83). Routledge.

Ankaralıgil, N., & Kartal, H. (2013). Game, Ideology and Consumption: The Transformation of Football from Entertainment to Consumption in the Context of Mass Media [Oyun, İdeoloji ve Tüketim: Kitle İletişim Araçları Bağlamında Eğlenceden Tüketime Futbolun Dönüşümü]. *New Thoughts Journal*, *7*(April), 125–144.

Antonovsky, A. (1987). *Unraveling the mystery of health.* Jossey-Bass.

Appave, G., & David, I. (2017). Integration that values diversity - exploring a model for current migration dynamics. In M. McAuliffe & M. Klein Solomon (Eds.), *Migration research leaders' syndicate: Ideas to inform international cooperation on safe, orderly and regular migration* (pp. 151–158). International Organization for Migration.

Appel, M., Krisch, N., Stein, J. P., & Weber, S. (2019). Smartphone zombies! Pedestrians' distracted walking as a function of their fear of missing out. *Journal of Environmental Psychology*, *63*, 130–133. doi:10.1016/j.jenvp.2019.04.003

Argan, M., Argan, M. T., & İpek, G. (2018). I wish i were! Anatomy of a foncumer. *Journal of Internet Applications and Management*, *9*(1), 43–57. doi:10.34231/iuyd.407055

Arı, K. (1991). The problem of transporting exchange immigrants to Turkey and the immigrants of Izmir (1923-1924) [Mübadele göçmenlerini Türkiye'ye taşıma sorunu ve İzmir göçmenleri (1923-1924)]. *Çağdaş Türkiye Tarihi Araştırmaları Dergisi, 1*(1), 13-46.

Arnold, M. J., & Reynolds, K. E. (2003). Hedonic shopping motivations. *Journal of Retailing*, *79*(2), 77–95. doi:10.1016/S0022-4359(03)00007-1

Aronson, E., Wilson, T. D., & Akert, R. M. (2010). *Social psychology* (7th ed.). Pearson Prentice Hall.

Arslan, Ü., & Gümüşçağlayan, G. (2018). Solution focused brief therapy: A brief overview [Çözüm odaklı kısa süreli terapiye kısa bir bakış]. *Mehmet Akif Ersoy Üniversitesi Eğitim Fakültesi Dergisi*, (47), 491–507. doi:10.21764/maeuefd.396228

Assael, H. (1992). *Consumer behavior and marketing action.* PWS-KENT Publishing Company.

Atabek, Y. (1992). Narrative by Theorists [Kuramcılara Göre Anlatı.]. *Kurgu Dergisi*, *11*, 339.

Atasay Jewelry. (2018, Dec 17). *Wear What Suits You* [Video]. YouTube. https://www.youtube.com/watch?v=gwrssbRWJfo

Axe Türkiye. (2019). *Put in Your Pocket; You'll Need It* [Video]. YouTube. https://www.youtube.com/watch?v=vygySn0T-8w

Aydın, C. & Aslıtürk G. E. (2017). Creation in the Framework of Mythology and the History of Religions: Reflections on the Sistine Chapel Ceiling Frescoes [Mitoloji ve Dinler Tarihi Çerçevesinde Yaratılış: Sistine Şapeli Tavan Freskolarına Yönelik Düşünceler]. *İdil Journal, 6*(30).

Aydin, D., Selvi, Y., Kandeger, A., & Boysan, M. (2021). The relationship of consumers' compulsive buying behavior with biological rhythm, impulsivity, and fear of missing out. *Biological Rhythm Research*, *52*(10), 1514–1522. doi:10.1080/09291016.2019.1654203

Aziz, A. (2006). *Television and Radio Broadcasting* [Televizyon ve Radyo Yayıncılığı]. Turhan Yayıncılığı.

Badham, C. (2020). Tales from the east end: Dialogic and confessional storytelling as therapy (?) in the plays of Philip Ridley. In W. C. Boles (Ed.), *After in-yer-face theatre* (pp. 185–200). Palgrave Macmillan. doi:10.1007/978-3-030-39427-1_12

Baker, Ç. (2012). *Culturel Studies, Theory and Practice*. Sage.

Baker, Z. G., Krieger, H., & LeRoy, A. S. (2016). Fear of missing out:Relationships with depression, mindfulness, and physical symptoms. *Translational Issues in Psychological Science*, *2*(3), 275–282. doi:10.1037/tps0000075

Bakhtin, M. (2005). Rabelais and His World: carnival and grotesque (Ç. Öztek, Trans.). Ayrıntı Publications.

Balcı, Ş., Bekiroğlu, O., & Karaman, S. Y. (2019). Self-Esteem as a Determinant of Social Media Addiction: A Study in the Case of Konya [Sosyal Medya Bağımlılığının Bir Belirleyicisi Olarak Öz Saygı: Konya Örneğinde Bir Araştırma]. *İletişim Kuram ve Araştırma Dergisi*, (48), 36-64.

Barad, K. (2007). *Meeting the universe halfway: Quantum physics and the entanglement of matter and meaning*. Duke University Press. doi:10.2307/j.ctv12101zq

Bardon, A. (2019). *A Brief History of the Philosophy of Time [Zaman Felsefesinin Kısa Tarihi]* (Ö. Yalçın, Trans.). Türkiye İş Bankası Kültür Publication.

Baron, I. Z. (2018). *How to save politics in a post-truth era*. Manchester University Press. doi:10.7765/9781526126832

Barthes, R. (2005). *Semiotic Adventure* [Göstergebilimsel Serüven] (R. Mehmet & R. Sema, Trans.). Yapı Kredi Yayınları.

Bartlett, J. C. (2020). Information Literacy and Science Misinformation. In K. Dalkir & R. Katz (Eds.), Navigating Fake News, Alternative Facts, and Misinformation in a Post-Truth World (pp. 1-17). IGI Global. doi:10.4018/978-1-7998-2543-2.ch001

Bateson, M. C. (1989). *Composing a life*. Atlantic Monthly Press.

Batista-Pinto Wiese, E. (2010). Culture and migration: Psychological trauma in children and adolescents. *Traumatology*, *16*(4), 142–152. doi:10.1177/1534765610388304

Bauloz, C., Vathi, Z., & Acosta, D. (2019). Migration, inclusion and social cohesion: Challenges, recent developments and opportunities. In M. McAuliffe & B. Khadria (Eds.), *World Migration Report 2020* (pp. 185–206). International Organization for Migration.

Bavelas, J., De Jong, P., Franklin, C., Froerer, A., Gingerick, W., & Kim, J. (2013). Solution focused therapy treatment manual for working with individuals (2nd ed.). Solution Focused Brief Therapy Association.

Bayrakcı, O. (2021). İktidar-Hegemonya İlişkisinde Algı Yönetimi [Perception Management in the Power-Hegemony Relationship]. *Yüzüncü Yıl Üniversitesi Sosyal Bilimler Enstitüsü Dergisi*, (52), 93–108.

Bayraktaroğlu, A. M. & Uğur, U. (2011). The Case of Magazineization in Television Journalism [Televizyon Haberciliğinde Magazinleşme Olgusu]. *Süleyman Demirel Üniversitesi Güzel Sanatlar Fakültesi Hakemli Dergisi*, *4*(7), 1–47.

BBC. (2022). *Ukraine-Russia crisis: What is the latest situation at the border, how did the tension escalate?* [Ukrayna-Rusya krizi: Sınırda son durum ne, gerilim nasıl tırmandı?]. Retrieved from https://www.bbc.com/turkce/haberler-dunya-60047078

Bekcan, U. (2019). Stalin Döneminde Sovyet Dış Politikası İdeolojiden Saptı mı? [Did Soviet Foreign Policy Under Stalin Deviate From Ideology?]. *Pamukkale Üniversitesi Sosyal Bilimler Enstitüsü Dergisi*, (36), 371–382.

Bekiroğlu, O., Kaya, S. & Yaman, D. (2019). Accumulations and Leaps of Media and Journalism in The Period of Digital Transformation [Dijital Dönüşümün Periyotlarında Medya ve Gazetecilik Alanındaki Birikim ve Sıçramalar]. *Uluslararası Türk Dünyası Basın Sempozyumu.*

Belge, M. (2018). *"If you want…": Essays on Populism* ["Siz isterseniz...": Popülizm Üzerine Yazılar]. İletişim Yayınları.

Benesch, K. (2021). Is the Relationship between Truth and Post-Truth a Relationship between Modernism and Postmodernism? Heidegger, the Humanities and the Death of Common Sense [*Hakikat ile Hakikat Sonrası İlişkisi Modernizm ile Postmodernizm İlişkisi midir? Heidegger, Beşeri Bilimler ve Sağduyunun Ölümü]. Cogito Journal, 104,* 49–66.

Berry, J. W. (2020). How shall we all live together? In S. Safdar, C. Kwantes, & W. Friedlmeier (Eds.), *Wiser world with multiculturalism: Proceedings from the 24th Congress of the International Association for Cross-Cultural Psychology.* Retrieved from https://scholarworks.gvsu.edu/iaccp_papers/284

Berry, J. W. (2001). A psychology of immigration. *The Journal of Social Issues*, *57*(3), 615–631. doi:10.1111/0022-4537.00231

Berry, J. W. (2006a). Contexts of acculturation. In D. L. Sam & J. W. Berry (Eds.), *The Cambridge handbook of acculturation psychology* (pp. 27–42). Cambridge University Press. doi:10.1017/CBO9780511489891.006

Berry, J. W. (2006b). Stress perspectives on acculturation. In D. L. Sam & J. W. Berry (Eds.), *The Cambridge handbook of acculturation psychology* (pp. 43–57). Cambridge University Press. doi:10.1017/CBO9780511489891.007

Berry, J. W. (2009). Living together in culturally-plural societies: Understanding and managing acculturation and multiculturalism. In S. Bekman & A. Aksu-Koç (Eds.), *Perspectives on human development, family, and culture* (pp. 227–240). Cambridge University Press. doi:10.1017/CBO9780511720437.017

Berry, J. W., Kim, U., Minde, T., & Mok, D. (1987). Comparative studies of acculturative stress. *The International Migration Review*, *21*(3), 491–511. doi:10.1177/019791838702100303

Berry, J. W., Phinney, J. S., Sam, D. L., & Vedder, P. (2006). Immigrant youth: Acculturation, identity, and adaptation. *Applied Psychology*, *55*(3), 303–332. doi:10.1111/j.1464-0597.2006.00256.x

Berry, T. (2015). *The Dream of the Earth.* Counterpoint Berkley.

Berry, T. M. (2000). *The Great Work: Our Way into the Future.* Bell Tower.

Besley, A. C. (2002). Foucault and the turn to narrative therapy. *British Journal of Guidance & Counselling*, *30*(2), 125–143. doi:10.1080/03069880220128010

Beyebach, M., Morejon, A. R., Palenzuela, D. L., & Rodriguez-Arias, J. L. (1996). Research on the process of solution-focused therapy. In S. D. Miller, M. A. Hubble, & B. L. Duncan (Eds.), *Handbook of solution-focused brief therapy* (pp. 299–334). Jossey-Bass Publishers.

Beyebach, M., Rodríguez-Sánchez, M. S., Arribas de Miguel, J., De Vega, M. H., Hernández, C., & Rodríguez-Morejón, A. (2000). Outcome of solution-focused therapy at a university family therapy center. *Journal of Systemic Therapies*, *19*(1), 116–128. doi:10.1521/jsyt.2000.19.1.116

Beyens, I., Frison, E., & Eggermont, S. (2016). "I don't want to miss a thing": Adolescents' fear of missing out and its relationship to adolescents' social needs, Facebook use, and Facebook related stress. *Computers in Human Behavior*, *64*, 1–8. doi:10.1016/j.chb.2016.05.083

Bezembinder, C. (2018). *Is Post-Truth Politics Really Post-Truth?* (Unpublished Master Thesis). Leiden: Leiden University Faculty of Humanities Institute for Philosophy.

Bezerra, M. S. M., de Souza, I. P., de Souza, S. P. S., & da Silva Barbosa, M. A. R. (2018). Experience of a young woman's cancer and the family care constellation. *Cienc Cuid Saude*, *17*(2), 1–8. doi:10.4025/cienccuidsaude.v17i2.42185

Bhaskaran, H., Mishra, H., & Nair, P. (2017). Contextualizing Fake News in Post-truth Era: Journalism Education in India. *Asia Pacific Media Educator*, *27*(1), 41–50. doi:10.1177/1326365X17702277

Bhattacharyya, A. (2006). Historical backdrop. In K. N. Dwivedi (Ed.), *The therapeutic use of stories* (pp. 1–18). Routledge.

Biehl, J. G., & Locke, P. A. (Eds.). (2017). *Unfinished: the anthropology of becoming*. Duke University Press. doi:10.1215/9780822372455

Bochner, A. P. (2016). Autoethnography's existential calling. In S. Holman Jones, T. E. Adams, & C. Ellis (Eds.), Handbook of autoethnography. (pp. 50-56). Routledge.

Bokerija, S. A., & Dieva, A. A. (2015). Opyt informacionnoj propagandy v SSSR kak instrument mjagkoj sily [The experience of information propaganda in the USSR as a tool of soft power]. *Vestnik Rossijskogo universiteta družby narodov Serija: Istorija Rossii*, (3), 81–89.

Bolat, N. (2019). Görsel Okuryazarlık Bağlamında Televizyon Dizilerindegeleneksel Mekânlar Üzerine Bir Çalışma [A Study On Tradıtıonal Spaces In Televısıon Serıes In The Context Of Vısual Lıteracy]. Uluslararası İletişim ve Yönetim Bilimleri Kongresi.

Bolat, N., & Çakın, Ö. (2018). Violence as a Marketing Motif in Television Series: The Example of the Black Sea Series You Tell. In Virtual Media Violence and Social Traumas. HEGEM Publications.

Bolat, N. (2016). Effect of Image Tekniks in The Fact that Feudal Content Series Do Not Reach High Audience in Modern Turkey: Karagül Series [Modern Türkiye'de Feodal İçerikli Dizilerin Yüksek İzleyiciye Ulaşmadında Görüntü Tekniklerinin Etkisi: Karagül Dizisi]. *Middle Black Sea Journal of Communication Studies*, *1*(2), 69–86.

Bolat, N. (2018). Erkek Egemen Bir Dünyada Kadının Medyada Temsiliyeti Üzerine Bir İnceleme: Eşkiya Dünyaya Hükümdar Olmaz Dizisi Örneği [An Analysis on the Representation of Women in the Media in a Male-Dominated World: The Example of the TV Series Bandit Does Not Rule the World]. *Gümüşhane Üniversitesi İletişim Fakültesi Dergisi*, *6*(2), 1676–1703.

Bolat, N. (2018). Erkek Egemen Bir Dünyada Kadının Medyada Temsiliyeti Üzerine Bir İnceleme: Eşkıya Dünyaya Hükümdar Olmaz Dizisi Örneği [An Analysis on the Representation of Women in the Media in a Male-Dominated World]. *Gümüşhane Üniversitesi İletişim Fakütesi Elektronik Dergisi*, *6*(2), 1676–1703.

Bolat, N. (2019). *Post-modernizm, inside: Communication in the Age of Posts [Post-modernizm içinde: Postlar Çağında İletişim]* (M. N. Erdem & N. K. Şener, Eds.). Literatürk Publication.

Bolat, N. (2019). The New Roadmap of Modernism: Post-Modernism [Modernizmin Yeni Yol Haritası: Post-Modernizm]. In M. N. Erdem & N. Kocabay Şener (Eds.), *Communication in the Age of Posts* [Postlar Çağında İletişim] (pp. 33–59). Literatürk Academia.

Bolat, N. (2020). The Impact of The Technical Transformation of Television on Content. Televizyonun Teknik Dönüşümünün İçeriğe Etkisi. In E. Sirer (Ed.), *Yeni İzlence Yeni İzlerkitle* (pp. 107–126). Literatürk.

Bolat, N., & Çakın, Ö. (2018). In N. Sargın (Ed.), *"Violence" as a Marketing Motif in Television Series: The Example of the Sen Anlat Karadeniz, Virtual Realm / Media Violence [Televizyon Dizilerinde Bir Pazarlama Motifi Olarak "Şiddet": Sen Anlat Karadeniz Dizisi Örneği, Sanal Alem / Medya Şiddeti]*. Hegem Publication.

Bolat, N., & Çakın, Ö. (2018). Violence as a Marketing Motif in Television Series: You Tell Black Sea Series Example. In *Virtual Realm/Media Violence and Social Conflict Traumas*. Hegem Publication.

Bolt, B. (2016). Artistic research: A performative paradigm. *Parse Journal*, *3*, 129–142.

Bourdieu, P. (2000). On Television (T. Ilgaz, Trans.). Cogito Publications.

Bourdieu, P. (1997). *On Television [Televizyon Üzerine]* (T. Ilgaz, Trans.). Yapı Kredi Publication.

Boyner. (2019, May 2). *Mother's Day Campaign* [Video]. YouTube. https://www.youtube.com/watch?v=gOMYQcPP_cw

Boztepe, V. (2017). Representation of Violence Against Women in Television News: An Analysis on the Murder of Özgecan Aslan [Televizyon Haberlerinde Kadınlara Yönelik Şiddetin Temsili: Özgecan Aslan Cinayeti Üzerinden Bir İnceleme]. *İstanbul Üniversitesi İletişim Fakültesi Dergisi*, *1*, 39-66.

Braun, V., & Clarke, V. (2006). Using thematic analysis in psychology. *Qualitative Research in Psychology*, *3*(2), 77–101. doi:10.1191/1478088706qp063oa

Brodziak, A., Wolinska, A., & Myrta, A. R. (2017). The Story Theory is a Key Element of Many Holistic Nursing Procedures. *Journal of Gerontology & Geriatric Research*, *6*(6). Advance online publication. doi:10.4172/2167-7182.1000454

Brooks, P. (2016). *Psychoanalysis and Storytelling* [Psikanaliz ve Hikâye Anlatıcılığı] (H. Demir Atay & H. Atayt, Trans.). Boğaziçi Üniversitesi Yayınları.

Browne, B. L., Aruguete, M. S., McCutcheon, L. E., & Medina, A. M. (2018). Social and emotional correlates of the fear of missing out. *North American Journal of Psychology*, *20*(2), 341–353.

Brown, J. (1997). Circular questioning: An introductory guide. *Australian and New Zealand Journal of Family Therapy*, *18*(2), 109–114. doi:10.1002/j.1467-8438.1997.tb00276.x

Brown, J. A. C. (1963). *Techniques of Persuasion: From Propaganda to Brainwashing*. Penguin.

Bülbül, A. R. (2001). *Anatomy of the News and Basic Approaches [Haberin Anatomisi ve Temel Yaklaşımlar]*. Nobel Publication.

Bulut, Ö. (2021). Philosophy, Truth and Beyond [Felsefe, Hakikat ve Sonrası]. In B. Özçelik (Ed.), *Post-truth Politics, Philosophy, Media, International Relations* [Hakikat Sonrası Siyaset, Felsefe, Medya, Uluslararası İlişkiler] (pp. 97–118). Nika Yayınevi.

Burns, G. W. (2016). *Çocuklar ve ergenler için 101 tedavi edici öykü* [101 healing stories for kids and teens] (N. Cihanşümül Maral, Trans.). Nobel Yaşam. (Original work published 2001)

Burrows, L. (2013). Transforming 'The Red Beast' within through mindfulness and therapeutic storytelling: A case study. *Australian Journal of Guidance & Counselling*, *23*(2), 172–184. doi:10.1017/jgc.2013.17

Burton, G. (1995). *More Than Looks [Görünenden Fazlası]* (N. Dinç, Trans.). Alan Publication.

Burwell, R., & Chen, C. P. (2006). Applying the principles and techniques of solution-focused therapy to career counselling. *Counselling Psychology Quarterly*, *19*(2), 189–203. doi:10.1080/09515070600917761

Bushman, B. J., & Huesmann, L. R. (2006). Short Termand Long-term Effects of Violent Media on Aggression in Children and Adults. *Arch Pediatr Adolesc Med, Vol*, *160*(4), 348–352. doi:10.1001/archpedi.160.4.348 PMID:16585478

Bush, S. (2018). Emergence, resonant felt sensing and the arts: With/in relational spaces of us. *ANZJAT Australia and Journal of Arts Therapy*, *13*(1 & 2), 125–129.

Cabas, M. (2019). Tell Me Sweet Little Lies [Bana Tatlı Küçük Yalanlar Söyle]. In L. Mcintyre (Ed.), *Post-Truth* [Hakikat Sonrası] (pp. 15–19). Tellekt.

Cabassa, L. J. (2003). Measuring acculturation: Where we are and where we need to go. *Hispanic Journal of Behavioral Sciences*, *25*(2), 127–146. doi:10.1177/0739986303025002001

Çakar Mengü, S. (2004). *Televizyon Reklamlarında Kadına Yönelik Oluşturulan Toplumsal Kimlik* [Social Identity Created for Women in Television Advertisements]. İstanbul Üniversitesi İletişim Faültesi Yayınları.

Çakın, Ö., & Bolat, N. (2018). *An Analysis of Violence and Violent Posts on Social Media, Virtual World / Media Violence [Sosyal Medyada Şiddet Ve Şiddet İçerikli Paylaşımlara Yönelik Bir Çözümleme, Sanal Alem / Medya Şiddeti]*. Hegem Publication.

Çakırer Özservet, Y., & Yurtsever, B. (2017). *Research on prejudice against immigrants.* (International Migration and Social Cohesion Research Series: 1) [*Göçmenlere yönelik önyargı araştırması.* (Uluslararası Göç ve Toplumsal Uyum Araştırmaları Serisi: 1)]. İstanbul: Marmara Üniversitesi Kent sorunları ve Yerel Yönetimler Uygulama ve Araştırma Merkezi. Retrieved from https://www.researchgate.net/publication/324834708_Gocmenlere_ Yonelik_Onyargi_Arastirmasi

Çakır, S. (2008). Media and Violence [Medya ve Şiddet]. *Doğu Batı Düşünce Dergisi*, (43), 161–180.

Campbell, J. (1976). *The Masks of God: Creative Mythology*. Penguin Books.

Campbell, J. (1995). *Reflections on the art of living: A Joseph Campbell companion*. Harpercollins.

Campbell, J. (2013). *Hero's Eternal Journey* [Kahramanın Sonsuz Yolculuğu] (S. Gürses, Trans.). Kabalcı Yayıncılık.

Carey, M., Walthers, S., & Russell, S. (2009). The absent but implicit: A map to support therapeutic enquiry. *Family Process*, *48*(3), 319–331. doi:10.1111/j.1545-5300.2009.01285.x PMID:19702920

Carlson, M. (2018). The Information Politics of Journalism in a Post-truth Age. *Journalism Studies*, *19*(13), 1879–1888. doi:10.1080/1461670X.2018.1494513

Carlson, R. (2001). Therapeutic use of story in therapy with children. *Guidance & Counseling*, *16*(3), 92–99.

Carlson, R., & Arthur, N. (1999). Play therapy and the therapeutic use of story. *Canadian Journal of Counselling*, *33*(3), 212–226.

Carr, E. H. (2011). Lenin'den Stalin'e Rus Devrimi 1917-1929 [Russian Revolution from Lenin to Stalin 1917-1929]. Yordam Kitap.

Carr, A. (2009). The effectiveness of family therapy and systemic interventions for child-focused problems. *Journal of Family Therapy*, *31*(1), 3–45. doi:10.1111/j.1467-6427.2008.00451.x

Castles, S., & Miller, J. M. (2008). *The age of migrations, international migration movements in the modern world* [Göçler çağı, modern dünyada uluslararası göç hareketleri]. İstanbul Bilgi Üniversitesi.

Çaus, N. (2010). Sovetskiye plakatı1917-1922 gg. Osnovnoye sredstvo propagandı sotsialistiçeskaya ideologii [Soviet Posters 1917-1922 Basic Propaganda and Social Ideology]. *Sotsial'no -ekonomçeskiye yavleniya i protsesı, 6*(22).

Çelenk, S. (2010). Representation of Women in the Media and Ethical Issues [Kadınların Medyada Temsili ve Etik Sorunlar]. *Academia (Caracas)*, 229–236.

Çelik, N. B. (2000). Introduction: Television, Women, and Violence. In Television, Women and Violence [Televizyon, Kadın ve Şiddet]. KİV Publication.

Çelik, H. (2017). Psikoterapide yeni soluk: Öyküsel terapi. *E-Kafkas Eğitim Araştırmaları Dergisi*, *4*(1), 34–50.

Cepeda, L. M., & Davenport, D. S. (2006). Person-centered therapy and solution-focused brief therapy: An integration of present and future awareness. *Psychotherapy (Chicago, Ill.)*, *43*(1), 1–12. doi:10.1037/0033-3204.43.1.1 PMID:22121955

Çetinkaya, F. Ö., & Şahbaz, R. P. (2019). Sosyal medyada gelişmeleri kaçırma korkusunun kişinin tatil satın alma niyetine etkisi [The effect of FoMO on the intention of buying a holiday on social media]. *Türk Turizm Araştırmaları Dergisi*, *3*(3), 383–402. doi:10.26677/TR1010.2019.168

Çetin, Z. (1999). *The Introduction of a Narrative Form, The Novel, to Cinema* [Bir Anlatı Formu Olan Romanın Sinemaya Uyarlanması]. Marmara Üniversitesi Sosyal Bilimler Enstitüsü Radyo Televizyon ve Sinema Anabilim Dalı Doktora Tezi.

Chandler, D., & Munday, R. (2018). *A Dictionary of Media and Communication* [Medya ve İletişim Sözlüğü] (B. Taşdemir, Trans.). İletişim Yayınları.

Chang, C. (2012). Advertisements and Narrative Processing. In Advertising Theory (pp. 241–254). Routledge.

Chang, C. (2009). Repetıtıon Varıatıon Strategıes For Narrative Advertising. *Journal of Advertising*, *38*(3), 51–65. doi:10.2753/JOA0091-3367380304

Charmaz, K. (2012). The power and potential of grounded theory. *Medical Sociology Online*, *6*(3).

Cheever, N. A., Rosen, L. D., Carrier, L. M., & Chavez, A. (2014). Out of sight is not out of mind: The impact of restricting wireless mobile device use on anxiety levels among low, moderate and high users. *Computers in Human Behavior*, *3*, 290–197. doi:10.1016/j.chb.2014.05.002

Chilton, G., & Scotti, V. (2014). Snipping, gluing, writing: The properties of collage as an arts-based research practice in art therapy. *Art Therapy: Journal of the American Art Therapy Association*, *31*(4), 163–171. doi:10.1080/07421656.2015.963484

Chogandaryan, M. G. (2013). Methods, methods and techniques of Soviet propaganda in the 1920-30s. XX century. *Theory and Practice of Social Development*, (4), 181-183.

Clandinin, J. D. (2013). *Engaging in Narrative Inquiry. Developing Qualitative Inquiry* (Vol. 9). Left Coast Press, Inc.

Clegg, S. (1978). *Power, Rule and Domination*. Routledge & Kegan Paul.

Clément, R., Noels, K. A., & Deneault, B. (2001). Interethnic contact, identity, and psychological adjustment: The mediating and moderating roles of communication. *The Journal of Social Issues*, *57*(3), 559–577. doi:10.1111/0022-4537.00229

Cloke, K. (2017). Thinking Locally, Acting Globally, Mediating beyond borders and integrated global capacity building. In A. Georgakopoulos (Ed.), *The Mediation Handbook, Research, Theory, and Practice* (pp. 293–304). Routledge.

Cobb, S. B. (2013). *Speaking of Violence: The Politics and Poetics of Narrative Dynamics in Conflict Resolution. In Explorations in Narrative Psychology*. Oxford University Press. doi:10.1093/acprof:oso/9780199826209.001.0001

Cobb, S. B., Federman, S., & Castel, A. (Eds.). (2020). *Introduction to conflict resolution: discourses and dynamics*. Rowman & Littlefield International.

Coffey, A. (1999). The ethnographic self. *Sage (Atlanta, Ga.)*.

Čogandarjan, M. G. (2013). Metody, sposoby i priemy sovetskoj propagandy v 1920-30-e gg. XX v [Methods, methods and techniques of Soviet propaganda in the 1920-30s. twentieth century]. *Teorija i praktika obŝestvennogo razvitija*, (4), 181-183.

Cohen, D. B. (2006). "Family constellations": An innovative systemic phenomenological group process from Germany. *The Family Journal (Alexandria, Va.)*, *14*(3), 226–233. doi:10.1177/1066480706287279

Coles, A. (2014). 'Being time': An exploration of personal experiences of time and implications for art psychotherapy practice. *International Journal of Art Therapy, 19*(2), 71–81. doi:10.1080/17454832.2013.844184

Combs, G., & Freedman, J. (2012). Narrative, poststructuralism, and social justice: Current practices in narrative therapy. *The Counseling Psychologist, 40*(7), 1033–1060. doi:10.1177/0011000012460662

Connelly, F. M., & Clandinin, D. J. (1990). Stories of experience and narrative inquiry. *Educational Researcher, 19*(5), 2–14. doi:10.3102/0013189X019005002

Connie, E., & Metcalf, L. (2009). *The art of solution focused therapy*. Springer Publishing Company.

Conserva, H. (2009). *Propaganda: A Question and Answer Approach*. AuthorHouse.

Cook, J. W., Taylor, L. A., & Silverman, P. (2004). The application of therapeutic storytelling techniques with preadolescent children: A clinical description with illustrative case study. *Cognitive and Behavioral Practice, 11*(2), 243–248. doi:10.1016/S1077-7229(04)80035-X

Çopuroğlu, F. (2021). Tüketicilerin sosyal medya kullanımı, fomo ve hedonik tüketim arasındaki ilişki [The relationship between consumers' use of social media, FoMO and hedonic consumption]. *OPUS International Journal of Society Researches, 17*(37), 4298–4326.

Corcoran, J. (2006). A comparison group study of solution-focused therapy versus "treatment-as-usual" for behavior problems in children. *Journal of Social Service Research, 33*(1), 69–81. doi:10.1300/J079v33n01_07

Corey, G. (2015). *Theory and practice of counseling and psychotherapy* (10th ed.). Cengage.

Cosentino, G. (2020). *Social Media and the Post-Truth World Order: The Global Dynamics of Disinformation*. Palgrave Macmillan. doi:10.1007/978-3-030-43005-4

Cottingham, J. (1995). Akılcılık [Rationalism]. Sarmal Yayınevi.

Crăciun, A. (2017). *New challenges of communication in the age of post truth*. ttps://euprera.org/2017/07/01/new-challenges-of-communication-in-the-age-of-post-truth/.

Crisp, J. (2004). *The local integration and local settlement of refugees: A conceptual and historical analysis* (New Issues in Refugee Research Working Paper No. 102). United Nations High Commissioner for Refugees.

Csikszentmihalyi, M. (2004). *Mihaly Csikszentmihalyi on flow*. https://www.ted.com/talks/mihaly_csikszentmihalyi_on_flow

Csikszentmihalyi, M. (1990). *Flow: The psychology of optimal experience*. Harper and Row.

Çuhadaroğlu, F. (2007). Psychological Dimension of Violence: Youth and Violence Studies. In *Symposium on Preventing Violence Against Children and Adolescents*. Aem Kitap.

D'ancona, M. (2017). *Post Truth The New War on Truth and How to Fight Back*. Ebury Press.

D'Cruz, K., Douglas, J., & Serry, T. (2020). Narrative storytelling as both an advocacy tool and a therapeutic process: Perspectives of adult storytellers with acquired brain injury. *Neuropsychological Rehabilitation, 30*(8), 1409–1429. doi:10.1080/09602011.2019.1586733 PMID:30822228

Dallos, R. (2006). *Attachment narrative therapy*. McGraw-Hill Education.

Danilova, J. J., & Nurieva, D. R. (2015). Sovetskie plakaty kak sredstvo vizual'no-verbal'noj političeskoj agitacii [Soviet posters as a means of vizual'no-verbal political agitation]. *Mir nauki, kul'tury, obrazovanija, 2*(51), 408-411.

Darmody, C. (2019). Narrative walks. *International Journal of Narrative Therapy and Community Work*, (1), 52–60.

Davies, B. (2000). *(In)scribing body/landscape relations*. Altamira Press.

De Mol, J., & Buysse, A. (2008). Understandings of children's influence in parental-child relationships: A Q-methodological study. *Journal of Social and Personal Relationships*, *25*(2), 359–379. doi:10.1177/0265407507087963

De Mol, J., & Rimé, B. (2017). Depression in young people: the family as a source of change and a place for sharing emotions with others or how my depression can also become my friend [Depressie bij jongeren: het gezin als bron van verandering en een plaats voor het delen van emoties met anderen of hoe mijn depressie ook mijn vriend kan worden]. In S. Vermeire & J. Sermijn (Eds.), *Wegen naar herverbinding. Narratieve, collaboratieve en dialogische praktijken*. Interactie-Academie VZW.

de Shazer, S. (1975). Brief therapy: Two's company. *Family Process*, *14*(1), 79–93. doi:10.1111/j.1545-5300.1975.00079.x

de Shazer, S. (1985). *Keys to solution in brief therapy*. Norton.

de Shazer, S., & Berg, I. K. (1997). 'What works?' Remarks on research aspects of solution-focused brief therapy. *Journal of Family Therapy*, *19*(2), 121–124. doi:10.1111/1467-6427.00043

de Shazer, S., Berg, I. K., Lipchik, E. V. E., Nunnally, E., Molnar, A., Gingerich, W., & Weiner-Davis, M. (1986). Brief therapy: Focused solution development. *Family Process*, *25*(2), 207–221. doi:10.1111/j.1545-5300.1986.00207.x PMID:3732502

de Shazer, S., & Dolan, Y. (2012). *More than miracles: The state of the art of solution-focused brief therapy*. Routledge. doi:10.4324/9780203836484

Debord, G. (1996). *Gösteri Toplumu* [Spectacle society]. Ayrıntı Yayınları.

Degot, E. (2000). *Russkoe iskusstvo XX. Veka* [Russian Art in the 20th Century]. M. Trilistnik.

Delal, Ö., & Abanoz, E. (2021). Information Sharing and Misinformation about Covid-19 on Social Media in the Context of New Media Literacy [Yeni Medya Okuryazarlığı Bağlamında Sosyal Medyada Covid-19 ile İlgili Bilgi Paylaşımı ve Misenformasyon]. In F. Ünal Çolak & O. Yıldırım (Eds.), *Pandemic, Research and Discussions in the Digital World* [Dijital Dünyada Pandemi, Araştırmalar ve Tartışmalar] (pp. 265–296). Literatürk Academia.

Deleuze, G. (1994). *Difference and repetition* (P. Patton, Trans.). Athlone.

Demir, Ö. (2018). *Philosophy of Science* [Bilim Felsefesi]. Sentez Yayıncılık.

Denborough, D. (2008). Responding to trauma / responding to social issues. In *Collective Narrative Practice*. Dulwich Centre Publications.

Denborough, D. (2014). *Retelling the stories of our lives: Everyday narrative therapy to draw inspiration and transform experience*. W. W. Norton.

Dentith, S. (2005). *Bakhtinian Thought: An Introductory Reader*. Routledge.

Denzin, N. K. (2013). The death of data? *Cultural Studies « Critical Methodologies*, *13*(4), 353-356. doi:10.1177/1532708613487882

Denzin, N. K. (2014). *Interpretive Autoethnography* (2nd ed.). SAGE. doi:10.4135/9781506374697

Dervişcemaloğlu, B. (2014). *Anlatıbilime Giriş* [Introduction to Narratology]. Dergah Publications.

Dervişcemaloğlu, B. (2016). *Introduction to Narrative Science* [Anlatıbilime Giriş]. Dergah.

Desmond, K. J., Kindsvatter, A., Stahl, S., & Smith, H. (2015). Using creative techniques with children who have experienced trauma. *Journal of Creativity in Mental Health, 10*(4), 439–455. doi:10.1080/15401383.2015.1040938

Dilmen, D. (2015). *Why 11 People, Why 90 Minutes [Neden 11 Kişi, Neden 90 Dakika]* (Vol. 4). Fitbol Journal.

Divinyi, J. (1995). Storytelling: An enjoyable and effective therapeutic tool. *Contemporary Family Therapy, 17*(1), 27–37. doi:10.1007/BF02249302

Dizdar, C. (2019). VAR is the funeral of football! [VAR, futbolun cenaze merasimidir!]. *TRT Academic Journal, 4*(8).

Doğan, İ. (2021). Sovyetler Birliği'nde Din Karşıtı Propaganda: 1917-1960 Dönemi Üzerine Bir Değerlendirme [Anti-Religious Propaganda in the Soviet Union: An Evaluation of the Period 1917-1960.]. *Selçuk İletişim, 14*(1), 408–431.

Dollard, J., Doob, L., Miller, N., Mowrer, O., & Sears, R. (1939). *Frustration and aggression.* Yale University Press. doi:10.1037/10022-000

Doui, A. (2019). Global and Arab Media in The Post-Truth Era: Globalization, Authoritarianism and Fake News. *IEMed: Mediterranean Yearbook, 2019*, 124–132.

Dovidio, J. F., & Esses, V. M. (2001). Immigrants and immigration: Advancing the psychological perspective. *The Journal of Social Issues, 57*(3), 375–387. doi:10.1111/0022-4537.00219

Duman, Ö. (2009). The settlement efforts of Balkan immigrants in Atatürk's era (1923-1938) [Atatürk döneminde Balkan göçmenlerinin iskân çalışmaları (1923-1938)]. *Ankara Üniversitesi Türk İnkılâp Tarihi Enstitüsü Atatürk Yolu Dergisi, 11*(43), 473–490. doi:10.1501/Tite_0000000299

Dündar, S. (2010). Representation of Women in Television News [Televizyon Haberlerinde Kadının Temsili]. *Erciyes İletişim Dergisi, 1*(4), 91–105.

Dursun, Ç. (2010). News Ethics Against Violence Against Women [Kadına Yönelik Şiddet Karşısında Haber Etiği]. *Fe Dergi, 2*(1), 19–32.

DW. (2022). *How did Russia and Ukraine come to the brink of war?* [Rusya ile Ukrayna savaşın eşiğine nasıl geldi?]. Retrieved from https://www.dw.com/tr/rusya-ile-ukrayna-sava%C5%9F%C4%B1n-e%C5%9Fi%C4%9Fine-nas%C4%B1l-geldi/60522203.

Eagleton, T. (1996). *İdeoloji* [Ideology]. Ayrıntı Yayınları.

Eco, U. (1992). The Open Work (Y. Şahan, Trans.). Kabalcı Publication.

Eco, U. (2012). *Turning Back the Clock: Hot Wars and Media Populism* [Yengeç Adımlarıyla: Sıcak Savaşlar ve Medyatik Popülizm] (S. Gezgin, Trans.). Doğan Kitap.

Elhai, J. D., Levine, J. C., Alghraibeh, A. M., Alafnan, A. A., Aldraiweesh, A. A., & Hall, B. J. (2018). Fear of missing out: Testing relationships with negative affectivity, online social engagement, and problematic smartphone use. *Computers in Human Behavior, 89*, 289–298. doi:10.1016/j.chb.2018.08.020

Elhai, J. D., Levine, J. C., Dvorak, R. D., & Hall, B. J. (2016). Fear of missing out, need for touch, anxiety and depression are related to problematic smartphone use. *Computers in Human Behavior, 63*, 509–516. doi:10.1016/j.chb.2016.05.079

Elhai, J. D., Yang, H., & Montag, C. (2021). Fear of missing out (FOMO): Overview, theoretical underpinnings, and literature review on relations with severity of negative affectivity and problematic technology use. *The British Journal of Psychiatry, 43*(2), 203–209. doi:10.1590/1516-4446-2020-0870 PMID:32401865

Elizabeth, V. (2008). Another string to our bow: Participant writing as research method. *FQS, 9*(1). https://www.qualitative-research.net/index.php/fqs/article/view/331

Ellis, J. (1992). *Visible Fictions Cinema Television Video*. Routledge.

Ellul, J. (1998). *The Fall of the Word [Sözün Düşüşü]* (H. Arslan, Trans.). Paradigma Publication.

Emir, İ. Y. (2003). *Image in Mass Communication* [Kitle İletişiminde İmaj]. İletiş-im Kitapları.

Ensonhaber. (2022). *Russia-Ukraine Tension Will Reflect on Fuel Prices* [Rusya-Ukrayna Gerilimi Akaryakıt Fiyatlarına Yansıyacak]. Retrieved from https://www.ensonhaber.com/ekonomi/rusya-ukrayna-gerilimi-pompaya-yansiyacak

Epston, D., & White, M. (1992). Consulting your consultants: 'The documentation of alternative knowledges. In *Experience, Contradiction, Narrative and Imagination*. Dulwich Centre Publications.

Erçevik, A. (2021). A comparative study regarding solution-focused brief counseling and narrative counseling approaches [Çözüm odaklı kısa süreli psikolojik danışma ve öyküsel psikolojik danışma yaklaşımlarına dair karşılaştırmalı bir inceleme]. *Humanistic Perspective, 3*(2), 400–419. doi:10.47793/hp.942378

Erciş, A., Deligoz, K., & Mutlu, M. (2021). Öğrencilerin FoMO ve plansiz satin alma davranişlari üzerine bir uygulama [A Study on FoMO and impulsıve purchasing behaviors of students]. *Atatürk Üniversitesi İktisadi ve İdari Bilimler Dergisi, 35*(1), 219–243.

Erdal, İ. (2006). Aid activities for Turk emigrant in Turkish-Greece exchange of population. [Türk Yunan nüfus değişiminde Türk mübadillere yapılan yardım faaliyetleri]. *Tarih Araştırmaları Dergisi, 25*(40), 203–214. doi:10.1501/Tarar_0000000255

Erdem, M. N. (2017). *Dijital Çağda Kültür, Yeni Tüketici Kapitalizmi ve Reklam Anlatısı* [Culture, New Consumer Capitalism and Advertising Narrative in the Digital Age] [Conference presentation]. 1st International Conference on New Trends in Communication, Istanbul, Turkey.

Erdem, M. N. (2020). An Argumentative Study on the Presentation of Violence in Media Content [Medya İçeriğinde Şiddetin Sunumu Üzerine Argümantatif Bir Çalışma]. *MANAS Journal of Social Studies, 9*(2), 1198–1217.

Erdem, M. N. (2020). An Argumentative Study on the Presentation of Violence in Media Content [Medya İçeriğinde Şiddetin Sunumu Üzerine Argümantatif Bir Çalışma]. *MANAS Sosyal Araştırmalar Dergisi, 9*(2), 1198–1217. doi:10.33206/mjss.526941

Erdoğan, İ. (2006). *Media and Ethics: A Critical Introduction* [Medya ve Etik: Eleştirel Bir Giriş]. İletişim Kuram ve Araştırma Dergisi.

Erdoğan, İ. (2008). On Studying Football [Futbolu İnceleme Üzerine]. *Journal of Communication Theory and Research*, (26), 1–57.

Eren, A. A. (1936, October 14). What will immigration policy bring to the country? [Göç politikası memlekete neler kazandıracaktır?]. *Tan Gazetesi*, p. 5. Retrieved from https://www.gastearsivi.com/gazete/tan/1936-10-14/5

Ergül, H. (2000). *Magazineization of News on Television [Televizyonda Haberin Magazinleşmesi]*. İletişim Publication.

Erten, Y., & Ardalı, C. (1996). *Psychosocial Structures of Aggression, Violence and Terrorism* [Saldırganlık, Şiddet ve Terörün Psikososyal Yapıları]. YKY Publication.

Escalas, J. E. (1998). Advertising Narratives: What are they and how do they work? In Representing Consumer: Voices, Views and Visions (pp. 241–254). Routledge. doi:10.4324/9780203380260_chapter_9

Escalas, J. E. (1998). Advertising narratives: What are they, and how do they work? *Journal of Consumer Psychology*, 267–289.

Escalas, J. E. (2004). Narrative Processing: Building Consumer Connections to Brands. *Journal of Consumer*, *12*(1&2), 168–180. doi:10.120715327663jcp1401&2_19

Escalas, J. E., & Bettman, J. (2003). You Are What The Eat: The Influence of Reference Groups on Consumers' Connections to Brands. *Journal of Consumer Psychology*, *13*(3), 339–348. doi:10.1207/S15327663JCP1303_14

Esikova, M. M. (2009). Rasprostranenie agronomičeskih znanij i povyšenie èffektivnosti sel′skohozjajstvennogo proizvodstva v gody nèpa. Istoričeskie, filosofskie, političeskie i juridičeskie nauki, kul′turologija i iskusstvovedenie [Dissemination of agronomic knowledge and increasing the efficiency of agricultural production during the NEP years. Historical, philosophical, political and legal sciences, cultural studies and art history. Questions of theory and practice]. *Voprosy teorii i praktiki*, (2), 41-43.

Eti. (2018, Oct 5). *"The Messy" Publicity Campaign* [Video]. YouTube. https://www.youtube.com/watch?v=m7WpFeZrLp8

Evans, B. (2018). Earthbound teaching nature connected arts therapy. *Creative Arts Education and Therapy*, *4*(2), 164–173. doi:10.15212/CAET/2018/4/26

Evre, B. (2009). Different Approaches to Discourse Analysis: A Classification Attempt [Söylem Analizine Yönelik Farklı Yaklaşımlar: Bir Sınıflandırma Girişimi]. In İ. Parlak (Ed.), Construction of Truth in the Media [Medyada Gerçekliğin İnşası] (pp. 107-152). Konya: Çizgi Kitabevi.

Facchini, G., & Mayda, A. M. (2008). From individual attitudes towards migrants to migration policy outcomes: Theory and evidence. *Economic Policy*, *23*(56), 651–713. doi:10.1111/j.1468-0327.2008.00212.x

Fedosov, E. A. (2016). S Sovetskim Soyuzom Navsegda Lozungi i obrazı vostoçnoevropeyskogo plakata 1948-1956 gg [İn With the Soviet Union forever, the slogans and images of the Eastern European poster of 1948-1956.gilizce başlık]. *Vestnik Tomskogo Gosudarstvennogo Universiteta*, (411), 171–176. doi:10.17223/15617793/411/23

Fenerbahce.org Archive. (2022). https://www.fenerbahce.org/haberler/arsiv/orumcek-kamera-stadimizda

Ferro, A. (2006). *Psychoanalysis as Therapy and Storytelling*. Routledge Taylor & Francis Group.

Feuerbach, L. (2008). Hıristiyanlığın Özü [Essence of Christianity]. Say Yayınları.

Finish Türkiye. (2018, Nov 21). *Let Bahar Smile* [Video]. YouTube. https://www.youtube.com/watch?v=BXyP-3s4Ubc

Finneran, M. (2013, October). Keynote presentation. In *Critical journeys in applied theatre*. University of Auckland.

Fischer, D. (2019). Storytelling as a nursing pedagogy. *The Midwest Quarterly*, *60*(3), 311–319.

Fish, B. J. (2012). Response art: The art of the art therapist. *Journal of the American Art Therapy Association*, *29*(3), 138–143. doi:10.1080/07421656.2012.701594

Fiske, J. (2011). İletişim Çalışmalarına Giriş [Introduction to Communication Studies]. Pharmakon.

Fiske, J. (2011). *İletişim çalışmalarına giriş* [Introduction to communication studies]. (S. İrvan, Trans.). Pharmakon Publications.

Fizer, J. (1957). The Irrationality of Soviet Behavior-* Gerhart Niemeyer with the assistance of John S. ReshetarJr.: An Inquiry into Soviet Mentality.(New York: Frederick A. Praeger, 1956. Pp. 113. $2.75.). *The Review of Politics*, *19*(3), 399–400. doi:10.1017/S0034670500012110

Foa, M. (2006). The Invisible Threat: How Spin Doctors Bypass Media Ethics Rules? [Görünmez Tehlike: Spin doktorları Medya ve Etik Kurallarını Nasıl Atlarlar?]. İletişim Kuram ve Araştırma Dergisi, 23.

Ford Trucks, T. R. (2018, Nov 16). *The Biggest Ford Trucks F-Max* [Video]. YouTube. https://www.youtube.com/watch?v=HmfS_ZlMh9Q

Ford, J. D., & Blaustein, M. E. (2013). Systemic self-regulation: A framework for trauma-informed services in residential juvenile justice programs. *Journal of Family Violence*, *28*(7), 665–677. doi:10.100710896-013-9538-5

Foss, B. (2012). Narration Techniques and Dramaturgy in Cinema and Television (M.K. Gerçeker, Trans.). Hayalperest Publication.

Foucault, M. (2001). *Fearles Speech* [Doğruyu Söylemek] (K. Eksen, Trans.). Ayrıntı Yayınları.

Francis. Laudato si. (2015). 1st ed.). Our Sunday Visitor Pub.

Fredman, G. (2004). *Transforming emotions*. Wurr Publishers Ltd.

Freud, S. (2000). *Metapsychology* [Metapsikoloji] (B. Büyükkal & M. Tura, Trans.). İdea Yayınevi.

Frolov, İ. (1991). *Dictionary of Philosophy* [Felsefe Sözlüğü] (A. Çalışlar, Trans.). Cem Yayınevi.

Fromm, E. (1984). *The Origins of Human Destructive [İnsandaki Yıkıcılığın Kökenleri]* (Ş. Alpagut, Trans.). Payel Publication.

Gammer, C. (2009). *The child's voice in family therapy. A systemic perspective*. W. W. Norton & Company.

Geçer, E. (2013). *Media and Popular Culture–TV Series, Television and Society [Medya ve Popüler Kültür–Diziler, Televizyon ve Toplum]*. Metamorfoz Publication.

Geçikli, F. (1999). Geçmişten Günümüze Propaganda Kavramı [The Concept of Propaganda from the Past to the Present]. *İstanbul Üniversitesi İletişim Fakültesi, 9*, 265-276.

Geerts, E., & van der Tuin, I. (2016). *Diffraction & Reading Diffractively.* https://newmaterialism.eu/almanac/d/diffraction.html

Gemicibasi, U., & Yilmaz, R. (2021). Meta-narrative of immigration: A study on migration and the presentation of immigration in Fatih Akin's films. In R. Yilmaz (Ed.), *Handbook of research on narrative interactions* (pp. 63–85). IGI Global. doi:10.4018/978-1-7998-4903-2.ch005

Gençtan, E. (2011). *Psychodynamic Psychiatry and Abnormal Behavior* [Psikodinamik Psikiyatri ve Normaldışı Davranışlar]. Metis Yayınları.

Gendlin, E. T. (1997). *Experiencing and the creation of meaning*. Northwestern University Press.

Geray, C. (1962). *Migration and resettlement of immigrants from and to Turkey (1923-1961), Turkish Economic Development Research Project* [Türkiye'den ve Türkiye'ye göçler ve göçmenlerin iskanı (1923-1961), Türk İktisadi Gelişmesi Araştırma Projesi]. Siyasal Bilimler Fakültesi Maliye Enstitüsü.

Gerber, N., Biffi, E., Biondo, J., Gemignani, M., Hannes, K., & Siegesmund, R. (2020). Arts-based research in the social and health sciences: Pushing for change with an Interdisciplinary Global Arts-Based Research Initiative. *FQS*, *21*(2). Advance online publication. doi:10.17169/fqs-21.2.3496

Gerbner, G. (1972). Violence in Television Drama: Trends and Symbolic Function, Television and Social Behavior: Media Content and Control. National Institute of Mental Health.

Gergen, K. J. (2015). From Mirroring To World-Making: Research As Future Forming. *Journal For The Theory Of Social Behaviour, 45*(3), 287-310. http://works.swarthmore.edu/fac-psychology/797

Gergen, K. (1999). *An invitation to social construction*. Sage Publications.

Gergen, K. (2009). *Relational being: beyond self and community*. Oxford University Press.

Gergen, K. J. (2009). *Relational Being: Beyond Self and Community*. Oxford University Press.

Gergen, K. J. (2021). *The Relational Imperative, Resources for a World on Edge*. Taos Institute Publications.

Gergen, K., & Gergen, M. (1988). Advances in Experimental Social Psychology: Vol. 21. *Narrative And The Self As Relationship*. Academic Press Inc.

Gergen, M. (2007). Life stories: pieces of a dream. In M. Gergen & K. Gergen (Eds.), *Social Construction, A Reader*. Sage Publications.

Gjunter, H. (1999). *Sčastlivaja Moskva" i arhetip materi v sovetskoj kul'ture 30-h godov." Strana filosofov" Andreja Platonova: problemy tvorčestva* [Happy Moscow" and the mother archetype in Soviet culture of the 1930s. Country of Philosophers" by Andrey Platonov: problems of creativity]. https://lit.wikireading.ru/45173

Gladding, S. T. (2019). Family therapy: History, theory and practice (7th ed.). Pearson.

Goal.com. (2018). *What is video referee application (VAR)?* [Video hakem uygulaması (VAR) nedir]. https://www.goal.com/tr/haber/video-hakem-uygulamasi-var nedir/1n1vfg3dgig3o18pdz6c7l142q

Gobble, C. (2009). The Value of Story Theory in Providing Culturally Sensitive Advanced Practice Nursing in Rural Appalachia. *Online Journal of Rural Nursing and Health Care: the Official Journal of the Rural Nurse Organization, 9*(1), 94–105. doi:10.14574/ojrnhc.v9i1.108

Gökçe, G. (1997). *Television Program Production and Directing [Televizyon Program Yapımcılığı ve Yönetmenliği]*. Derin Publication.

Goldberg, S. H. (2015). Transference, the Interpersonal Field, and Psychological Transformation in the Work of Antonino Ferro. *Psychoanalytic Inquiry, 35*(5), 495–511. doi:10.1080/07351690.2015.1044407

Good, B. (1994). Medicine, rationality, and experience: an anthropological perspective. In The Lewis Henry Morgan lectures 1990. Cambridge University Press.

Good, M. C., & Hyman, M. R. (2020). 'Fear of missing out': Antecedents and influence on purchase likelihood. *Journal of Marketing Theory and Practice, 28*(3), 330–341. doi:10.1080/10696679.2020.1766359

Good, M. C., & Hyman, M. R. (2021). Direct and indirect effects of fear-of-missing-out appeals on purchase likelihood. *Journal of Consumer Behaviour, 20*(3), 564–576. doi:10.1002/cb.1885

Goodman, S. (2010). Integration requirements for integration's sake: Identifying, categorising and comparing civic integration policies. *Journal of Ethnic and Migration Studies, 36*(5), 753–772. doi:10.1080/13691831003764300

Görgün, A. (2006). A New Communication Trend in Turkey: Spin Doctor [Türkiye'de Yeni Bir iletişim Eğilimi: Spin Doctor]. *21. Yüzyılda Halkla İlişkilerde Yeni Yönelimler, Sorunlar ve Çözümler Sempozyumu.*

Gray, B. (2011). Autoethnography and arts therapy: The arts meet healing. *Australia and New Zealand Journal of Arts Therapy, 6*(1), 67–80.

Green, D. (2015a). *Quake destruction/arts creation: arts therapy and the Canterbury earthquakes* (Unpublished doctoral thesis). University of Auckland, New Zealand.

Green, D. (2018). Arts therapy, imagical play, and trauma: Exploring arts therapy during the canterbury earthquakes. *The International Journal of the Arts in Society: Annual Review, 13*(1). doi:10.18848/1833-1866/CGP

Green, D. (2018b). Reclaiming messy-mudpies & magic through poiesis, education & arts therapy. *The International Journal of Arts in Education,* 31-57.

Green, D. & Evans, Bettina. (2018). Kites and shaking hearts in the rubble. *Australia and New Zealand Journal of Arts Therapy*, *13*(1&2), 35–46.

Green, D. (2015). Exploring and sharing arts therapy experiences through fiction-based research. *Australia and New Zealand Journal of Arts Therapy*, *10*(1), 33–42.

Green, D. (2017). Imagical play: arts therapy and trauma. In P. O'Connor & C. R. Gómez (Eds.), *Playing with possibilities* (pp. 200–222). Cambridge Scholars.

Green, D. (2017a). Quake destruction/arts creation: Arts therapy and the Canterbury earthquakes. *Australia and New Zealand Journal of Arts Therapy*, *12*(1), 40–45.

Green, D. (2018a). Making-sense of poietic presense in arts therapy and education. *Creative Arts in Education and Therapy*, *4*(2), 139–148. doi:10.15212/CAET/2018/4/21

Green, D. (2019). Communitas and soul-healing: arts therapy within the loss-upon-loss of natural disaster. In M. J. M. Wood, B. Jacobson, & H. Cridford (Eds.), *The international handbook of art therapy in palliative and bereavement care* (pp. 340–356). Routledge. doi:10.4324/9781315110530-35

Green, D., Levey, A., Evans, B., Lawson, W., & Marks, K. (2022). The arts of making-sense in uncertain times: arts-based research and autoethnography. In H. Kara & S. Khoo (Eds.), *Qualitative and digital research in times of crisis: methods, reflexivity, and ethics* (pp. 59–77). Policy Press.

Green, D., Pears-Scown, N., Weir, M., Csata, I., Heney, R., McGeever, M., Lambert, R., Marks, K., & Wang, I. (2018). The arts of making sens/e. *Australia and New Zealand Journal of Arts Therapy*, *12*(1), 112–130.

Greenwood, J. (2012). Arts-based research: Weaving magic and meaning. *International Journal of Education & the Arts*, *13*(1). http://www.ijea.org/v13i1/

Greer, G.-H., & Blair, L. (2018). Arts-based research and the discourse of danger. *Studies in Art Education*, *59*(3), 243–255. doi:10.1080/00393541.2018.1479824

Groot, D. S. (2002). *Shifting gears: An integration of solution-focused therapy and experiential therapy in couples counselling* (Master's thesis, University of Manitoba). Retrieved from https://mspace.lib.umanitoba.ca/xmlui/handle/1993/22624

Guenon, R. (2012). Niceliğin Egemenliği ve Çağın Alametleri [The Sovereignty of Quantity and the Signs of the Age]. İz Yayıncılık.

Gültekin, Z. (2006). Before Iraq: The Valley of the Wolves [Irak'dan önce: Kurtlar Vadisi Dizisi]. *İletişim Kuram ve Araştırma, 22*, 9-36.

Günay, N. (2015). *The Role of Spin Doctors in Persuasion Process of Public Relations* [Halkla İlişkiler Çalışmalarında İkna Açısından Döngü Yönetiminin (Spin Doctors) Rolü] [Unpublished Master Thesis]. Ege Üniversitesi Sosyal Bilimler Enstitüsü.

Günay, M. A., & Çakın, Ö. (2021). Changes in Consumer Behaviors in the Covid 19 Pandemic Process. In G. Çalışır & E. Diker (Eds.), *The Changing Face of Communication Covid-19 Process [Covid 19 Pandemi Sürecinde Tüketici Davranışlarında Yaşanan Değişimler, içinde: Covid-19 Sürecinde İletişimin Değişen Yüzü]* (pp. 10–334). Eğitim Publications.

Güner, O. (2014). *The solution is hidden in me* [Çözüm bende saklı]. Eflatun.

Gürdin, B. (2019). Sosyal medyanın hedonik tüketimi ve FoMO'nun gücü [Hedonic Consumption Of Social Media And FoMO's Power]. *Üçüncü Sektör Sosyal Ekonomi Dergisi, 54*(3), 1259-1278.

Gürer, M. (2016) Narrative Structure of Television and Hybridization In Television Programs [Televizyonun anlatı Yapısı ve Televizyon Programlarında Hibritleşme Süreci]. *International Peer-Reviewed Journal of Communication and Humanities Research*, 69-94.

Gürer, S. Z., & Gürer, M. (2017). The Sunumu of "Pretentious Consumption" on the Axis of Lives Designed on Television: An Example of a Bold and Beautiful Series [Televizyonda Tasarlanan Hayatlar Ekseninde "Gösterişçi Tüketimin" Sunumu: Cesur ve Güzel Dizisi Örneği]. *Uluslararası Sosyal Araştırmalar Dergisi, 10*(51), 1160–1173.

Gurtan, K. (1982). *Statistics and Research Methods* [İstatistik ve Araştırma Metodları]. İstanbul Üniversitesi Yayınları.

Güven, A. (2020). Post-Truth as the Loss of the Truth: A Conceptualization Attempt [Hakikatin Yitimi Olarak Post-Truth: Bir Kavramsallaştırma Denemesi]. *İnsan ve İnsan, 7*(23), 20-36.

Gu, Y. (2018). Narrative, life writing, and healing: The therapeutic functions of storytelling. *Neohelicon, 45*(2), 479–489. doi:10.100711059-018-0459-4

Güz, H. (2007). Violence and Youth Perception of Violence. In *Prevention of Violence Against Children and Adolescents Symposium.* Aem Kitap.

Güz, N. (2007). The Role of the Media in Preventing Violence. In *Child and Adolescent Symposium on the Prevention of Violence Against.* Aem Kitap.

Habermas, J. (1993). Technique and Science as Ideology (M. Tüzel, Trans.). Yapı Kredi Publications.

Habertürk. (n.d.). *The 'hand of God' story was a symbolic 'revenge'* [Tanrı'nın eli" hikayesi, sembolik bir 'intikam'dı]. https://www.haberturk.com/tanri-nin-eli-hikayesi-sembolik-bir-intikam-di-maradona-1986-dunya-kupasi-ndaki-golu-anlatti-2882076-spor

Hall, C. S. (2010). *Introduction to Freudian Psychology* [Freudyen Psikolojiye Giriş] (E. Delvrim, Trans.). Kaknüs Yayınları.

Halprin, D. (2003). *The expressive body in life, art and therapy. Working with movement, metaphor and meaning.* Jessica Kingsley.

Hansen, T. (2020). Critical Conflict Resolution Theory and Practice. In An Introduction to Conflict Resolution, Discourses and Dynamics (pp. 759-777). Academic Press.

Haraway, D. (2016). *Staying with the trouble: Making kin in the Chthulucene.* Duke University Press.

Harjuniemi, T. (2021). Post-Truth, Fake News and The Liberal 'Regime of Truth' – The Double Movement Between Lippmann and Hayek. *European Journal of Communication*, 1–15. doi:10.1177/02673231211046784

Harsin, J. (2018). Post-Truth and Critical Communication Studies. In Oxford Research Encyclopedia of Communication (pp. 1–32). Oxford University Press. doi:10.1093/acrefore/9780190228613.013.757

Haseman, B. (2006). A manifesto for performative research. *Media International Australia Incorporating Culture and Policy, Theme Issue Practice-led Research*, (118), 98–106.

Hawk-eye innovations. (2022). https://www.hawkeyeinnovations.com/about

Hawkins, D. I., Best, R. J., & Coney, K. A. (2004). *Consumer behavior*. McGraw-Hill.

Hayran, C., Anik, L., & Gurhan-Canli, Z. (2016). Exploring the antecedents and consumer behavioral consequences of. ACR North American advances. In P. Moreau & S. Puntoni (Eds.), *NA - Advances in Consumer Research* (Vol. 44, pp. 468–468). Association for Consumer Research.

Hayran, C., Anik, L., & Gürhan-Canli, Z. (2020). A threat to loyalty: Fear of missing out (FOMO) leads to reluctance to repeat current experiences. *PLoS One*, *15*(4), 1–17. doi:10.1371/journal.pone.0232318 PMID:32353059

He Kicked His Ex-Wife Many Times In Front Of His Child! (2021). https://www.youtube.com/watch?v=_GcZ0ggens8

Hedges, F. (2010). *Reflexivity in Therapeutic Practice*. Bloomsbury. doi:10.1007/978-1-137-12293-3

Hedtke, L. (2014). Creating stories of hope: A narrative approach to illness, death and grief. *Australian and New Zealand Journal of Family Therapy*, *35*(1), 4–19. doi:10.1002/anzf.1040

Hegeman, S. (2015). A sociological imagination. *Studia Neophilologica*, *87*(sup1), 97–103. doi:10.1080/00393274.2014.981960

Heidegger, M. (1935/1975). *Poetry, language, thought* (A. Hofstadter, Trans.). Harper & Row, Perennial Library.

Herman, D. (2019). *The Fear of Missing Out*. http://fomofearofmissingout.com/fomo

Herman, D., Jahn, M., & Ryan, M. L. (Eds.). (2005). *Routledge Encylopedia of Narrative Theory*. Routledge.

Hernandez, M. Y. (2009). Psychological theories of immigration. *Journal of Human Behavior in the Social Environment*, *19*(6), 713–729. doi:10.1080/10911350902910898

Hillman, J. (1983). *InterViews: Conversations with Laura Pozzo on psychology, biography, love, soul, the gods, animals, dreams, imagination, work, cities, and the state of the culture*. Spring Publications.

Hinton, D., & Kirmayer, L. J. (2017). The Flexibility Hypothesis of Healing. *Culture, Medicine and Psychiatry*, *41*(1), 3–34. doi:10.100711013-016-9493-8 PMID:27142641

Hinz, L. D. (2009). *Expressive therapies continuum: A framework for using art in therapy*. Routledge. doi:10.4324/9780203893883

Hloponina, O. O. (2017). Censkiy mir v sovetskom plakate 1910-1930-x godov: evolutsiya mifologiçeskix konstrujtov [The World of Women in Soviet Posters 1910-1930]. *Znanie, Ponimanie, Umenie, 4*(25), 287-295.

Hodkinson, C. (2016). 'Fear of Missing Out'(FOMO) marketing appeals: A conceptual model. *Journal of Marketing Communications*, *25*(1), 1–24.

Holman Jones, S., Adams, T. E., & Ellis, C. (2016). *Handbook of autoethnography*. Left Coast Press Inc.

Horton, J. L. (2008). *Publicity Stunts, What Are They? Why Do Them?* http://online pr.com/Holding/PRStuntsarticle.pdf

Hoşgör, H., Koç Tütüncü, S., Gündüz Hoşgör, D., & Tandoğan, Ö. (2017). Üniversite öğrencileri arasında sosyal medyadaki gelişmeleri kaçırma korkusu yaygınlığının farklı değişkenler açısından incelenmesi [Examination in terms of different variables of prevalence of fear of missing out among college students]. *International Journal of Academic Value Studies.*, *3*(17), 213–223.

Howell, R. (1975). The USSR: Sport and Politics Intertwined. *Comparative Education, 11*(2), 137–145. doi:10.1080/0305006750110204

Hsieh, H. F., & Shannon, S. E. (2005). Three Approaches to Qualitative Content Analysis. *Qualitative Health Research, 15*(9), 1277–1288. doi:10.1177/1049732305276687 PMID:16204405

Hurriyet. (2022). *The blood pressure is too high... Biden: If we enter Ukraine, there will be a world war* [Tansiyon çok yüksek... Biden: Ukrayna'ya girersek dünya savaşı çıkar]. Retrieved from https://www.hurriyet.com.tr/dunya/tansiyon-cok-yuksek-biden-ukraynaya-girersek-dunya-savasi-cikar-42002279

Hurtado, A., Gurin, P., & Peng, T. (1994). Social identities-A framework for studying the adaptations of immigrants and ethnics: The adaptations of Mexicans in the United States. *Social Problems, 41*(1), 129–151. doi:10.2307/3096846

İçişleri Bakanlığı, Müdürlüğü, Politika, & Başkanlığı. (2017). *2016 Turkey migration report* [2016 Türkiye göç raporu] (Publication No. 40). Retrieved from https://www.goc.gov.tr/kurumlar/goc.gov.tr/YillikGocRaporlari/2016_yiik_goc_raporu_haziran.pdf

Iglesias, A., & Iglesias, A. (2016). Hypnotic mediated therapeutic storytelling with over-involved children. *Contemporary Hypnosis & Integrative Therapy, 31*(1), 6–12.

İlerialkan, D., & Yılmaz, R. (2015). *How to Write a Script, How Do They Write?* [Senaryo Nasıl Yazılır? Nasıl Yazıyorlar?]. Alfa Yayınları.

İlerialkan, D., & Yılmaz, R. (2015). Script: How to Write? How Do They Write? [Senaryo: Nasıl Yazılır? Nasıl Yazıyorlar?]. *Alfa.*

İlerialkan, D., & Yılmaz, R. (2015). Script: How to Write? How They Write [Senaryo: Nasıl Yazılır? Nasıl Yazıyorlar?]. *Alfa.*

İnal, U. & Şevik E. (2017). Facebook Usage of Turkey's 10 Most Listened Radios. [Türkiye'nin En Çok Dinlenen 10 Radyosunun Facebook Kullanımı]. *Ulakbilge Sosyal Bilimler, 5*(9), 199-230.

İnal, A. (1999). *Television, Genre and Representation [Televizyon, Tür ve Temsil].* Mahmut Tali Öngören'e Armağan.

İnal, M. A. (1996). *Reading the News [Haberi Okumak].* Temuçin Publication.

İnal, R. (2008). *Globalization and Sports [Küreselleşme ve Spor].* Evrensel Publication.

İnal, U. (2016). An Investigation into Film 'Good Night and Good Luck' within Theories of Journalism ['Good Night and Good Luck' Filminin Gazetecilik Kuramları Çerçevesinde İncelenmesi]. *Middle Black Sea Journal of Communication Studies, 1*(2), 87–96.

İnal, U., & Şevik, E. (2019). Survive in Rating Battles. In R. Yılmaz, M. N. Erdem, & F. Resuloglu (Eds.), *Handbook of Research on Transmedia Storytelling and Narrative Strategies* (pp. 190–208). IGI Global. doi:10.4018/978-1-5225-5357-1.ch010

İpek, N. (2000). *Exchange and Samsun* [Mübadele ve Samsun]. Türk Tarih Kurumu.

İpek, N. (2012). *Exchanged people from Thessaloniki to Samsun* [Selanik'ten Samsun'a mübadiller] (2nd ed.). Samsun Büyükşehir Belediyesi, Kültür ve Sosyal İşler Daire Başkanlığı.

İstanbul Kültür Sanat Vakfı. (2018 Sep 26). *Despite This Advertisement* [Video]. YouTube. https://www.youtube.com/watch?v=C_Kzw768hfw

Iveson, C. (2002). Solution-focused brief therapy. *Advances in Psychiatric Treatment, 8*(2), 149–157. doi:10.1192/apt.8.2.149

Jahn, M. (2015). *Anlatıbilim* [The Narratology] (B. Dervişcemaloğlu, Trans.). Dergah Publications.

Jahn, M. (2015). *Narrative Theory Handbook* [AnlatıBilim Anlatı Teorisi El Kitabı] (B. Dervişcemaloğlu, Trans.). Dergah.

Jarskoj-Smirnovoj, E. R., & Romanova, P. V. (2009). *Vizual'naja antropologija: režimy vidimosti pri socializme* [Visual anthropology: visibility regimes in socialism]. Moskva: BBK 60.5 V 76.

Jenkins, A. (2009). Becoming ethical. A parallel, political journey with men who have abused. Rusell House Publishing Ltd.

Jolly, K., Weiss, J. A., & Liehr, P. (2007). Understanding Adolescent Voice as a Guide for Nursing Practice and Research. *Issues in Comprehensive Pediatric Nursing, 30*(1–2), 3–13. doi:10.1080/01460860701366518 PMID:17613138

Jood, T. E. (2017). *Missing the present for the unknown: the relationship between fear of missing out (fomo) and life satisfaction* [Unpublished doctoral dissertation]. University of South Africa, Pretoria.

Joyce, L., & Liamputtong, P. (2017). Acculturation stress and social support for young refugees in regional areas. *Children and Youth Services Review, 77*, 18–26. doi:10.1016/j.childyouth.2017.03.016

Jung, C. G., & Chodorow, J. (1997). *Jung on active imagination*. Princeton University Press. doi:10.1515/9781400866854

Jung, C. G., & Shamdasani, S. (2009). *The Red Book = Liber Novus* (1st ed.). W.W. Norton & Co.

Kaçik, S., & Acar, F. (2020). Üniversite öğrencilerinin gelişmeleri kaçirma korkusu (GKK) ve yaşam doyumu düzeylerinin demografik değişkenler açisindan incelenmesi [The evaluation of fear of missing out (FoMO) and the level of life satisfaction of university students in terms of demographic variables]. *Kayseri Üniversitesi Sosyal Bilimler Dergisi, 2*(1), 74–90.

Kağıtçıbaşı, Ç., & Cemalcılar, Z. (2014). *Human and people from past to present: Introduction to social psychology* [Dünden bugüne insan ve insanlar: Sosyal psikolojiye giriş] (16th ed.). Evrim.

Kakutani, M. (2018). *The Death of Truth: Notes on Falsehood in the Age of Trump* [Hakikatin Ölümü: Trump Çağında Yalancılık Sanatı] (C. Mizrahi, Trans.). Doğan Kitap.

Kandinsky, W. (1977). *Concerning the Spiritual in Art*. Dover Publications.

Kang, I., Cui, H., & Son, J. (2019). Conformity consumption behavior and FoMO. *Sustainability, 11*(17), 1–18. doi:10.3390u11174734

Kapitan, L. (2013). Editorial. Reexamining the map: Extending and disrupting art therapy assumptions of representation. *Art Therapy: Journal of the American Art Therapy Association, 30*(3), 96–97. doi:10.1080/07421656.2013.819548

Kapitan, L. (2014). *Introduction to art therapy research*. Routledge.

Kapitan, L., Litell, M., & Torres, A. (2011). Creative Art Therapy in a Community's Participatory Research and Social Transformation. *Art Therapy: Journal of the American Art Therapy Association, 28*(2), 64–73. doi:10.1080/07421656.2011.578238

Karadağ, Ç. (2019). *Post-truth kavramı üzerinden medya ve siyaset ilişkisinin The Post, Spotlight ve Truth filmleri çerçevesinde incelenmesi* [Examining the relationship between media and politics through the concept of post-truth within the framework of The Post, Spotlight and Truth films] [Master's thesis]. İstanbul Gelişim Üniversitesi Sosyal Bilimler Enstitüsü.

Karadut, İ. C. (2020). Telling the Truth in the Post-Truth Age: Two Cases of Parrhesia [Hakikat-Ötesi Çağda Hakikati Söylemek: İki Parrhesia Vakası]. *Pasajlar Sosyal Bilimler Dergisi, 4*, 125–140.

Kara, H., & Khoo, S. (Eds.), *Qualitative and digital research in times of crisis: methods, reflexivity, and ethics*. Policy Press. doi:10.2307/j.ctv2321kdr

Karakuş, S. (2017). *Lived 79 years ago: The first football match to be televised live* [79 yıl önce naklen: Televizyondan canlı yayınlanan ilk futbol maçı]. https://www.gzt.com/zpor/79-yil-once-naklen-televizyondan-canliyayinlanan-ilk-futbol-maci-2798065

Kars, N. (2003). *Let's Make a TV Program, Let Everyone Watch [Televizyon Programı Yapalım, Herkes İzlesin]*. Derin Publication.

Kars, N. (2012). *Let's Make a TV Program for Everyone to Watch [Televizyon Programı Yapalım Herkes İzlesin]*. Derin Publication.

Kars, N. (2015). *History, Theories, Discourse and Radio-Television Journalism of the News, [Haberin Tarihi, Kuramları, Söylemi ve Radyo-Televizyon Haberciliği]*. Derin Publication.

Kaufmann, E. (2017). Why values, not economics, hold the key to the populist right-and to crafting new migration narratives. In M. McAuliffe & M. Klein Solomon (Eds.), *Migration research leaders' syndicate: Ideas to inform international cooperation on safe, orderly and regular migration* (pp. 183–188). International Organization for Migration.

Kaya, R. (2021). An Old Truth A New Concept: The Trivialization of Truth or Post-Truth [Eski Bir Hakikat Yeni Bir Kavram: Hakikatin Önemsizleşmesi ya da Post-Truth]. *Isparta Okulu Dergisi*, *1*(1), 25–35.

Keane, B. (2007). Taniwha. *Te Ara - the Encyclopedia of New Zealand*. http://www.TeAra.govt.nz/en/taniwha

Kelly, M. S., Kelly, M. S., Kim, J. S., & Franklin, C. (2008). *Solution focused brief therapy in schools: A 360 degree view of research and practice*. Oxford University Press. doi:10.1093/acprof:oso/9780195366297.001.0001

Kemp, S. (2021, Jan). *Digital 2021: The latest insights into the 'state of digital'*. https://wearesocial.com/uk/blog/2021/01/digital-2021-the-latest-insights-into-the-state-of-digital/

Ker Dinçer, M., & Başok, N. (2014). Public Relations Spin Doctor Management Public Relations Practitioners are also not Spin Doctors [Halkla İlişkiler Döngü Yönetimi, Halkla İlişkiler Uygulamacıları da Döngü Uzmanı Değildir]. In What Public Relations Is Not [Halkla İlişkiler Ne Değildir?] (pp. 297-328). Say Yayınları.

Kernberg, O. F. (2019). *Border Situations and Pathological Narcissism* [Sınır Durumlar ve Patolojik Narsisizm]. Metis Yayınları.

Keyes, R. (2021). The Post-Truth Era, Lying and Deception in Today's World (D. Özçetin, Trans.). Tudem Publication.

Keyes, R. (2017). *Hakikat Sonrası Çağ: Günümüz Dünyasında Yalancılık ve Aldatma* [The Post-Truth Age: Lying and Deception in Today's World]. Tudem Yayın Grubu.

Keyes, R. (2017). *The Post-Truth Era: Dishonesty and Deception in Contemporary Life* [Hakikat Sonrası Çağ: Günümüz Dünyasında Yalancılık ve Aldatma] (D. Özçetin, Trans.). Delidolu Yayınları.

Kılıç, L. (2003). *Image Aesthetics [Görüntü Estetiği]*. İnkılâp Publication.

Kılınç, U. (2017). Create It! Extend It!: Evolution of Comics Through Narrative Advertising. In R. Yılmaz (Ed.), *Narrative Advertising Models and Conceptualization in the Digital Age* (pp. 117–132). IGI Global. doi:10.4018/978-1-5225-2373-4.ch007

Kim, D., Lee, Y., Lee, J., Nam, J. K., & Chung, Y. (2014). Development of Korean smartphone addiction proneness scale for youth. *PLoS One*, *9*(5), e97920. doi:10.1371/journal.pone.0097920 PMID:24848006

Kim, J. S., & Franklin, C. (2009). Solution-focused brief therapy in schools: A review of the outcome literature. *Children and Youth Services Review*, *31*(4), 464–470. doi:10.1016/j.childyouth.2008.10.002

Kim, J., Lee, Y., & Kim, M. L. (2020). Investigating 'fear of missing out'(FOMO) as an extrinsic motive affecting sport event consumer's behavioral intention and FOMO-driven consumption's influence on intrinsic rewards, extrinsic rewards, and consumer satisfaction. *PLoS One*, *15*(12), e0243744. doi:10.1371/journal.pone.0243744

Kim, K. S., Loring, S., & Kwekkeboom, K. (2018). Use of art-making intervention for pain and quality of life among cancer patients a systematic review. *Journal of Holistic Nursing*, *36*(4), 341–353. doi:10.1177/0898010117726633 PMID:28836473

Kiser-Larson, N. (2000). The Concepts of Caring and Story Viewed from Three Nursing Paradigms. *International Journal for Human Caring*, *4*(2), 26–32. doi:10.20467/1091-5710.4.2.26

Kleinman, A. (1989). *The Illness Narratives: Suffering, Healing, and the Human Condition*. Basic Books.

Knill, P. (2011). Communal art-making and conflict transformation. In E. Levine & S. K. Levine (Eds.), *Art in Action* (pp. 53–77). Jessica Kingsley.

Knill, P. J., Levine, E. G., & Levine, S. K. (2005). *Principles and practice of expressive arts therapy, toward a therapeutic aesthetics*. Jessica Kingsley.

Koban, K., Neureiter, A., Stevic, A., & Matthes, J. (2022). The COVID-19 infodemic at your fingertips. Reciprocal relationships between COVID-19 information FOMO, bedtime smartphone news engagement, and daytime tiredness over time. *Computers in Human Behavior*, *130*, 1–8. doi:10.1016/j.chb.2021.107175 PMID:35035063

Koç Holding. (2019, Sep 12). *Biennial 2019* [Video]. YouTube. https://www.youtube.com/watch?v=oJ6-ZNtrBk8

Koç, A. A. (1993). Conceptual and Linguistic Development of Narrative Structure [Anlatı Yapısının Kavramsal ve Dilsel Gelişimi]. *Dilbilim Araştırmaları Dergisi*, *4*, 51–60.

Kocabay Şener, N. (2019). Post-Truth If You Want Lies, Let Me Lies [Post-Hakikat (Post-Truth) Yalanlar İstiyorsan Yalanlar Söyleyeyim]. In M. N. Erdem & N. Kocabay Şener (Eds.), *Communication in the Age of Posts* [Postlar Çağında İletişim] (pp. 383–416). Literatürk Academia.

Kohut, H. (2020-a). *Self-Resolution* [Kendiliğin Çözümlenmesi] (O. Cebeci, Trans.). Metis Yayınları.

Kohut, H. (2020-b). *Self-Restructuring* [Kendiliğin Yeniden Yapılanması] (O. Cebeci, Trans.). Metis Yayınları.

Köknel, Ö. (2000). *Individual and Community Violence [Bireysel ve Toplumsal Şiddet]*. Altın Kitaplar Publication.

Kotler, S. (2015). *The Neurochemistry of flow states*. Think Big. https://www.youtube.com/watch?v=aHp2hkue8RQ

Kreitner, R. (2016). *Post-Truth and Its Consequences: What a 25-Year-Old Essay Tells Us About the Current Moment*. Retrieved from https://www.thenation.com/article/archive/post-truth-and-its-consequences-what-a-25-year-old-essay-tells-us-about-the-current-moment/

Kress, V. E., Adamson, N. A., & Yensel, J. (2010). The use of therapeutic stories in counseling child and adolescent sexual abuse survivors. *Journal of Creativity in Mental Health*, *5*(3), 243–259. doi:10.1080/15401383.2010.507657

Kronick, R., Rousseau, C., & Cleveland, J. (2018). Refugee children's sandplay narratives in immigration detention in Canada. *European Child & Adolescent Psychiatry*, *27*(4), 423–437. doi:10.100700787-017-1012-0 PMID:28643110

Küçükerdoğan, R. (2016). Anlatısal Yapı Çözümlemesi ve Reklam İletişimde "Anlatı Yerlemleri" ['Narrative Locations' in Narrative Structure Analysis and Advertising Communication]. *Dilbilim Dergisi*, *2*(30), 5–18.

Küçükkömürler, S., & Sakallı-Uğurlu, N. (2017). Social contact theories to regulate intergroup relations: Intergroup, extended, imagined contact [Gruplar arası ilişkileri düzenlemede sosyal temas kuramları: Gruplar arası, yayılmacı ve hayali temas]. *Nesne Psikoloji Dergisi*, *9*(5), 1–31. doi:10.7816/nesne-05-09-01

Kuczynski, L., & De Mol, J. (2015). Dialectical Models of Socialization. In W. F. Overton & P. C. M. Molenaar (Eds.), Theory and Method. Volume 1 of the Handbook of Child Psychology and Developmental Science (7th ed.). Wiley. doi:10.1002/9781118963418.childpsy109

Kundakçı, E. (2011). Politics, Media and Spin Doctor [Siyaset, Medya ve Spin Doctor]. In M. Ü. Erzen (Ed.), *Politics with its Historical, Cultural and Social Paradigms* [Tarihi, Kültürel ve Sosyal Paradigmaları ile Siyaset] (pp. 275–328). Der Yayınları.

Kuper, S. (2014). Football is Never Just Football (S. Gürtunca, Trans.). İthaki Publication.

KurumuT. D.SözlükG. T. (n.d.). *Propaganda* [Propaganda]. https://sozluk.gov.tr/

Laing, C. M., Moules, N. J., Sinclair, S., & Estefan, A. (2019). Digital storytelling as a psychosocial tool for adult cancer survivors. *Oncology Nursing Forum*, *46*(2), 147–154. doi:10.1188/19.ONF.147-154 PMID:30767963

Landau, L. B. (2017). Southern urbanism, legalization, and the limits of migration law. In M. McAuliffe & M. Klein Solomon (Eds.), *Migration research leaders' syndicate: Ideas to inform international cooperation on safe, orderly and regular migration* (pp. 33–36). International Organization for Migration. doi:10.1017/aju.2017.39

Langdridge, D. (2006). Solution focused therapy A way forward for brief existential therapy? *Journal of the Society for Existential Analysis*, *17*(2), 359–370.

Larkin, D. M., & Zabourek, R. P. (1988). Therapeutic storytelling and metaphors. *Holistic Nursing Practice*, *2*(3), 45–53. doi:10.1097/00004650-198802030-00009 PMID:3366805

Lasch, C. (2006). *Narcissism Culture* [Narsisizm Kültürü] (S. Öztürk & Ü. H. Yolsal, Trans.). Bilim ve Sanat.

Leavy, P. (2013). *Fiction as research practice: Short stories, novellas, and novels (Developing qualitative inquiry).* Left Coast Press.

Leavy, P. (2018). *Handbook of arts-based research.* The Guildford Press.

Lederach, J. P. (2010) *The Moral Imagination: The Art and Soul of Building Peace*. Oxford University.

Lederach, J. P. (2020) An Integrated Framework for Peacebuilding. In An Introduction to Conflict Resolution, Discourses and Dynamics (pp. 481-491). Academic Press.

Lederach, J. P. (1999). *The journey toward reconciliation.* Herald Press.

Lee, E., Bristow, J., Faircloth, C., & MacVarish, J. (2014). *Parenting culture studies.* Palgrave Macmillan. doi:10.1057/9781137304612

Lee, H., Fawcett, J., & DeMarco, R. (2016). Storytelling/narrative theory to address health communication with minority populations. *Applied Nursing Research*, *30*, 58–60. doi:10.1016/j.apnr.2015.09.004 PMID:27091254

Lee, J. A., Bright, L. F., & Eastin, M. S. (2021). Fear of missing out and consumer happiness on instagram: A serial mediation of social media influencer-related activities. *Cyberpsychology, Behavior, and Social Networking*, *24*(11), 762–766. doi:10.1089/cyber.2020.0431 PMID:33877908

Lee, S. Y., Oh, S., & Jung, S. (2018). Influence of scarcity claims on product evaluation: The role of reversibility of decision. *Social Behavior and Personality*, *46*(2), 281–292. doi:10.2224bp.6576

Leight, S. B. (2002). Starry night: Using story to inform aesthetic knowing in women's health nursing. *Journal of Advanced Nursing*, *37*(1), 108–114. doi:10.1046/j.1365-2648.2002.02050.x PMID:11784404

Lenin, V. (1969). Polnoye sobraniye soçineniy [Complete collection of compositions]. T. 26, Gospolitizdat.

Lenin, V. (2011). Ne Yapmalı? [What to do?]. Evrensel Basım Yayın.

Lethem, J. (2002). Brief solution focused therapy. *Child and Adolescent Mental Health*, *7*(4), 189–192. doi:10.1111/1475-3588.00033 PMID:33158321

Levine, E. G., & Levine, S. K. (2017). *New developments in expressive arts therapy: The play of poiesis*. Jessica Kingsley.

Levine, P. A. (2010). *In an unspoken voice: How the body releases trauma and restores goodness*. North Atlantic Books.

Levine, S. K. (2009). *Trauma, tragedy, therapy: The arts and human suffering*. Jessica Kingsley.

Liehr, P. (2000). Using Story Theory to Guide Nursing Practice. *International Journal for Human Caring*, *4*(2), 13–18. doi:10.20467/1091-5710.4.2.13

Liehr, P. R., & Smith, M. J. (2018). Story Theory. In M. J. Smith & P. R. Liehr (Eds.), *Middle Range Theory for Nursing* (pp. 241–264). Springer Publishing Company. doi:10.1891/9780826159922.0011

Liehr, P., & Smith, M. J. (2020). Claiming the Narrative Wave With Story Theory. *Advances in Nursing Science*, *43*(1), 15–27. doi:10.1097/ANS.0000000000000303 PMID:32015246

Ligtv.com Archive. (2022). *The hawk's eye is being tried for football* [Şahin gözü futbol için deneniyor]. http://www.ligtv.com.tr/haber/sahin-gozufutbol-icin-deneniyor

Lilleker, D. G. (2013). *Siyasal İletişim: Temel Kavramlar* [Political Communication: Basic Concepts]. Kaknüs Yayınları.

Lincoln, Y. S., & Denzin, N. K. (2003). *Turning points in qualitative research: tying knots in a handkerchief*. Altamira Press.

Lindforss, L., & Magnusson, D. (1997). Solution-focused therapy in prison. *Contemporary Family Therapy*, *19*(1), 89–103. doi:10.1023/A:1026114501186

Lipchik, E. (1994). The rush to be brief. *The Family Therapy Networker*, *18*(2), 35–39.

Llorente, J. A. (2017). *The post-truth era: Reality vs. perception*. UNO Developing Ideas.

Lodge-Guttery, C. (2004). *The impact of narrative storytelling on cognitive re-composition in individuals struggling with eating disorders* (Order No. 3138725) [Unpublished doctoral dissertation]. University of Oklahoma, Norman, Oklahoma, United States. ProQuest Dissertations & Theses Global.

Long, N. (2013). *Therapeutic storytelling in a pupil referral unit: The story of intersubjectivity* [Unpublished doctoral dissertation]. The University of Manchester, Manchester, UK.

Lučšev, E. M. (2016). Antireligioznaja propaganda v SSSR: 1917-1941 gg [Anti-religious propaganda in the USSR: 1917-1941]. *Informatsionno-tekhnicheskoe agentstvo Ritm, 2*(20), 167-172.

Lutz, A. B. (2013). *Learning solution-focused therapy: An illustrated guide*. American Psychiatric Pub. doi:10.1176/appi.books.9781615370986

Macmillan Contemporary Dictionary. (1988). ABC Publication.

Madigan, S., & Epston, D. (1998). From 'Spy-chiatric Gaze' to communities of concern. From professional monologue to dialogue. In D. Epston (Ed.), *Catching up with David Epston: A collection of narrative practice-based papers published between 1991 & 1996* (pp. 127–148). Dulwich Centre Publications.

Madsen, W. C. (2007). *Collaborative Therapy With Multi-Stressed Families* (2nd ed.). The Guilford Press.

Mager, B. (2019). Storytelling contributes to resilience in older adults. *Activities, Adaptation and Aging*, *43*(1), 23–36. doi:10.1080/01924788.2018.1448669

Magomedov, R., & Çogandaryan, M. (2013). İstoriko-psihologiçeskiye osnovaniya obraza vneşnogo vraga SSSR v Pervoy Polovine 1930 godov [Historical and psychological foundations of the image of the external enemy of the USSR in the first half of the 1930s]. *Vestnik OGU, 3*(152).

Manders, E., & Chilton, G. (2013). Translating the essence of dance: Rendering meaning in artistic inquiry of the creative arts therapies. *International Journal of Education & the Arts*, *14*(16). http://www.ijea.org/v14n16/

Man-Kwong, H. (2004). Overcoming craving: The use of narrative practices in breaking drug habits. *International Journal of Narrative Therapy & Community Work*, (1), 17–24. doi:10.3316/informit.228689124056043

Manners, B. (2017). Being Adventist in A Post-Truth World. *Advntist Record,* 14-15.

Marie, A., & Grybś, M. (2013). Modern trends in consumer behaviour in era of ecommunication. *Studia Ekonomiczne*, *151*, 263–273.

Marshall, H., & Drieschova, A. (2018). Post-Truth Politics in the UK's Brexit Referendum. *New Perspectives*, *26*(3), 89–105. doi:10.1177/2336825X1802600305

Masgoret, A. M., & Ward, C. (2006). Culture learning approach to acculturation. In D. L. Sam & J. W. Berry (Eds.), *The Cambridge handbook of acculturation psychology* (pp. 58–77). Cambridge University Press. doi:10.1017/CBO9780511489891.008

Mavioğlu, E. (2012). *Turkey is in a Deserted State in Terms of Journalism* [Türkiye, Habercilik Açısından Çölleşmiş Bir Durumda]. http://www.yurtsuz.net/News.aspx?newsid=1355#.UXsEjrXIZF4

Mazhari, S. (2012). Association between problematic ınternet use and ımpulse control disorders among Iranian university students. *Cyberpsychology, Behavior, and Social Networking*, *15*(5), 270–273. doi:10.1089/cyber.2011.0548 PMID:22489545

Mazzoleni, G. (2015). *Media Logic*. http://www.communicationencyclopedia.com/public/tocnode?id=g9781405131995_yr2013_chunk_g978140513199518_ss40-1

Mbaye, L. (2017). Supporting communities under migration pressure: the role of opportunities, information and resilience to shocks. In M. McAuliffe & M. Klein Solomon (Eds.), *Migration research leaders' syndicate: Ideas to inform international cooperation on safe, orderly and regular migration* (pp. 91–96). International Organization for Migration.

McAuliffe, M., & Triandafyllidou, A. (Eds.). (2021). *World migration report 2022*. International Organization for Migration.

McColl, D., & Legorburu, G. (2019). *Story Design* [Hikâye Tasarımı] (M. Benveniste, Trans.). Kapital Medya.

McConeghey, H. (2017). Art and soul (2nd ed.). Spring.

McCracken, G. (1986). Culture and Consumption: A Theoretical Account of the Structure and Movement of the Cultural Meaning of Consumer Goods. *The Journal of Consumer Research*, *13*(1), 71–84. doi:10.1086/209048

McIntyre, L. (2019). *Post-truth* [Hakikat-Sonrası] (M. F. Biçici, Trans.). Tellekt.

McKee, R. (2003). Storytelling that moves people. A conversation with screenwriting coach Robert McKee. *Harvard Business Review*, *81*(6), 51–55. PMID:12800716

McKergow, M., & Korman, H. (2009). Inbetween-neither inside nor outside: The radical simplicity of solution-focused brief therapy. *Journal of Systemic Therapies*, *28*(2), 34–49. doi:10.1521/jsyt.2009.28.2.34

McLean, L., & Tuite, E. (2016). Stories and their value: Exploring the role of storytelling in social care practice. *Scottish Journal of Residential Child Care*, *15*(2), 29–45.

McNamee, S., & Hosking, D. M. (2012). *Research and social change: a relational constructionist approach.* Routledge. doi:10.4324/9780203127537

McNiff, S. (1998). *Art based research.* Shambhala.

McNiff, S. (2004). *Art heals: How creativity cures the soul.* Shambhala.

McNiff, S. (2013). Art as research: Opportunities and challenges. *Intellect.*

McNiff, S. (2015). *Imagination in action: secrets for unleashing creative expression.* Shambhala.

McQuillin, J., & Welford, E. (2013). How many people are gathered here? Group work and family constellation theory. *Transactional Analysis Journal*, *43*(4), 352–365. doi:10.1177/0362153713519743

Michael, L. A. (2007). *The Principles of Existence & Beyond.* Lulu Enterprises.

Micozzi, M. S. (2018). *Fundamentals of complementary, alternative, and integrative medicine* (6th ed.). Elsevier.

Millerson, G. (2009). *Production and Management on Television* [Televizyonda Yapım ve Yönetim]. Tur-Gen Yayınları.

Milyavskaya, M., Saffran, M., Hope, N., & Koestner, R. (2018). Fear of missing out: Prevalence, dynamics, and consequences of experiencing FOMO. *Motivation and Emotion*, *42*(5), 725–737. doi:10.100711031-018-9683-5

Mirzoeff, N. (1998). *The Visual Culture Reader.* Routledge.

Molnar, A., & de Shazer, S. (1987). Solution-focused therapy: Toward the identification of therapeutic tasks. *Journal of Marital and Family Therapy*, *13*(4), 349–358. doi:10.1111/j.1752-0606.1987.tb00716.x

Moon, B. (2016). *Art-based group therapy: Theory and practice.* Charles C Thomas Ltd.

Moore, T. (1992). Introduction. In *Archetypal Imagination (Introduction).* Lindisfarne Press.

Moore, T. (2017). Strengths-based narrative storytelling as therapeutic intervention for refugees in Greece. *World Federation of Occupational Therapists Bulletin*, *73*(1), 45–51. doi:10.1080/14473828.2017.1298557

Morgan, A. (2000). *What is narrative therapy? An easy-to-read introduction.* Dulwich Centre Publications.

Morrison, J. (2016). *Diagnostic Guide for Clinicians Facilitating DSM-5* [DSM-5'i Kolaylaştıran Klinisyenler için Tanı Rehberi]. Nobel Akademik.

Moustakas, C. (1990). Heuristic Research: Design, methodology and applications. *Sage (Atlanta, Ga.).*

Mui, A. C., & Kang, S. Y. (2006). Acculturation stress and depression among Asian immigrant elders. *Social Work*, *51*(3), 243–255. doi:10.1093w/51.3.243 PMID:17076122

Mukba, G. (2020). *Yas olgusu yaşayan çocukların yaşantılarının sistemik müdahale içeren hikâye anlatıcılığı tekniği ile incelenmesi: Vaka çalışması* [Unpublished doctoral dissertation]. Çukurova University, Adana, Turkey.

Mukba, G., Sanberk, İ., & Akbaş, T. (2019). An eclectic intervention involving systemic intervention with storytelling. *Psikiyatride Güncel Yaklasimlar*, *11*(3), 386–401. doi:10.18863/pgy.452521

Murdock, N. L. (2013). Narrative therapy [Anlatımsal terapi]. In F. Akkoyun (Ed.), *Psikolojik danışma ve psikoterapi kuramları: Olgu sunumu yaklaşımıyla* (pp. 490–513). Nobel Yayıncılık.

Murphy, J. J. (1994). Working with what works: A solution-focused approach to school behavior problems. *The School Counselor*, *42*, 59–65.

Murphy, J. J. (2015). *Solution-focused counseling in schools*. John Wiley & Sons.

Mutlu, E. (1991). *Understanding Television [Televizyonu Anlamak]*. Gündoğan Publication.

Mutlu, E. (1999). *Television and Society [Televizyon ve Toplum]*. Türkiye Radyo ve Televizyon Kurumu Publication.

Nalçaoğlu, H. (2003). A Framework for Understanding the Media and Society Relationship. In S. Alankuş (Ed.), *Media and Society* (pp. 43–57). İletişim Vakfı Publication.

Narin, B. (2018). The Examination Of Personalized News Feed in The Context Of Echo Chamber Effect, Filter Bubble And Cyberbalcanization Concepts [Kişiselleştirilmiş Çevrimiçi Haber Akışının Yankı Odası Etkisi, Filtre Balonu ve Siberbalkanizasyon Kavramları Çerçevesinde İncelenmesi]. *Selçuk İletişim*, *11*(2), 232–251.

Nel, F. (2005). *Writing For the Media*. Oxford University Press.

Nelson, H. L. (2020) Narrative Repair, Reclaiming Moral Agency. In Introduction to Conflict Resolution, Discourses and Dynamics. (pp. 730-757). Roman & Littlefield.

Nescafe 3ü1 Arada. (2018, Oct 22). *More Famous Than the Celebrity* [Video]. YouTube. https://www.youtube.com/watch?v=iAR-zcIFhOQ

Newman, E. J., Garry, M., Bernstein, D. M., Kantner, J., & Lindsay, D. S. (2012). Nonprobative photographs (or words) inflate truthiness. *Psychonomic Bulletin & Review*, *19*(5), 969–974. doi:10.375813423-012-0292-0 PMID:22869334

Newsome, W. S. (2005). The impact of solution-focused brief therapy with at-risk junior high school students. *Children & Schools*, *27*(2), 83–90. doi:10.1093/cs/27.2.83

Nguyen, A. M., & Benet-Martinez, V. (2013). Biculturalism and Adjustment: A Meta-analysis. *Journal of Cross-Cultural Psychology*, *44*(1), 122–159. doi:10.1177/0022022111435097

Nichols, M. P., & Davis, S. D. (2012). *Family therapy: Concepts and methods*. Pearson.

Nicolaides, A., Eschenbacher, S., Buergelt, P. T., Gilpin-Jackson, Y., Welch, M., & Misawa, M. (2022). *The Palgrave Handbook of Learning for Transformation*. doi:10.1007/978-3-030-84694-7

Nightingale, S. J., Wade, K. A., & Watson, D. G. (2017). Can people identify original and manipulated photos of real-world scenes? *Cognitive Research: Principles and Implications*, *2*(1), 1–21. doi:10.118641235-017-0067-2 PMID:28776002

Nikolaeva, M. F. (2012). Dinamika Obraza Vraga V Sovetskom Plakate (1917-1941) İ Modeli İdentifikatsii Sovetskogo Çeloveka [Dynamics of the image of the enemy in the Soviet poster (1917-1942) and models of identification of the Soviet person]. *Jurnal Dialog so vremenem*, (39), 372-386.

Nikolaeva, M. F. (2012). Sovetskij plakat (1917-1941): Meždu iskusstvom i medijnoj tehnologiej. Obŝestvo [Soviet Posters with Art and Technology (1917-1941)]. *Razvitie*, (3), 129–132.

Nisan, F., & Tuncel, I. (2020). Presentation of Violence Against Women in the News: Emine Cloud Example [Kadına Yönelik Şiddet Olgusunun Haberlerde Sunumu: Emine Bulut Örneği]. *International Journal of Cultural and Social Studies*, *6*(1), 104–123.

O'Connor, N. (2018). Visual whakapapa: An arts therapy experiential. *Australia and New Zealand Journal of Arts Therapy*, *13*(1&2), 63–66.

O'Connor, P., & Anderson, M. (2015). *Applied theatre: research: radical departures.* Bloomsbury. doi:10.5040/9781472513489

Oberst, U., Wegmann, E., Stodt, B., Brand, M., & Chamarro, A. (2017). Negative consequences from heavy social networking in adolescents: The mediating role of fear of missing out. *Journal of Adolescence*, *55*(1), 51–60. doi:10.1016/j.adolescence.2016.12.008 PMID:28033503

Odabaşı, Y. (2019). *Consumption Culture From Content society to consuming society* [Tüketim Kültürü Yetinen Toplumdan Tüketen Topluma]. Agora Kitaplığı.

Oh, Y., Koeske, G. F., & Sales, E. (2002). Acculturation, stress, and depressive symptoms among Korean immigrants in the United States. *The Journal of Social Psychology*, *142*(4), 511–526. doi:10.1080/00224540209603915 PMID:12153126

Öksüz, G. Sovyet Rusya'da Bir Propaganda Aracı Olarak Din Karşıtı Alfabe [The Anti-Religious Alphabet as a Propaganda Tool in Soviet Russia]. *International Science Technology Conference.*

Oktay, M. (2002). *Public Relations in Politics* [Politikada Halkla İlişkiler]. Derin Yayınları.

Öngören, M. T., Yanık, F., İşcan, C., & Demirergi, N. (1994). *What Violence Is This [Bu Ne Şiddet].* Kitle Publication.

Oxford Advanced Learner's Dictionaries. (2021a). *Oxford Advanced Learner's Dictionaries.* https://www.oxfordlearnersdictionaries.com/definition/english/posttruth? q=post+truth

Oxford Advanced Learner's Dictionary. (2016). *Post* [Dictionary]. https://www.oxfordlearnersdictionaries.com/definition/english/post_2?q=post

Oxford Dictionary. (2021). *Post-Truth.* Retrieved from https://www.oxfordlearnersdictionaries.com/definition/english/posttruth?q=post-truth

Oxford Learner's Dictionaries. (2016). https://www.oxfordlearnersdictionaries.com/definition/english/post-truth?q=post-truth

Özbay, M. (2005). Writing as a Science and Culture Transceasor [Bilim ve Kültür Aktarıcısı Olarak Yazı]. *Hacettepe Üniversitesi Türkiyat Araştırmaları Dergisi*, *2*, 67–74.

Özçelik, B. (2021a). Religion in the Post-Truth and Public Space [Hakikat Sonrası ve Kamusal Alanda Din]. In B. Özçelik (Ed.), *Post-truth Politics, Philosophy, Media, International Relations* [Hakikat Sonrası Siyaset, Felsefe, Medya, Uluslararası İlişkiler] (pp. 185–198). Nika Yayınevi.

Özçelik, B. (2021b). Presentation: To Defend the Truth [Sunuş: Hakikati Savunmak İçin] In B. Özçelik (Ed.), *Post-truth Politics, Philosophy, Media, International Relations* [Hakikat Sonrası Siyaset, Felsefe, Medya, Uluslararası İlişkiler] (pp. 1–12). Nika Yayınevi.

Özdemir, F. (2019). Post-Truth Çağda Görsel İletişim Aracı Olarak Fotoğraf [Photography as a Visual Communication Tool in the Post-Truth Age]. *Uluslararası İletişim ve Yönetim Bilimleri Kongresi*, 1056-1068.

Özel, S., & Durmaz, T. (2021). Next Generation Monitoring Practices: Watching [Yeni Nesil İzleme Pratikleri: Tıkınırcasına İzlemek]. *Marmara Üniversitesi Öneri Dergisi*, *16*(55), 363–388.

Özen, A. & Ortaç, S. (2020). Gelişmeleri takip edememe kaygısı (fear of missing out) ve piyasa örneklemleri [Fear of missing out and market samples]. *İzmir Sosyal Bilimler Dergisi, 2*(2), 92-97.

Özer, Ö. (2011). *News Discourse Ideology* [Haber Söylem İdeoloji]. Literatürk.

Özgen, E., & Bayraktar, N. (2016). Public Relation is under the Threat of Spin Doctoring [Spin Doctor Kavramının Tehdidi Altında Halkla İlişkiler]. *Marmara İletişim Dergisi, 0*(21), 1–17.

Özmen, S. (2014). *Radio and Television Readings [Radyo ve Televizyon Okumaları].* Derin Publication.

Pace, S. (2012). *Writing the self into research: Using grounded theory analytic strategies in autoethnography. Creativity: Cognitive.* Social and Cultural Perspectives.

Palabıyıkoğlu, R. (1997). Media and Violence [Medya ve Şiddet]. *Kriz Dergisi, 5*(2), 123–126.

Palmer, H., & Hunter, V. (2018). *Worlding.* https://newmaterialism.eu/almanac/w/worlding.html

Park, C., & Lee, T. M. (2009). Antecedents of online reviews' usage and purchase influence: An empirical comparison of U.S. and Korean consumers. *Journal of Interactive Marketing, 23*(4), 332–340. doi:10.1016/j.intmar.2009.07.001

Parry, A., & Doan, R. E. (1994). *Story re-visions: Narrative therapy in the postmodern world.* The Guilford Press.

Parsa, S. (1993). *Television Journalism and Theories [Televizyon Haberciliği ve Kuramları].* Ege Üniversitesi İletişim Fakültesi Publication.

Parsa, S. (1999). Television Semiotics [Televizyon Göstergebilimi]. *Editing Journal., 16,* 15–28.

Paşin, V. P., Bogdanov, S. V., & Bogdanova, Y. S. (2011). Antialkogolhaya Kampaniya 1985-1987 gg. V. SSCP [Anti-Alcohol Campaign 1985-1987 V. SSCP]. *Po Sovetskim Arhivnım Dokumentam i Rassekreçennım Materialam TSRU.*

Patton, M. Q. (2014). *Qualitative research & evaluation methods: Integrating theory and practice* (4th ed.). Sage.

Peros Temizlik. (2018, Oct 28). *Maids' Choice, Not Celebrities* [Video]. YouTube. https://www.youtube.com/watch?v=nZTXWX1li8E

Petters, M. A. (2018). *Education in a Post-truth World. In Truth, Fake News.* Springer.

Phipps, W. D., & Vorster, C. (2011). Narrative therapy: A return to the intrapsychic perspective? *Journal of Family Psychotherapy, 22*(2), 128–147. doi:10.1080/08975353.2011.578036

Picciotto, R. (2019). Is Evaluation Obsolete in a Post-Truth World? *Evaluation and Program Planning, 73,* 88–96. doi:10.1016/j.evalprogplan.2018.12.006 PMID:30562668

Pısch, A. (2016). *Stalın in Sovıet posters, 1929–1953 archetypes, inventıons & fabrıcatıons.* Anu Press.

Platon. (2005). *State* [Devlet] (S. Eyüboğlu & M. A. Cimcoz, Trans.). Türkiye İş Bankası Publication.

Pocheptsov, G. (2015). *Fenomen Sovetskoy Propagandi* [The Phenomenon of Soviet Propaganda]. https://ms.detector.media/manipulyatsii/post/13750/2015-07-19-fenomen-sovetskoy-propagandy/

Polkinghorne, D. E. (2004). Narrative therapy and postmodernism. In L. E. Angus & J. McLeod (Eds.), *The handbook of narrative and psychotherapy: Practice, theory and research* (pp. 53–67). Sage.

Polkinghorne, D. E. (2013). Narrative identity and psychotherapy. In C. A. Ingemark (Ed.), *Therapeutic uses of storytelling* (pp. 21–41). Nordic Academic Press.

Polonskij, V. (1925). *Russkij revoljucionnyj plakat* [Russia Regime posters]. Gosudarstvennoe izdatel′stvo.

Porgham, S. (2020). *Why Is the Truth of the News Worthless in the Era of Post-Truth?* [Post-Truth Çağında Haberin Gerçekliği Neden Değersiz?]. Retrieved from https://gergedan.press/abd-baskanlik-secimleri-yaklasirken-post-truth-caginda-haberin-gercekligi-neden-degersiz-8150/

Porter, L. (2006). Narrative therapy: An introduction for counsellors. *Journal of Family Studies*, *12*(2), 294–310.

Pösteki, N., & Kaplan, N. (2005). Illusional Lives. In Media Reviews. Beta Publication.

Postman, N. (1994). Amusing Ourselves to Death (O. Akınhay, Trans.). Ayrıntı Publication.

Postman, N. (2003). *Amusing Ourselves to Death Public Discourse in The Age Of Show Business [Televizyon Öldüren Eğlence]* (O. Akınhay, Trans.). Ayrıntı Publication.

Poynton, M. (2012). "We should be playing, not talking": Play, self-agency and moving towards depressive moments. *Journal of Child Psychotherapy*, *38*(2), 185–198. doi:10.1080/0075417X.2012.684488

Prado, C. G. (2018). *America's Post-Truth Phenomenon*. ABC-Clio, LLC.

Pratchett, T. (1998). *Reaper man*. Transworld, Ltd.

Profilo. (2020, May 20). *Profilo XXL Refrigerator Advertising* [Video]. YouTube. https://www.youtube.com/watch?v=3xB8IEIPQvo

Proudlock, S. (2017). *The solution focused way: Incorporating solution focused therapy tools and techniques into your everyday work*. Routledge. doi:10.4324/9781315145433

Przybylski, A. K., Murayama, K., DeHaan, C. R., & Gladwell, V. (2013). Motivational, emotional, and behavioral correlates of fear of missing out. *Computers in Human Behavior*, *29*(4), 1814–1848. doi:10.1016/j.chb.2013.02.014

Quiroga, A., Jimenez, J. V., Beltran, G. A., Casas, V., & Lopez, B. N. (2016). A narrative approach to addressing pain in hospitalised paediatric patients: Handicraft and digital interventions. *International Journal of Narrative Therapy & Community Work*, *4*, 77–85.

Radecki, T. (1986). Violent Entertainment. In *Mass Media and Violence*. Hürriyet Vakfı Eğitim Publication.

Ramaekers, S., & Suissa, J. (2012). *The claims of parenting: reasons, responsibility and society*. Springer. doi:10.1007/978-94-007-2251-4

Rambo Ronai, C. (1995). Multiple reflections of child sex abuse: An argument for a layered account. *Journal of contemporary ethnography, 23*, 395-426.

Randall, W. L., & McKim, A. E. (2008). *Reading Our Lives: The Poetics of Growing Old*. Oxford Univ. Press. doi:10.1093/acprof:oso/9780195306873.001.0001

Rankin, J. (2002). What is Narrative? Ricoeur, Bakhtin, and Process Approaches. Concrescence. *The Australasian Journal of Process Thought*, *3*, 1–12. Retrieved June 20, 2020, from http://citeseerx.ist.psu.edu/viewdoc/download;jsessionid=D1CCBE62D6C8DC41942C868A2FA1D76E?doi=10.1.1.452.6099&rep=rep1&type=pdf

Rappaport, L. (2008). *Focusing-oriented art therapy: Accessing the body's wisdom and creative intelligence*. Jessica Kingsley.

Rappaport, L. (2013). Trusting the felt sense in art-based research. In S. McNiff (Ed.), *Art as research: Opportunities and challenges* (pp. 201–208). Intellect. doi:10.1386/9781783200016_24

Rappaport, L. (2014). Focusing-orientated arts therapy: Cultivating mindfulness and compassion, and accessing inner wisdom. In L. Rappaport (Ed.), *Mindfulness and the arts therapies: Theory and practice* (pp. 193–207). Jessica Kingsley.

Ratner, H., George, E., & Iveson, C. (2012). *Solution focused brief therapy: 100 key points and techniques*. Routledge. doi:10.4324/9780203116562

Reeves, N. (2004). *Power of Film Propaganda: Myth of Reality?* Continuum.

Resuloğlu, F., & Yılmaz, R. (2017). A Model for Interactive Advertising Narration. In R. Yılmaz (Ed.), *Narrative Advertising Models and Conceptualization in The Digital Age* (pp. 1–20). IGI Global. doi:10.4018/978-1-5225-2373-4.ch001

Reynolds, J., & Bove, K. B. (2016, February 27). *The power of mutual storytelling in play therapy* [Workshop presentation]. Colorado Association for Play Therapy.

Rhodes, J., & Ajmal, Y. (1995). *Solution focused thinking in schools: behaviour, reading and organisation*. BT Press.

Ricci, R. J. (2003). Autoethnographic verse: Nicky's boy: A life in two worlds. *Qualitative Report*, *8*(4), 591–596. http://www.nova.edu/sss/QR/QR8-4/ricci.pdf

Ricks, L., Kitchens, S., Goodrich, T., & Hancock, E. (2014). My story: The use of narrative therapy in individual and group counseling. *Journal of Creativity in Mental Health*, *9*(1), 99–110. doi:10.1080/15401383.2013.870947

Rifkin, J., Cindy, C., & Kahn, B. (2015). FoMO: how the fear of missing out leads to missing out. In K. Diehl & C. Yoon (Eds.), *ACR North American Advances* (Vol. 43, pp. 244–248). Duluth, MN: Association for Consumer Research.

Riley, S., & Malchiodi, C. A. (2003). Solution-focused and narrative approaches. In C. A. Malchiodi (Ed.), *Handbook of art therapy* (pp. 82–92). The Guilford Press.

Riordan, B. C., Flett, J. A. M., Hunter, J. A., Scarf, D., & Conner, T. S. (2015). Fear of missing out (FoMO): The relationship between FoMO, alcohol use, and alcohol-related consequences in college students. *Journal of Psychiatry and Brain Functions*, *2*(9), 1–7.

Riva, S. (2019). Linkedness: Relational transformation and narrative conflict resolution. In Togetherness and Its Discontents (pp. 497-513). Pensa MultiMedia Editore s.r.l.

Riva, S. K. M. (2015). Creating Dialogical Space In Generative Research Using Professional's Narratives. Nova Perspectiva Sistémica, 33-51.

Riva, S. M. (2020). Homing in: An Adopted Child's Story Mandala of Connecting, Reunion, and Belonging. WriteLife Publishing.

Riva, S. M. (2021) From Life-o-grams to Transformagrams: Storying Transformational Processes and Pedagogies. *Interdisciplinary Studies in Education & Society, 23*(89).

Riva-Mossman, S. K. (2009). *Conflict Narratives: Mediation Case Studies in an Intercultural Context.* Tilburg University. https://www.taosinstitute.net/Websites/taos/files/Content/5693761/Susi_Riva_-_Conflict_Narratives.pdf

Riva-Mossman, S., & Verloo, H. (2017). Explorative healthy aging processes fostering social innovation: Thematizing life course narratives for older adult women participating in a documentary film. *Qualitative Research in Medicine & Healthcare*, *1*(1), 14–22. doi:10.4081/qrmh.2017.6199

Riva, S. K. M. (2019). Writing to Transform Relations. In E. Alegre-Agis & S. Fernandez-Garrido (Eds.), *Autoetnografias, Cuerpos Y Emociones (1) Perspectivas metodologicas en la investigacion en salud* (pp. 47–70). Publications URV.

Rogers, N. (1999). The creative connection: A holistic expressive arts process. In S. K. Levine & E. G. Levine (Eds.), *Foundations of expressive arts therapy theoretical and clinical perspectives* (pp. 113–131). Jessica Kingsley.

Rolbiecki, A. J., Washington, K. T., & Bitsicas, K. (2019). Digital storytelling as an intervention for bereaved family members. *Omega*, *0*(0), 1–17. doi:10.1177/0030222819825513 PMID:30678536

Romanyshyn, R. D. (2013). *The wounded researcher: research with soul in mind.* Spring Journal, Inc.

Roosa, L. W. (1981). The family drawing / storytelling technique: An approach to assessment of family dynamics. *Elementary School Guidance & Counseling*, *15*(3), 269–272.

Rose, J. (2017). Brexit, Trump, and Post-truth Politics. *Public Integrity*, *19*(6), 555–558. doi:10.1080/10999922.2017.1285540

Roux, M. (2013). Socrate en Crampons (B. Yanık, Trans.). Tekin Publication.

Rowley, A. (2006). Sport in the Service of The State: Images of Physical Culture and Soviet Women, 1917–1941. *The International Journal of the History of Sport*, *23*(8), 1314–1340. doi:10.1080/09523360600922246

Russo, M. F., Vernam, J., & Wolbert, A. (2006). Sandplay and storytelling: Social constructivism and cognitive development in child counseling. *The Arts in Psychotherapy*, *33*(3), 229–237. doi:10.1016/j.aip.2006.02.005

RVD. (2019). *Türkiye'deki Effie Ödüllü TV Reklamlarının 10 Yıllık Toplumsal Cinsiyet Eşitliği Karnesi Özet Bulgular.* https://www.rvd.org.tr/uploads/2019/02/effie-kisa-arastirma-raporu.pdf

Ryan, M. L. (2004). Metaleptic Machine. *Semiotica*, *1*(4), 439–469. doi:10.1515emi.2004.055

Ryan, R., & Deci, E. (2000). Self – Determination theory and the facilitation of intrinsic motivation, social development and well- being. *The American Psychologist*, *55*(1), 68–78. doi:10.1037/0003-066X.55.1.68 PMID:11392867

Safire, W. (1996). *The Spinner Spun.* https://www.nytimes.com/1996/12/22/magazine/the-spinner-spun.html

Sağır, A., & Aktaş, Z. (2019). The sociological analysis of the relationship between Turkish immigrants from Romania and the Turkish community: The period of 1934-1938 in the Turkish newspapers [Romanya'dan Türkiye'ye gelen göçmenlerle Türk toplumu arasındaki ilişkinin sosyolojik çözümlemesi: Türk yazılı basınında 1934-1938 dönemi]. *Atatürk Araştırma Merkezi Dergisi*, *35*(1), 141–214.

Sakaki, T., Ji, Y., & Ramirez, S. Z. (2007). Clinical application of color inkblots in therapeutic storytelling. *The Arts in Psychotherapy*, *34*(3), 208–215. doi:10.1016/j.aip.2007.01.007

Salgado, S. (2018). Online Media Impact on Politics. Views on Post-truth Politics and Post Postmodernism. *International Journal of Media and Cultural Politics*, *14*(3), 317–331. doi:10.1386/macp.14.3.317_1

Sam, D. L. (2006). Acculturation: Conceptual background and core components. In D. L. Sam & J. W. Berry (Eds.), *The Cambridge handbook of acculturation psychology* (pp. 11–26). Cambridge University Press. doi:10.1017/CBO9780511489891.005

Sam, D. L., & Berry, J. W. (2006). Introduction. In D. L. Sam & J. W. Berry (Eds.), *The Cambridge handbook of acculturation psychology* (pp. 1–7). Cambridge University Press. doi:10.1017/CBO9780511489891.003

Sam, D. L., & Berry, J. W. (2010). Acculturation: When individuals and groups of different cultural backgrounds meet. *Perspectives on Psychological Science*, *5*(4), 472–481. doi:10.1177/1745691610373075 PMID:26162193

Saraç, H. (2019). *Sovyet Propaganda Dili* [Soviet Propaganda Language]. Değişim Yay.

Sarder, Z. (2010). *Welcome to postnormal times.* https://ziauddinsardar.com/2011/03/welcome-to-postnormal-times/

Sarınay, Y. (2011). Migrations from the Balkan countries to Ankara during the republican period (1923-1990) [Cumhuriyet döneminde Balkan ülkelerinden Ankara'ya yapılan göçler (1923-1990)]. *Atatürk Araştırma Merkezi Dergisi, 27*(80), 351–388.

Satir, M. (2018). İdeoloji ve Sanat İlişkisi Bağlamında Sovyet Anıtsal Propagandası [Soviet Monumental Propaganda in the Context of the Relationship between Ideology and Art]. *Manas Sosyal Araştırmalar Dergisi, 7*(3), 565–583.

Şavlyutova, Z. (2011). Bor'ba sovetskoy vlasti s religioznım soznaniyem naseleniya Zaural'ya v 1920-e gg [The struggle of Soviet power with the religious consciousness of the population of the Trans-Urals in the 1920 ss]. *Vestnik Arheologii, antropologii i etnografii, 1*(14).

Sawyer, M. E. (2018). Post-Truth, Social Media, and The "Teal" as Phantasm. In M. Stenmark, S. Fuller, & U. Zackariasson (Eds.), Relativism and Post-Truth in Contemporary Society (pp. 55-69). Palgrave Macmillan.

Sawyer, R. D., & Norris, J. (2013). *Duoethnography. Understanding qualitative research.* Oxford University Press.

Saygın, S., & Hasta, D. (2018). Migration, acculturation and adaptation [Göç, kültürleşme ve uyum]. *Psikiyatride Güncel Yaklasimlar, 10*(3), 312–333. doi:10.18863/pgy.364115

Schaubroeck, K. (2010). *Een verpletterend gevoel van verantwoordelijkheid. Waarom ouders zich altijd schuldig voelen* [A crushing sense of responsibility. Why parents always feel guilty]. De Geus.

Seıtel, F. P. (1998). *The Practice of Public Relation* (7th ed.). Prentice Hall.

Şeker, M., & Gölcü, A. (2008). Reproduction of Football on Television [Futbolun Televizyonda Yeniden Üretimi]. *Communication Theory and Research Journal., 26*, 111–129.

Selekman, M. D. (1997). *Solution-focused therapy with children: Harnessing family strengths for systemic change.* Guilford Press.

Semmler, P. L., & Williams, C. B. (2000). Narrative Therapy: A Storied Context for Multicultural Counseling. *Journal of Multicultural Counseling and Development, 28*(1), 51–62. doi:10.1002/j.2161-1912.2000.tb00227.x

Şen, O. (2021) Robot Journalism [Robot Gazetecilik]. In Gazetecilikte Uzmanlaşma alanları (pp. 57-75). Pelikan Yayınevi.

Şen, O. (2021). Robot Journalism [Robot Gazetecilik]. In M. Şahin & E. İlhan (Eds.), *Specialization Areas in Journalism* [Gazetecilikte Uzmanlaşma Alanları] (pp. 57–76). Pelikan Yayınları.

Sergeyeva, O. (2017). Vizual'nyy yazyk «krasnykh» i «belykh» plakatov perioda Grazhdanskaya voyny v Rossii [The visual language of the "red" and "white" posters of the period of the Civil War in Russi]. *Zhurnal sotsiologii i sotsialnoy antropologii, 20*(4), 210–229.

Serim, Ö. (2014). *Football Art [Futbol Sanatı].* Bence Book.

Serneels, A. (2013). Picturing stories: Drawings in narrative family therapy with children. *International Journal of Narrative Therapy & Community Work, 4*, 21–29.

Sezerer Albayrak, E. (2015). Televizyon Reklamlarında Kadın İmgesi Kullanımı [Using the Image of Women in Television Ads]. In G. Ağrıdağ (Ed.), Türkiye'de ve Dünya'da Kadın Araştırmaları. Çukurova Üniversitesi Basımevi.

Shabo, M. E. (2008). *Techniques of Propaganda and Persuasion.* Prestwick House.

Shankar, S. (2020). *Emotions as the new ethical turn in social research.* https://items.ssrc.org/covid-19-and-the-social-sciences/social-research-and-insecurity/emotions-as-the-new-ethical-turn-in-social-research/

Shapiro, J., & Ross, V. (2002). Applications of narrative theory and therapy to the practice of family medicine. *Family Medicine*, *34*(2), 96–100. PMID:11874032

Shepler, R. (2008). *The Bolshevik campaign against religion in Soviet Russia: 1917-1932* (Unpublished Doctoral Dissertation). The Ohio State University.

Shoshitaishvili, B. (2021). From Anthropocene to Noosphere: The Great Acceleration. *Earth's Future, 9*. doi:10.1029/2020EF001917

Siegel, D. J. (2020). *The developing mind: How relationships and the brain interact to shape who we are* (3rd ed.). Guilford Press.

Sim, Ş., (1996). Media and Violence [Medya ve Şiddet]. *İletişim Fakültesi, 3*, 127-131.

Şimşek, M., & Yalı, S. (2019). Did It Real (Really) Happen: Representation of History in Post-Truth Times [Gerçekte(N) Öyle Mi Olmuş: Post Truth Zamanlarda Tarihin Temsili]. İstanbul: Yeni İnsan Yayınevi.

Şimşek, V. (2018). Post-truth and New Media: A Study on Social Media Groups [Post-truth ve Yeni Medya: Sosyal Medya Grupları Üzerinden Bir İnceleme]. *Global Media Journal TR Edition*, *8*(16), 1–14.

Sirer, E. (2020). *New Curriculum New Audience [Yeni İzlence Yeni İzlerkitle]*. Literatürk Publication.

Sirer, E. (2020). *The Language of the Image in Football Broadcasts [Futbol Yayınlarında Görüntü Dili]*. Kriter Publication.

Sirer, E. (2020). Violence Aestheticized in Sports Publications and Broadcasts. In *Handbook of Research on Aestheticization of Violence, Horror, and Power*. IGI Global.

Sırgy, M. J. (1982). Self-Concept in Consumer Behavior: A Critical Review. *The Journal of Consumer Research*, *9*(3), 287–300. doi:10.1086/208924

Skovholt, T. M. (2012). *Becoming a therapist: On the road to mastery*. John Wiley & Sons, Inc.

Slivinske, J., & Slivinske, L. (2014). *Therapeutic storytelling for adolescents and young adults*. Oxford University Press.

Smith, M. J., & Liehr, P. (1999). Attentively Embracing Story: A middle-range theory with practice and research implications. *Scholarly Inquiry for Nursing Practice*, *13*(3), 187–210. PMID:10628236

Smith, M. J., & Liehr, P. (2005). Story theory: Advancing nursing practice scholarship. *Holistic Nursing Practice*, *19*(6), 272–276. doi:10.1097/00004650-200511000-00008 PMID:16269946

Smith, S. (2010). A preliminary analysis of narratives on the impact of training in solution-focused therapy expressed by students having completed a 6-month training course. *Journal of Psychiatric and Mental Health Nursing*, *17*(2), 105–110. doi:10.1111/j.1365-2850.2009.01492.x PMID:20465754

Solodovnik, L.V. (2012). *Faktor ideologii v sovetskom obschestve: retrospektivnyi analiz v koordinatah ideologicheskoi bezopasnosti gosudarstva i obschestva* [The Ideological Factor in Soviet Society: A Retrospective Analysis in the Coordinates of the Ideological Security of the State and Society]. UDK 323.

Solovev, Z., Strasul, İ. (1926). *Alkogolizm* [Alcoholism]. BSE, T.2.

Sozcu. (2022). *Russia-Ukraine tension: Putin to invade on Wednesday* [Rusya-Ukrayna gerilimi: Putin, Çarşamba günü işgal edecek]. Retrieved from https://www.sozcu.com.tr/2022/dunya/rusya-ukrayna-gerilimi-putin-carsamba-gunu-isgal-edecek-6947902/

Sözen, E. (2008). *Icon Usage, Media Sensitivity to Violence Panel [Simge Kullanımı, Medyada Şiddete Duyarlılık Paneli]*. RTÜK Publication.

Sparrer, I. (2012). *Introduction to the solution-oriented approach and systemic structural alignment* [Çözüm odaklı yaklaşıma ve sistemik yapısal dizime giriş]. Pan Yayıncılık.

Speed, E., & Mannion, R. (2017). The Rise of Post-truth Populism in Pluralist Liberal Democracies: Challenges for Health Policy. *International Journal of Health Policy and Management*, *6*(5), 249–251. doi:10.15171/ijhpm.2017.19 PMID:28812811

Spencer-Thomas, S. (2020). Phoenix rising: The power of storytelling in suicide prevention. In S. Shahtahmasebi & H. A. Omar (Eds.), *The broader view of suicide* (pp. 379–399). Cambridge Scholars Publishing.

Springgay, S., Irwin, R. L., Leggo, C., & Gouzouasis, P. (Eds.). (2008). *Being with a/r/tography*. Sense. doi:10.1163/9789087903268

Springgay, S., Irwin, R. L., & Wilson Kind, S. (2005). A/r/tography as living inquiry through art and text. *Qualitative Inquiry*, *11*(6), 897–912. doi:10.1177/1077800405280696

Stalin, J., (1978). *Leninizmin İlkeleri* [Principles of Leninism]. Ankara: Sol yayınları.

Stern, S., Doolan, M., Staples, E., Szmukler, L., & Eisler, I. (1999). Disruption and reconstruction: Narrative insights into the experience of family members caring for a relative diagnosed with serious mental illness. *Family Process*, *38*(3), 353–369. doi:10.1111/j.1545-5300.1999.00353.x PMID:10526771

Stevens, A. (2014). *Jung* (N. Örge, Trans.). Dost Publication.

Stewart, K. (2010). Worlding refrains. In M. Gregg & G. J. Siegworth (Eds.), *The affect theory reader* (pp. 339–353). Duke University Press. doi:10.1215/9780822393047-015

Suh, S., Yang, H. C., Kim, N., Yu, J. H., Choi, S., Yun, C. H., & Shin, C. (2017). Chronotype differences in health behaviors and health-related quality of life: A population-based study among aged and older adults. *Behavioral Sleep Medicine*, *15*(5), 361–376. doi:10.1080/15402002.2016.1141768 PMID:27148632

Sullivan, G. (2006). Research acts in art practice. *Studies in Art Education*, *48*(1), 19–35. doi:10.1080/00393541.2006.11650497

Sunderland, M. (2017). *Using story telling as a therapeutic tool with children*. Speechmark Publishing. doi:10.4324/9781315148830

Taggart, P. (2004). *Populism* [Popülizm] (B. Yıldırım, Trans.). Bilgi Üniversitesi Yayınları.

Tajfel, H., & Turner, J. C. (1979). An integrative theory of intergroup conflict. In W. Austin, & S. Worchel (Eds.), The social psychology of intergroup relations (pp. 33-48). Brooks/Cole.

Talimciler, A. (2009). Within the (un)changing) States of Male Identity: The Overlooked Area in: Formation of Male Identity in Turkey: Sports/Football [Erkek Kimliği'nin Değiş(meye)n Halleri içinde: Türkiye'de Erkek Kimliğinin Oluşumunda Göz Ardı Edilen Alan: Spor/Futbol]. Beta Publications.

Tanyolaç Öztokat, N. (2005). *Yazınsal Metin Çözümlemesinde Kuramsal Yaklaşımlar* [Theoretical Approaches to Literary Text Analysis]. Multilingual.

Tapper, H. (2021). Uninvited guests, soul-filled skies and universes beneath my toes: Exploring poiesis at the confluence of the arts and self for arts therapy research. *Journal of Creative Arts Therapies*, *16*(2), 52–67.

Taşkıran, N. Ö., & Bolat, N. (2013). Ad and Perception Relationship: A Review of the Functions of Sensory Organs in The Acquisition of Advertising Texts [Reklam ve Algı İlişkisi: Reklam Metinlerinin Alımlanmasında Duyu Organlarının İşlevleri Üzerine Bir İnceleme]. *Beykent University Journal of Social Sciences*, *6*(1), 49–69.

Taş, O., & Taş, T. (2018). Fake News in Social Media and Syrian Refugee Crisis in the Post-truth Era [Post-Hakikat Çağında Sosyal Medyada Yalan Haber ve Suriyeli Mülteciler Sorunu]. *Galatasaray Üniversitesi İletişim Dergisi, 29*, 183–208. doi:10.16878/gsuilet.500943

Taylor, R. M. (2003). *Munitions of the Mind: A History of Propaganda*. Manchester University Press.

Terzi, A. (2020). On the Concept of Post-Truth and Its Turkish Equivalents [Post-Truth Kavramı ve Türkçe Karşılıkları Üzerine]. *Türk dili, 69*(820), 80–86.

Tesich, S. (2021). The Regime of Lies. *Cogito Journal, 104,* 23–28.

TFF. (2018). *Hawk-Eye CEO Carter: TFF VAR Center is one of the best in the world* [Hawk-Eye CEO'su Carter: TFF VAR Merkezi dünyanın en iyilerinden biri]. https://www.tff.org/default.aspx?pageID=248&ftxtID=29704

TFF. (2020). *VAR (Video Assistant Referee) Handbook*. https://www.tff.org/Resources/TFF/Images/MHK/VAR.pdf

TFF. (2022). *İş Ortakları. FIFA Fédération Internationale de Football Association.* Work Partners. https://www.tff.org/default.aspx?pageID=356

The Economist. (2016). *The Post-Truth World: Yes, I'd Lie to You.* https://www.economist. com/briefing/2016/09/10/yes-id-lie-to-you

The Guardian. (2016). *The scoreboard never lies: why sport in a post-truth world matters more than ever.* https://www.theguardian.com/sport/2016/dec/05/sports-distraction-post-truth-world

The UN Refugee Agency. (2021). *Figures at a glance*. Retrieved February 18, 2022, from https://www.unhcr.org/en-us/figures-at-a-glance.html

Thomson, J. (2019). Working with death through art and story: A collective biography. *ANZJAT, 14*(1), 77–90.

Tilley-Lubbs, G. A. (2016). Critical autoethnography and the vulnerable self as researcher. In G. A. Tilley-Lubbs & S. Bénard Calva (Eds.), *Re-telling our stories: Critical autoethnographic narratives* (pp. 3–5). doi:10.1007/978-94-6300-567-8_1

Timotijevic, L., & Breakwell, G. M. (2000). Migration and threat to identity. *Journal of Community & Applied Social Psychology, 10*(5), 355–372. doi:10.1002/1099-1298(200009/10)10:5<355::AID-CASP594>3.0.CO;2-Y

Tokgöz, O. (1981). *Basic Journalism [Temel Gazetecilik]*. Anakara Üniversitesi Siyasal Bilgiler Fakültesi Publication.

Tolstaya, T. (2006). *Russkiy plakat: kniga -albom* [Russia poster Album]. Kontakt- Kultura.

Trend, D. (2008). *The Myth of Violence in the Media [Medyada Şiddet Efsanesi]* (G. Bostancı, Trans.). YKY Publication.

Trepper, T. S., Dolan, Y., McCollum, E. E., & Nelson, T. (2006). Steve De Shazer and the future of solution-focused therapy. *Journal of Marital and Family Therapy, 32*(2), 133–139. doi:10.1111/j.1752-0606.2006.tb01595.x PMID:16676891

Turkcell. (2018, Nov 6). *The Cat Dripping from Upstairs* [Video]. YouTube. https://www.youtube.com/watch?v=5o-SANBtkAg

Turkcell. (2019, May 30). *Just Look at the Road When on Road* [Video]. YouTube. https://www.youtube.com/watch?v=n_p9pfu9LWc

Türkdoğan, O. (1996). *Social Violence and the Reality of Turkey [Sosyal Şiddet ve Türkiye Gerçeği]*. Timaş Publication.

Türker, D., & Yıldız, A. (2015). Socio-psychological integration analysis of immigrants [Göçmenlerde sosyo-psikolojik entegrasyon analizi]. In B. D. Şeker, İ. Sirkeci, & M. M. Yüceşahin (Eds.), *Göç ve uyum* (pp. 23–34). Transnational Press London.

Turkey Stands! Violence Against Women Aroused Indignation in Samsun. (2021). https://www.youtube.com/watch?v=aXq_O7P2s3k

Turkish Association of Advertising Agencies. (2019). *Türkiye'de Tahmini Medya ve Reklam Yatırımları Raporu.* https://www2.deloitte.com/content/dam/Deloitte/tr/Documents/technology-media-telecommunications/turkiyede-tahmini-medya-ve-reklam-yatirimlari-2019-ilk-6-ay-raporu.pdf

Türkiye İstatistik Kurumu (TÜİK). (2019). *International Migration Statistics, 2018* [Uluslararası Göç İstatistikleri, 2018]. Retrieved February 17, 2022, from https://data.tuik.gov.tr/Bulten/Index?p=Uluslararasi-Goc-Istatistikleri-2018-30711

Türkiye'nin Reklamları. (2018, Oct 15). *A101 E Cheap Campaign* [Video]. YouTube. https://www.youtube.com/watch?v=W_-MbqiFELo

Türkoğlu, N. (2010). *Social Communication [Toplumsal İletişim].* Urban Publication.

Türköne, M. (1995). *Gender Culture of the Old Turkish Society [Eski Türk Toplumunun Cinsiyet Kültürü].* Ark Publication.

Turner, V. W. (1995). The ritual process: structure and anti-structure. In The Lewis Henry Morgan lectures 1966. Aldine de Gruyter.

Turner, L. (Ed.). (2018). *International Perspectives on Autoethnographic Research and Practice*. Routledge. doi:10.4324/9781315394787

Turner, V. W. (1969). *The ritual process: Structure and antistructure.* Aldine.

Twenge, J. M., & Campbell, W. K. (2015). *Plague of the Century: The Plague of Narcissism* [Asrın Vebası: Narsisizm İlleti] (Ö. Korkmaz, Trans.). Kaknüs.

Uğurlu, H. (2008). *Constructing the Concept of Time in Live Broadcasts on Television [Televizyondaki Canlı Yayınlarda Zaman Kavramının Yapılandırılması].* Galatasaray Üniversitesi İleti-ş-im Journal.

Uğurlu, S. (2007). *"Interaction of Social Fabric with TV Programs", on Media Studies ["Sosyal Dokunun TV Programlarıyla Karşılıklı Etkileşimi", Medya üzerine Çalışmalar].* Beta Publication.

Uluk, M. (2018). *New Media and Fake News in the Post-Truth Age* [Hakikat Sonrası Çağda Yeni Medya ve Yalan Haber]. Dorlion Yayınları.

Uluk, M. (2018). *New Media and Fake News in the Post-Truth Era* [Hakikat Sonrası Çağda Yeni Medya ve Yalan Haber]. Dorlion.

Ulus Gazetesi. (1938, January 19). *Muhajir* [Muhacir]. Retrieved from https://www.gastearsivi.com/gazete/ulus/1938-01-19/1

Ulusal, D. (2007). Women in Violence and Violent News Presentation in the Written Media positioning [Yazılı Basında Şiddet Ve Şiddet İçerikli Haber Sunumunda Kadının Konumlandırılışı] [Master Thesis]. *Erciyes Üniversitesi, Sosyal Bilimler Enstitüsü, Gazetecilik Anabilim Dalı.*

Ünal, S. (2008). *An evaluation on the Balkans migrants in Turkey in the context of social integration and identity (a sample from İzmir)* [Sosyal bütünleşme ve kimlik bağlamında Türkiye'deki Balkan göçmenleri üzerine bir değerlendirme (İzmir'den bir örneklem)] [Master's thesis]. Retrieved from Council of Higher Education Thesis Center. (Thesis No. 219894)

Ünal, R., & Taylan, A. (2017). *The Fake News-False Enformatıon Problem in Health Communıcatıon And The Verıfıcatıon Platforms* [Sağlık İletişiminde Yalan Haber-Yanlış Enformasyon Sorunu ve Doğrulama Platformları]. Atatürk İletişim Dergisi.

Undurraga, J. K. A. S. (2021). What if reflexivity and diffraction intra-act? *International Journal of Qualitative Studies in Education*, 1–14. Advance online publication. doi:10.1080/09518398.2021.1900622

Ünlü, S. B., Uluyağcı, N., Uzoğlu, C., & Bayçu, S. (2009). Violence Against Women: A Study on Violence Against Women in TV Series [Kadına Yönelik Şiddet: TV Dizilerinde Kadına Yönelik Şiddet Üzerine Bir Araştırma]. *Selçuk İletişim, 5*(4), 95–104.

Ünsal, A. (1996). An Extended Typology of Violence, Violence [Genişletilmiş Bir Şiddet Tipolojisi, Şiddet]. *Cotigo, 6-7*, 29–36.

Uysal, M. (2006). *Media and Violence, Violence as a Social Problem Symposium* [Medya ve Şiddet, Toplumsal Bir Sorun Olarak Şiddet Symposium. Ankara, Turkey: Academic Press.

Uzun, R. (2002). Entertainment Industry and Television Journalism [Eğlence Endüstrisi ve Televizyon Haberciliği]. *Kocaeli, 1/2*, 9–27.

Van den Berge, L. (2017) *Parenting support revisited: retrieving an ethics of hermeneutics. A philosophical investigation inspired by the viewpoints of Heidegger, Wittgenstein and Taylor* [Doctoral dissertation]. KU Leuven, Belgium.

Van den Berge, L. (2013). Parenting Support and the Role of Society in Parental Self-Understanding: Furedi's Paranoid Parenting Revisited. *Journal of Philosophy of Education, 47*(3), 391–406. doi:10.1111/1467-9752.12008

Van den Berge, L. (2016). From fiction to friction: Towards an ethics of hermeneutics in parent counselling. *Ethics and Education, 11*(3), 259–273. doi:10.1080/17449642.2016.1242041

Van den Berge, L., & Ramaekers, S. (2014). Figures of Disengagement: Charles Taylor, Scientific Parenting and the Paradox of Late Modernity. *Educational Theory, 64*(6), 607–625. doi:10.1111/edth.12086

Van Dijk, T. (2003). Discourse and Ideology: A Multi-domain Approach [Söylem ve İdeoloji: Çok Alanlı Bir Yaklaşım]. In B. Çoban & Z. Özarslan (Eds.), *Mythology, Religion, Ideology* [Mitoloji, Din, İdeoloji] (AteşN., Trans., pp. 13–112). Su Yayınları.

Van Oudenhoven, J. P., Ward, C., & Masgoret, A. M. (2006). Patterns of relations between immigrants and host societies. *International Journal of Intercultural Relations, 30*(6), 637–651. doi:10.1016/j.ijintrel.2006.09.001

Van Reybrouck, T. (2007). *Mijn kind en drugs. Antwoorden voor ouders* [My child and drugs. Answers for parents]. Houtekiet.

Van Rooyen, H., & d'Ablon, R. (2020). Transforming Data into Poems: Poetic Inquiry Practices for Social and Human Sciences. *Education as Change, 24*(8103). https://upjournals.co.za/index.php/EAC

Vargas Delgado, J. J. (2019). Storytelling mindfulness: Storytelling program for meditations. In B. Peña-Acuña (Ed.), *Narrative transmedia* (pp. 1–18). IntechOpen. doi:10.5772/intechopen.86778

Vassilieva, J. (2016). *Narrative psychology: Identity, transformation and ethics*. Springer. doi:10.1057/978-1-137-49195-4

Vaughan, K. (2009). A home in the arts: From research/creation to practice or The story of a dissertation in the making, in action – so far! *International Journal of Education & the Arts, 10*(13). http://www.ijea.org/v10n13/

Ventriglio, A., Ayonrinde, O., & Bhugra, D. (2016). Culture-bound syndromes in 21st century. *Psychiatry and Clinical Neurosciences, 70*(1), 3–6. doi:10.1111/pcn.12359 PMID:26332813

Vermeire, S. & Van Reybrouck, T. (2013). Een zoektocht naar sprankeltjes hoop en toekomst [A search for sparkles of hope and a future]. *Tijdschrift voor ouderschapskennis, 16*(1), 59-75.

Vermeire, S. (2012). Ouders en schuldgevoelens: een hefboom tot verandering [Parents and guilt: a lever for change]. *Tijdschrift voor ouderschapskennis, 15*(1), 36-49.

Vermeire, S. (2011). Narratieve wegen tot herstel, het interview als therapeutische methode [Narrative paths to recovery, the interview as a therapeutic method]. *Systeemtheoretisch Bulletin, 29*(2), 123–142.

Vermeulen, T., & van den Akker, R. (2010). Notes on metamodernism. *Journal of Aesthetics & Culture, 2*. http://aestheticsandculture.net/index.php/jac/article/viewArticle/5677

Vincent, A. (2018) is there a definition? Ruminating on poetic inquiry, strawberries, and the continued growth of the field. *Art/Research International: A Transdisciplinary Journal, 3*(2), 48-76. doi:10.18432/ari29356

Violence Against Women! (2021). https://www.youtube.com/watch?v=qR2wdLCyliY

Vlasić Manaia, A. (2017). Kaupapa Māori arts therapy. *Australia and New Zealand Journal of Arts Therapy, 12*(1), 27–39.

Vygotskij, L. S. (1981). *Mind in Society: The Development of Higher Psychological Processes.* Harvard Univ. Press.

Wade, K. A., Garry, M., Read, J. D., & Lindsay, D. S. (2002). A picture is worth a thousand lies: Using false photographs to create false childhood memories. *Psychonomic Bulletin & Review, 9*(3), 597–603. doi:10.3758/BF03196318 PMID:12412902

Waller, D., & Sibbett, C. H. (Eds.). (2008). Art therapy and cancer care. KakJiSa/OUP.

Walsh, A. (2022). Beyond extraction: co-creating a decolonial and feminist research practice in post-conflict Guatemala. In H. Kara & S. Khoo (Eds.), *Qualitative and digital research in times of crisis: methods, reflexivity, and ethics* (pp. 235–246). Policy Press.

Walsh, F. (2006). *Strengthening Family Resilience.* The Guilford Press.

Wang, I., & Green, D. (2017). Stitching East and West. *Creative Arts in Education and Therapy – Eastern and Western Perspectives, 3*(1). https://caet.quotus.org/article/2017/1/4

Wang, C. C., & Geale, S. K. (2015). The power of story: Narrative inquiry as a methodology in nursing research. *International Journal of Nursing Sciences, 2*(2), 195–198. doi:10.1016/j.ijnss.2015.04.014

Ward, C. (1997). Culture learning, acculturative stress, and psychopathology: Three perspectives on acculturation. *Applied Psychology, 46*(1), 58–62. doi:10.1111/j.1464-0597.1997.tb01094.x

Ward, C., & Kennedy, A. (1993). Where's the "culture" in cross-cultural transition? Comparative studies of sojourner adjustment. *Journal of Cross-Cultural Psychology, 24*(2), 221–249. doi:10.1177/0022022193242006

Ward, C., & Masgoret, A. M. (2008). Attitudes toward immigrants, immigration, and multiculturalism in New Zealand: A social psychological analysis. *The International Migration Review, 42*(1), 227–248. doi:10.1111/j.1747-7379.2007.00119.x

Watson, W. H., & McDaniel, S. H. (2000). Relational therapy in medical settings: Working with somatizing patients and their families. *Journal of Clinical Psychology, 56*(8), 1065–1082. doi:10.1002/1097-4679(200008)56:8<1065::AID-JCLP6>3.0.CO;2-S PMID:10946733

Weakland, J. H., Fisch, R., Watzlawick, P., & Bodin, A. M. (1974). Brief therapy: Focused problem resolution. *Family Process, 13*(2), 141–168. doi:10.1111/j.1545-5300.1974.00141.x

Wenger, E., McDermott, R. A., & Snyder, W. (2002). *Cultivating communities of practice: a guide to managing knowledge*. Harvard Business School Press.

White, M. (2006a). Working with people who are suffering the consequences of multiple trauma: a narrative perspective. In Narrative responses to traumatic experience. Adelaide: Dulwich Centre Publications.

Whitehouse, M. (1963). The Tao of the body. In P. Pallaro (Ed.), Moving the body, moving the self, being moved: A collection of essays (2nd ed., pp.51-57). Jessica Kingsley.

White, M. (2006b). Children, Trauma and Subordinate Storyline Development. In D. Denborough (Ed.), *Trauma: Narrative responses to traumatic experience* (pp. 143–165). Dulwich Centre Publications.

White, M. (2006c). Working with Children who have Experienced Significant Trauma. In M. White & A. Morgan (Eds.), *Narrative therapy with children and their families* (pp. 85–97). Dulwich Centre Publications.

White, M. (2007). *Maps of narrative practice*. W. W. Norton & Company.

White, M., & Epston, D. (1990). *Narrative Means to Therapeutic Ends*. Norton.

White, M., & Epston, D. (1990). *Narrative means to therapeutic ends*. W.W. Norton & Company.

Whiting, A., & Williams, D. (2013). Why people use social media: Uses and gratifications approach. *Qualitavite Market Research: An International Journal, 16*(4), 362-369.

Whyte, D. (2006). *River flow: new and selected poems*. Many Rivers Press.

Wilbur, S. (1949, Sept.). The Nature of News. *Journalizm Quarterly*, 259 – 269.

Wılcox Dennis, L., Ault Philip, H., Agee Warren, K., & Cameron Glen, T. (2000). *Public Relations Strategies and Tactics* (6th ed.). Longman.

Wilkinson, R. G., & Pickett, K. (2018). *The inner level: how more equal societies reduce stress, restore sanity and improve everyone's well-being*. Allen Lane.

Williams, R. (2003). Television, Technology and Cultural Form (A. Ulvi Türkbağ, Trans.). Dost Publication.

Williams, C. L., & Berry, J. W. (1991). Primary prevention of acculturative stress among refugees: Application of psychological theory and practice. *The American Psychologist, 46*(6), 632–641. doi:10.1037/0003-066X.46.6.632 PMID:1952422

Williams-Reade, J., Freitas, C., & Lawson, L. (2014). Narrative-informed medical family therapy: Using narrative therapy practices in brief medical encounters. *Families, Systems & Health, 32*(4), 416–425. Advance online publication. doi:10.1037/fsh0000082 PMID:25329755

Wilson, R., & Magam, L. (2018). Frustration-aggression, afrophobia and the psycho-social consequences of corruption in South Africa. In A. O. Akinola (Ed.), *The Political Economy of Xenophobia in Africa* (pp. 93–107). Springer. doi:10.1007/978-3-319-64897-2_8

Winnicott, D. W. (1977). *Playing and reality*. Tavistock.

Winslade, J. & Williams, M. (2012). *Safe and Peaceful Schools. Addressing Conflict and Eliminating Violence*. Corwin, a Sage Publications Company.

Winslade, J. (2014). *Time travel and narrative practice using Deleuze's time machine*. Presentation at the 3rd European Narrative Conference, Iasi, Romania.

Winslade, J. (2017). Narrative Mediation of Family Conflict. In A. Georgakopoulos (Ed.), *The Mediation Handbook, Research, Theory, and Practice* (pp. 87–96). Routledge. doi:10.4324/9781315648330-10

Winslade, J., & Monk, G. (2008). *Practicing narrative mediation: loosening the grip of conflict* (1st ed.). Jossey-Bass.

Wiretna, C. D., Saputra, W. N. E., Muarifah, A., & Barida, M. (2020). Effectiveness of solution-focused brief counseling to reduce online aggression of student. *Universal Journal of Educational Research*, *8*(3), 1092–1099. doi:10.13189/ujer.2020.080344

Wolniewicz, C. A., Tiamiyu, M. F., Weeks, J. W., & Elhai, J. D. (2018). Problematic smartphone use and relations with negative affect, fear of missing out, and fear of negative and positive evaluation. *Psychiatry Research*, *262*, 618–623. doi:10.1016/j.psychres.2017.09.058 PMID:28982630

Wolter, J. A., DiLollo, A., & Apel, K. (2006). A narrative therapy approach to counseling: A model for working with adolescents and adults with language-literacy deficits. *Language, Speech, and Hearing Services in Schools*, *37*(3), 168–177. doi:10.1044/0161-1461(2006/019) PMID:16837440

Yapı Kredi. (2018, Nov 9). *How Great It Is to Love You* [Video]. YouTube. https://www.youtube.com/watch?v=cR_HbU52Svk

Yardley, A. (2008). Piecing together—A methodological bricolage. *FQS*, *9*(2). https://www.qualitative-research.net/index.php/fqs/article/view/416/902

Yeh, C. J. (2003). Age, acculturation, cultural adjustment, and mental health symptoms of Chinese, Korean, and Japanese immigrant youths. *Cultural Diversity & Ethnic Minority Psychology*, *9*(1), 34–48. doi:10.1037/1099-9809.9.1.34 PMID:12647324

Yıldırım, E. (2014). Sovyetler Birliği'nde Propaganda ve Proleter Hegemonik İdeolojinin Kurulumu Üzerine [On Propaganda and the Establishment of Proletarian Hegemonic Ideology in the Soviet Union]. *Doğu-Batı Dergisi, 69*, 271-293.

Yıldırım, A., & Şimşek, H. (2016). *Sosyal bilimlerde nitel araştırma yöntemleri* [Qualitative research methods in the social sciences]. Seçkin Publications.

Yıldırım, S., & Kişioğlu, A. N. (2018). Teknolojinin getirdiği yeni hastaliklar: Nomofobi, Netlessfobi, Fomo [New diseases due to technology: Nomophobia, netlessphobia, FoMO]. *Sdü Tıp Fakültesi Dergisi*, *25*(4), 473–480.

Yılmaz, G. E. (2014). The Power without Responsibility in Political Communication: Spin Doctor [Siyasal İletişimde Sorumluluğu Olmayan Güç: Spin Doctor]. Düşünen Siyaset, 197-222.

Yılmaz, R. (2014). *Anlatı Yoluyla Dünyanın Zihinsel Yeniden Kurulumu: ''Palto'', ''Dönüşüm'' ve ''Hayvan Çiftliği'' Romanlarının Alımlama Pratikleri Üzerine Bir İnceleme* [Mental Reconstruction of the World through Narrative: A Study on Reception Practices of "The Overcoat", "The Metamorphosis" and "The Animal Farm"] [Unpublished doctoral dissertation]. Kocaeli Üniversitesi Sosyal Bilimler Enstitüsü İletişim Bilimleri Anabilim Dalı.

Yılmaz, R. (2017) Typology of Metaleptic Uses in Television Advertisements [Televizyon Reklamlarında Metaleptik Kullanımların Tipolojisi]. E-gifder, 5(2), 691[704.

Yılmaz, R. (2017). Reklamlarda Bir Anlatı Öğesi Olarak Kadın İmgesinin Kullanımı [The Use of the Image of Woman as a Narrative Element in Advertisements]. In M. Talas & E. Yalçınkaya (Eds.), *4th International Congress on Social Sciences, China to Adriatic*. Academic Press.

Yılmaz, R. (2017). *Türkiye'de Reklam Anlatısının Dijital Çağdaki Yapısal Dönüşümü* [Structural Transformation of Advertising Narrative in Turkey in the Digital Age] [Conference presentation]. 1st International Conference on New Trends in Communication, İstanbul, Turkey.

Yılmaz, R. (2017). *Narrative Advertising Models and Conceptualization in the Digital Age*. IGI-Global. doi:10.4018/978-1-5225-2373-4

Yılmaz, R. (2017). Televizyon Reklamlarında Metaleptik Kullanımlarının Tipolojisi [Typology of Metaleptic Uses in TV Commercials]. *Gümüşhane Üniversitesi İletişim Fakültesi Elektronik Dergisi*, *5*(2), 691–704.

Yılmaz, R., & Çakın, Ö. (2017). A Review of Sulphur Coding in Advertising [Reklamda Süblatif Kodlama Üzerine Bir İnceleme]. *MANAS Journal of Social Studies*, *6*(4), 531–539.

Yılmaz, R., & Çakın, Ö. (2017). Reklamda Süblatif Kodlama Üzerine Bir İnceleme [A Study on Sublative Coding in Advertising]. *MANAS Journal of Social Studies*, *6*(4), 531–539.

Yılmaz, R., Çakır, A., & Resuloğlu, F. (2017). Historical Transformation of the Advertising Narration in Turkey: From Stereotype to Digital Media. In R. Yılmaz (Ed.), *Narrative Advertising Models and Conceptualization in the Digital Age* (pp. 133–152). IGI-Global. doi:10.4018/978-1-5225-2373-4.ch008

Yılmaz, R., & Erdem, M. N. (2016). *Traditional and Digital Advertising in 150 Questions* [150 Soruda Geleneksel ve Dijital Reklamcılık]. Umuttepe Yayınları.

Yılmaz, R., & Erdem, M. N. (2018). *An Analysis on Coding Violence in Advertising, Virtual Realm / Media Violence [Reklamda Şiddet Kodlamaları Üzerine Bir İnceleme, Sanal Alem / Medya Şiddeti]*. Hegem Publication.

Yılmaz, R., & Taskiran, N. Ö. (2015). A Modal For Mind- Device Dialectic and the Future of Advertising in the Social Age. In N. Ö. Taskıran & R. Yılmaz (Eds.), *Handbook of Research on Effective Advertising Strategies in Social Media Age* (pp. 1–16). IGI Global Publications.

Yılmaz, R., & Taskiran, N. O. (2015). A Model for Mind-Device Dialectic and The Future of Advertising in The Social Media Age. In M. N. Taskiran & R. Yılmaz (Eds.), *Handbook of Research on Effective Advertising Strategies in The Social Media Age* (pp. 1–16). IGI Global. doi:10.4018/978-1-4666-8125-5.ch001

Yücel, T. (1988). *Summer and Life* [Yazın ve Yaşam]. Yol Yayınları.

Yüksel, E., & Gürcan, H. İ. (2005). *News Gathering and Writing* [Haber Toplama ve Yazma]. Tablet Kitabevi.

Zabcı, F. (2021). Truth, Rhetoric and Politics [Hakikat, Retorik ve Siyaset]. In B. Özçelik (Ed.), *Post-truth Politics, Philosophy, Media, International Relations* [Hakikat Sonrası Siyaset, Felsefe, Medya, Uluslararası İlişkiler] (pp. 13–29). Nika Yayınevi.

Zhang, Z., Jiménez, F. R., & Cicala, J. E. (2020). Fear of missing out scale: A self-concept perspective. *Psychology and Marketing*, *37*(11), 1619–1634. doi:10.1002/mar.21406

Zimmerman, T. S., Jacobsen, R. B., MacIntyre, M., & Watson, C. (1996). Solution-focused parenting groups: An empirical study. *Journal of Systemic Therapies*, *15*(4), 12–25. doi:10.1521/jsyt.1996.15.4.12

Zinoviev, A. (2008). İdeologija Partii Buduŝego [Party ideology in the future]. Moskva: Litres.

Ziraat Bankası. (2018, Dec 25). *''Yeşilçam'' Advertising* [Video]. YouTube. https://www.youtube.com/watch?v=bm63JYzlGfA

Zorlu, Y. (2016). Violence in the Media and Its Effects [Medyadaki Şiddet Ve Etkileri]. *Humanities Sciences*, *11*(1), 13–32.

About the Contributors

Recep Yilmaz, Ph.D., has been working as Associate Professor at Ondukuz Mayis University, Public Relations and Publicity Department since August 15, 2018. He authored ten books (Handbook of Research on Narrative Interactions, Handbook of Research on Narrative Advertising, Handbook of Research on Transmedia Storytelling and Narrative Strategies, Narrative Advertising Models and Conceptualization in the Social Media Age, Traditional and Digital Advertising in 150 Questions, Handbook Research on Effective Advertising Strategies in the Social Media Age, Advertising in 99 Questions, Keywords in Advertising, Scenarios: How is it written? How are they writing?, Leadership and its Contemporary Dimensions), and he published numerous papers in several journals, conference proceedings, and chapters in edited books. The author also has a published novella (a philosophical horror story) called "Çerçici." His majors are Narrative Theory and Advertising. He also studies Theoretical Communication. Some of the courses he teaches Narrative in Literature, Cinema and Advertisement, Advertising Scriptwriting, Creative Writing.

Bozkurt Koç is a Professor in the Psychology Department at the Ondokuz Mayıs University since 2010. Koç completed his B.Sc. (1995) at Ondokuz Mayıs University; his M.Sc. (1997) and his PhD (2003) studies at Atatürk University. He currently is a head of Psychology Department Ondokuz Mayıs University. He became a professor in 2016. He is particularly interested in violence, aggression, interpersonal relations, and intercultural relations.

* * *

Betül Başer started Cumhuriyet University, Faculty of Communication, Public Relations and Publicity Department in 2013 and graduated in 2017. In the same year, she started her graduate degree at Marmara University, Social Science Institute, Public Relations and Publicity Department and completed this program in 2020 with "The Role of Social Media Phenomena on Purchasing Decision of Z Generation Consumers: The Example of Youtubers" thesis. In the same year, she started her doctorate education at İstanbul University, Social Science Institute, Public Relations and Publicity Department and she continues her education and works as a research assistant at Ondokuz Mayıs University, Faculty of Communication, Public Relations and Publicity Department. Study fields: Public relations, new media, digital games and consumer behavior.

Nursel Bolat graduated from Kocaeli University Radio, TV and Cinema Department in 2006. After completing his master's degree in the Social Sciences Institute Radio-TV Cinema of the same university, he started his doctorate in Istanbul University Social Sciences Institute Radio-TV Cinema in 2013. She completed his doctorate on January 4, 2017. Between 2010 and 2015, he worked as a lecturer and assistant director of Vocational School at Istanbul Arel University Vocational School. On September 2, 2015, he started to work as an expert in Ondokuz Mayıs University, Faculty of Communication, Radio, TV and Cinema Department. She served as a lecturer. In 2019, Assoc. Dr. Bolat, who received the title, is still at the same university as Assoc. Dr. and as the Head of the Department of Radio, Television and Cinema.

Ömer Çakın was born in 1983. In 2007 he received his master's degree from Kyrgyzstan Manas University Journalism Department and in 2009 he received his master's degree from the same university's communication sciences program. In 2013, he received his doctorate degree in the field of Communication Sciences by defending his doctoral thesis titled "Kyrgyzstan Localization of International Advertisement". Assoc. Dr. Ömer Çakın has been working as an assistant professor at Ondokuz Mayıs University, Department of Radio, TV and Cinema since 2014. works as.

Ozlem Delal is a PhD candidate in department of Journalism at Selcuk University. She completed MA degree with thesis title "Representation practices of social media in traditional media: The case of Arab Spring and Gezi Park events". Delal has worked as a research assisttant in department of journalism, faculty of communication at Ondokuz Mayıs University since 2018. Her research interest subjects are in the intersection of social media, woman representation, post-truth, fact-checking and parasocial interaction.

Deborah Green, PhD, MAAT, MEd, PGDip(Adult Ed), BA(Hons), Registered Clinical Arts Therapist (AThR), is Co-Head of School and Research Coordinator within the School of Creative Arts Therapies at Whitecliffe, Aotearoa New Zealand. Her academic/practitioner career encompasses educational/community theatre, adult education, community development, lifeskills/AIDS education and counselling (South Africa 1990-2004), and creative arts therapy (New Zealand 2006-). A passionate therapist, educator, and arts-based researcher, she's published and presented in/at several international journals/books and conferences/symposia.

Aysu Gül Şanli is a Teaching Assistant in the Psychology Department at the Ondokuz Mayıs University since 2018. Gül Şanli completed his M.Sc. (2016) and her undergraduate (2014) studies at Ondokuz Mayıs University. She is particularly interested in altruism, communication, and interpersonal relations.

Ufuk Inal has received undergraduate and master's degree from Radio, Television and Cinema department in Kocaeli University. He has started PHD study in communication sciences departmant in Kocaeli University. He's currently working in Radio, Television and Cinema department in Ondokuz Mayıs University. His current research interest are Radio Broadcasting and New Media Studies.

Aybike Tuba Özden is an associate professor in the Department of Marketing and Advertising at Ondokuz Mayıs University. She is also the Head of Marketing and Advertising she. She received her BS degree from Uludağ University in 2002, her MS degree from Ondokuz Mayıs University in 2013, and her PhD from Başkent University in 2017. Marketing communication, service marketing and consumer behavior are her research areas. She has several publications in the mentioned areas.

Susan Riva received her doctorate in the Social Sciences from the University of Tilburg in the Netherlands, in conjunction with the Taos Institute. She is a scholar practitioner using an interdisciplinary approach that connects narrative conflict resolution, social psychology, and medical anthropology. She teaches within the Department of Social and Cultural Studies at Creighton University in Omaha, Nebraska. She lives in the French-speaking Alps in Switzerland where she practices narrative mediation, narrative inquiry, and autoethnography.

Sena Şahin was born in Samsun. She graduated from Ondokuz Mayıs University, Faculty of Communication, Department of Public Relations and Publicity in 2018. In the same year, she started her graduate education in the Media and Communication Sciences program of Ondokuz Mayıs University Social Sciences Institute and continues her education.

Onur Şen was born on February 16, 1994, in Samsun. He completed his primary and secondary education in his hometown. Higher education, i.e., Ondokuz Mayıs University, Faculty of Communication, Journalism (Bachelor - Graduate), Ondokuz Mayıs University, Department of Public Law (Master - Graduate, with the study "Crimes Against Private Life and the Secret Area of Life through Media") Ondokuz Mayıs University, Department of Communication Sciences (Master - Graduate, with his study "Perception of Reliability Towards Local Media: A Study in the Example of Samsun Local Media"). Şen graduated from Ondokuz Mayıs University, Faculty of Communication (Department of Journalism), with a first degree from the department and the second degree from the faculty. Şen works as a lecturer at Ondokuz Mayıs University, Faculty of Communication, Department of Journalism.

Elif Şevik İnal is a PhD Student at Marmara University.

Esennur Sirer graduated from Istanbul University Press and Broadcasting School, Radio and Television Department in 1990. In 2010, he received his master's degree from Istanbul University, Institute of Social Sciences, Radio-TV Cinema, with his thesis titled "The Developing and Changing Formal Structure of Television Journalism". In 2018, with her thesis titled "Football as a Popular Cultural Product: Image Editing in terms of Production Elements in Broadcasting", she was awarded the title of doctorate in Istanbul University Social Sciences Institute Radio-TV Cinema Branch. Since August 2021, she has the title of associate professor. Between 1992 and 2018, she worked in the Istanbul Directorate of the TRT News and Sports Broadcasting Department. In addition to his duty as a Director at TRT, she has been continuing her academic studies since 2007 as a doctoral faculty member at Üsküdar University, Radio and Television Cinema Department, since October 2018.

Güven Soner currently works at the Department of Public Health Nursing, Ondokuz Mayis University. His current research interest is 'Vulnerable Populations'.

Nilay Tan Çakır has been working as Research Assistant at Ondokuz Mayis University, Public Relations and Publicity Department since March 1, 2019. She graduated from Bahcesehir University Public Relations Department in 2013 with a full scholarship of OSYM (Student Selection and Placement Centre). Also she completed her minor program in Strategic Advertising Planning in the same year. She studied communication at the University of Antwerp, Belgium for a semester with Erasmus exchange program. After graduation, she worked as a copywriter at a digital advertising agency in Istanbul 3 years.

Then she received her masters degree from Media and Communication Sciences program at Ondokuz Mayis University. She is doing her PhD in the Department of Public Relations and Publicity at Istanbul University.

Doğan Güneş Temli is a Research Assistant in the Psychology Department at the Ondokuz Mayıs University since 2017. Temli completed his M.Sc. (2016-2019) and his undergraduate (2012-2016) studies at Ondokuz Mayıs University. He currently is a second-year doctoral student in Social Psychology at the Bursa Uludağ University. He is particularly interested in social contact theories. His other major research interests are aggression and violence.

Eren Trabzon is a Teaching Assistant in the Psychology Department at the Ondokuz Mayıs University since 2019. Trabzon completed his M.Sc. (2016) at Beykent University and his undergraduate (2013) studies at Ondokuz Mayıs University. He is particularly interested in coping with stress, anger management, and attention deficit hyperactivity disorder.

Luc Van den Berge works as a systemic and narrative practitioner in a child and adolescent mental health service (Adentro VZW in Ghent, Belgium) and is visiting professor at Ghent University where he teaches systemic therapy. He did his PhD in educational sciences on parenting and parenting support.

Tomas Van Reybrouck is systemic and narrative psychotherapist, trainer, supervisor. He works in a mental health service with parents of addicted children (Adentro VZW in Ghent Belgium).

Sabine Vermeire is a systemic and narrative psychotherapist, trainer and supervisor in therapy and family counseling at Interactie-academie vzw, Antwerp, Belgium. She published many articles, book chapters and books on systemic and narrative therapy, especially with children and youngsters.

Index

T

W

www.ingramcontent.com/pod-product-compliance
Lightning Source LLC
Chambersburg PA
CBHW080501051126
54379CB00005B/143